Childhood Language Disorders

CURRENT THERAPY OF COMMUNICATION DISORDERS

Series Editor
William H. Perkins, Ph.D.

Childhood Language Disorders

Michael D. Smith, Ph.D.

MGH Institute of Health Professions
Graduate Program in Communication Sciences and Disorders
Boston, Massachusetts
and
The Reich College of Education
Appalachian State University
Boone, North Carolina

Jack S. Damico, Ph.D.

Department of Communicative Disorders
University of Southwestern Louisiana
Lafayette, Louisiana

1996
THIEME MEDICAL PUBLISHERS, INC. New York
GEORG THIEME VERLAG Stuttgart · New York

Thieme Medical Publishers, Inc.
381 Park Avenue South
New York, New York 10016

Library of Congress Cataloging-in-Publication Data

Childhood language disorders / [edited by] Michael D. Smith, Jack S. Damico
p. cm. — (Current therapy of communication disorders)
Includes bibliographical references and index.
ISBN 0-86577-501X (hard cover). — ISBN 3-13-10141-6 (hard cover)
1. Language disorders in children. I. Smith, Michael D. (Michael Douglas), 1942– . II. Damico, Jack Samual. III. Series.
[DNLM: 1. Language Disorders—in infancy & childhood. WL 340.2 C536 1995]
RJ496.L35C485 1995
618.92'855—dc20
DNLM/DLC
for Library of Congress 95-3583
CIP

Important note: Medicine is an ever-changing science. Research and clinical experience are continually broadening our knowledge, in particular our knowledge of proper treatment and drug therapy. Insofar as this book mentions any dosage or applications, readers may rest assured that the authors, editors, and publishers have made every effort to ensure that such references are strictly in accordance with the state of knowledge at the time of production of the book. Nevertheless, every user is requested to carefully examine the manufacturers' leaflets accompanying each drug to check on his own responsibility whether the dosage schedules recommended therein or the contraindications stated by the manufacturers differ from the statements made in the present book. Such examination is particularly important with drugs that are either rarely used or have been newly released on the market.

Some of the product names, patents, and registered designs referred to in this book are in fact registered trademarks or proprietary names even though specific reference to this fact is not always made in the text. Therefore, the appearance of a name without designation as proprietary is not to be construed as a representation by the publisher that it is in the public domain.

Printed in the United States of America.

5 4 3 2 1

TMP ISBN 0-86577-501-X
GTV ISBN 3-13-101141-6

We would like to dedicate the book to

Herbert Koepp-Baker
Priest
Scholar
ASHA Founder

Hula Halle Damico
Teacher
Mother
Best Friend

Stanley Dale Smith
Native American
Father
Risk-Taker

Other Volumes in the Series

General Principles of Therapy

Dysarthria and Apraxia

Language Handicaps in Adults

Voice Disorders

Phonologic-Articulatory Disorders

Hearing Disorders

Language Handicaps in Children

Stuttering Disorders

Aphasia and Related Neurogenic Language Disorders

Stuttering and Related Disorders of Fluency

Child Phonology: Characteristics, Assessment, and Intervention with Special Populations

Contents

Contributors

Lloyd E. Augustine, Ph.D.
Department of Communicative Disorders
University of Southwestern Louisiana
Lafayette, Louisiana

Anthony S. Bashir, Ph.D.
Freshman Academic Studies Program and
Division of Communication Disorders
Emerson College
100 Beacon Street
Boston, Massachusetts

David F. Bjorklund, Ph.D.
Department of Psychology
P.O. Box 3091
Florida Atlantic University
Baco Raton, Florida

Michael W. Casby, Ph.D.
Audiology and Speech Sciences
Michigan State University
378 Communication Arts and Sciences
East Lansing, Michigan

Holly K. Craig, Ph.D.
Communicative Disorders Clinic
University of Michigan
1111 E. Catherine Street
Ann Arbor, Michigan

Jack S. Damico, Ph.D.
Department of Communicative Disorders
University of Southwestern Louisiana
Lafayette, Louisiana

Carol M. Frattali, Ph.D.
Director, Health Services Division
American Speech-Language-Hearing
Association
10801 Rockville Pike
Rockville, Maryland

Jill Geschwint-Rabin, M.S.
Audiology, Speech and Swallowing Services,
Pediatric Division
Illinois Masonic Medical Center
Chicago, Illinois

Yvonne Gillette, Ph.D.
The University of Akron
School of Communicative Disorders
181 Polsky Building
Akron, Ohio

Alan G. Kamhi, Ph.D.
Department of Audiology and Speech Pathology
Memphis State University
807 Jefferson Avenue
Memphis, Tennessee

Diane M. Kirchner, Ph.D.
Private Practice
Suite 115, 2550 Ninth Street
Berkeley, California

Lesley A. Maxwell, M.S.
Graduate Program in Communication Sciences
and Disorders
Massachusetts General Hospital
Institute of Health Professions
Boston, Massachusetts

John M. Panagos
Department of Communication Disorders
Wayne State University
555 Manoogian Hall
Detroit, Michigan

Mary Ann Romski, Ph.D.
Department of Communication
Language Research Center
Georgia State University
Atlanta, Georgia

Richard G. Schwartz, Ph.D.
Program in Speech and Hearing Sciences
City University of New York
Graduate School and University Center
33 West 42nd Street
New York, New York

Rose A. Sevcik, Ph.D.
Department of Psychology
Language Research Center
Georgia State University
Atlanta, Georgia

Michael Smith, Ph.D.
MGH Institute of Health Professions
101 Merrimac Street
Boston, Massachusetts

Ann Z. Strominger, Sc.D.
Department of Otolaryngology
Children's Hospital
Boston, Massachusetts

Anne van Kleeck
Program in Communication Sciences and Disorders
Department of Speech Communication
University of Texas at Austin
Austin, Texas

Alice Richardson Vigil, Ph.D.
Program in Communication Sciences and Disorders
Department of Speech Communication
University of Texas at Austin
Austin, Texas

Preface

Of all the acts of cooperative behavior observed anywhere in nature, I can think of nothing to match *human language*. When we speak to each other, it is not like the social insects laying out chemical trails; human language contains the two most characteristic and accommodating human traits, ambiguity, and amiability. Almost every message in human communication can be taken in two or more ways. There are various choices to be made in the sending of messages and in their reception. We are, in this respect, unlike the ants and bees; we are obliged to listen more carefully, to edit whatever we hear, and to recognize uncertainty when we hear or read it.

Lewis Thomas, *The Fragile Species* (1992)

Childhood Language Disorders is *not* a book about the clinical equivalent of linguistic *correctness*, compliant normalization nor what Howard Goldstein (1990) cautiously referred to as the "stiff tests" of clinical significance. Optimistically, it *is* a book about linguistically fragile children—perhaps the most challenged of Lewis Thomas' the *fragile species*. More than adults, these children are capable of persisting—and engagingly so—in uncertain attempts to edit and make sense of complex linguistic affairs. It is a book on the resolution of nonmainstream variation and heightened ambiguity in language learning, and the clinician's obligatory search for *adaptive* responses.

Childhood Language Disorders comes to you with ambitious intent: To extend and to refine our *clinical* concept of native-speaker capability and accommodate child-as-client moves into the elusive mainstream of communicative behavior. We want to encourage reciprocity and enlarge on naturally occurring variations (adaptive client behaviors) in communicative behavior. We want to shed ourselves of *linguistic prescriptions* and study disordered sounding developments in and on their own terms, as nominal behaviors with an integrity and persistence of their own.

Clinicians, children, and books do come with attitudes, and they are mostly positive. *Childhood Language Disorders* comes with an attitude reminiscent of Carl Gustav Jung's thinking: "If there is anything that we wish to change in the child, we should first *examine it* and see whether it is not something that could better be changed in ourselves." When approaching children with language disorders, we understand that *relevant change* occurs only to the extent that the participant behaviors examined and the goals identified appropriately achieve the communicative needs of individual children and no one else (i.e., the linguistic status quo).

Over the past twenty years, we have run the course of conceptualizing and acting on childhood language disorders within our theory-driven, normal developmental models (J. Miller, 1991). On behalf of children, if we want to take behavior that is *different enough sounding* to be labeled "disordered" and make it *work better,* why not relax our preoccupation with overly *normalized* targets—typically those missed by no less than 5% of aspiring native speakers—and "stiff tests" of clinical significance?

Following the persuasive arguments of Thomas Moore (1992), we can avail ourselves of the abundant opportunities to "go with the symptoms" and avoid initial temptations to "*compensate,* to be drawn toward the opposite of what is presented. The move into opposites is deceptive. Oddly, it keeps the [child] in the same problem, only from the opposite side."

And because we willingly engage in *therapy,* Moore's suggestion is that we act on the Socratic dictum. Therapy begins by *cultivating* what is present by taking care of the practical elements, and by bringing *imagination* to areas seemingly devoid of it.

Much to our advantage in the pursuit of *best clinical practices* and the cultivation of existing behavior, as clinicians we qualify as "infallible" native-speakers and members of what Thomas (1972) called the "articulate generation." From the vantage point of a "biology watcher," Thomas observed that:

> We have been working at [language] for what seems an eternity, generation after articulate generation, and we still have no notion how it is done, nor what it will be like when it is finished, if it is ever to be finished. It is the most compulsively collective, genetically programmed, species-specific, and autonomic of the things we do, and we are *infallible* at it. (p. 152)

The native advantage to us may oddly serve as the distinct disadvantage to those individuals who aspire for intelligible language but encounter seemingly insurmountable barriers. We identify their language as being inarticulate and disordered. Like us, they have no notion how language is done. Unlike us, they audibly face the day-to-day reality of unfinished business: The *if it is ever to be finished* conditions placed on language development. Through therapy, our role is to work *collectively* with them in efforts to bring to the surface *how language is done* and practical communication is achieved. There is little to be gained here in attempts to jump-start systems or to accelerate the process of linguistic change.

Childhood Language Disorders begins with a study of *Perspectives* and Carol Frattali's persuasive Chapter 1, a probing essay on the value of seeking *socially adaptive* clinical outcomes—not allowing the "perfect" to become the enemy of the "good." According to Frattali, from a public policy perspective, academic and scientific concerns pale in comparison to the looming sociopolitical pressures to improve children's access to responsive treatment and education (as legislated under *America 2000* and *Healthy People 2000*).

David Bjorklund and Richard Schwartz follow in Chapter 2 with a compelling study of the nature and advantages of *developmental immaturity.* Bjorklund and Schwartz make the penetrating argument that clinical efforts to force more advanced cognitive and linguistic behavior on developmentally immature children may lead to appropriate sounding behavior, while not yielding *optimal* levels of performance.

Looking directly at clinical treatment perspectives and speech therapy discourse in Chapter 3, John Panagos asks why therapy is so often highly structured, adult centered, and simultaneously maladaptive. According to Panagos, therapy can be highly structured without *aggressive* speech correction wherein the child is treated as the *error maker,* with the risks of linguistic confusion and lowered self-esteem. Applying the logic of Alice Richardson and Anne van Kleeck in Chapter 4, the linguistic behavior of these *error makers* actually conforms to simple everyday wisdom: by its very nature, learning language involves the making of multiple, but not misguided, mistakes. No less common-sensed, they emphasize that if correct responses were always accessible to clinicians able to elicit them, we would have to question whether learning had in fact occurred at all.

Alan Kamhi concludes *Perspectives* in Chapter 5 with a revealing exposition of the linguistic and cognitive properties of childhood language disorders, and especially as related to conditions of *specific language impairment.* In Kamhi's typically lucid terms, what continues to frustrate our efforts to make coherent sense out of language spoken-in-error is our failure to identify specific cognitive limitations underlying the processing inefficiencies typical of childhood language disorders. We are reminded here of George Miller's (1989) observations made in his keynote address to the First Annual Convention of the American Psychological Society: "We already know far more about language than we *understand."*

To come to more workable terms with the dilemma of *childhood language disorders,* we move into *Practices and Populations.* In Chapter 6, Anthony Bashir and Ann Strominger take the lead with a thorough depiction of the personal, social, and academic vulnerability of children with developmental language disorders. They chronicle those obstacles faced by the most fragile members of our articulate species, and convey what it means to be faced with the life-long need to acquire language—the *if it is ever to be finished* condition placed on language development.

With thoroughness, the contributing authors attend to individuals who, in their need to acquire language, operate on the literal fringes of *admissible linguistic hypotheses.* If we consent that our clinical raison d'etre is to accommodate clients (however "approximate" they at first appear) into the mainstream of communicative activity, we must devote more time to reflective decision making. And in the context of what follows in *Childhood Language Disorders,* we can devote increasingly more time to *population-specific* characteristics and needs.

In Chapter 7, Holly Craig begins with a thought-provoking documentary on individuals with *specific language impairment.* And with equally well fashioned insight, in Chapter 8, Diane Kirchner presents the case for children with *pervasive developmental disorders.* Next, Michael Casby offers in Chapter 9 an account of *truly acquired* childhood language disorders. Mary Ann Romski and Rose Sevcik follow in Chapter 10 with a presentation of clinical profiles of children with *severe disabilities.*

Lesley Maxwell and Jill Geschwint-Rabin, in Chapter 11, offer a careful accounting of the *teratogenic effects* of substance abuse on language development. In Chapter 12, Jack Damico, Michael Smith, and Lloyd Augustine address the ever-pressing question, "How can speech–language pathologists best serve the needs of individuals from multicultural backgrounds who are suspected of exhibiting childhood language disorders?" And of no less urgency in Chapter 13, Yvonne Gillette presents the case for *collaborative family-centered* services to meet the needs of infant and toddlers who are at risk for developmental delay.

We are convinced rewarding consequences are gained from population-specific inquiries into childhood language disorders. In the words of Diane Kirchner (this volume), "We must begin to formulate intervention programs for children which are based on their own unique profiles and backed by theoretical weight. . . . Such approaches take advantage of children's strengths while minimizing their deficits."

As contributing authors of the sequel to William H. Perkins' original volume, *Current Therapy of Communication Disorders: Language Handicaps in Children* (1984), we want to acknowledge the significant contributions made by the "founding" authors. We indeed hope that they will receive the contents of this volume as a meaningful extension of their original work and commitment to serving the needs of children with language disorders.

The Editors

References

Goldstein, H. (1990). Assessing clinical significance. In L. Olswang, C. Thompson, S. Warren, and N. Minghetti (Eds.), *Treatment efficacy research in communication disorders.* Rockville, MD: American Speech-Language-Hearing Foundation.

Miller, J.F. (1991). Research on language disorders in children: A progress report. In J.F. Miller (Ed.), *Research on child language disorders: A decade of progress.* Austin, TX: Pro-Ed.

Moore, T. (1992). *Care of the soul: A guide to cultivating depth and sacredness in everyday life.* New York: Harper Collins Publishers.

Perkins, W. (Ed.) (1984). *Current therapy of communication disorders: Language handicaps in children.* New York: Thieme Stratton.

Thomas, L. (1992). *The fragile species.* New York: Macmillan.

Language clinicians know at least implicitly that they cannot teach everything about language that the child needs to learn to become a competent language user. They also know that most language impaired children have the capacity to learn at least some language on their own. . . . Consequently, the most efficient intervention program would be one aimed at positively influencing the child's language learning and utilization processes rather than to teach the child to make use of certain specific language behaviors.

(Marc E. Fey, Understanding and narrowing the gap between research and clinical practice with language-impaired children. In C. M. Shewan (Ed.), ASHA Reports 20: The Future of Science and Services Seminar. Rockville, MD: The American Speech-Language-Hearing Association, 1990).

Part I

Perspectives

1

Childhood Language Disorders
Clinical Outcome Perspectives

CAROL M. FRATTALI, PH.D.

Introduction

What is a clinical outcome? It can be described simply as a behavioral change resulting from a clinical intervention. Outcomes can be targeted or serendipitous. They can be *intermediate* (outcomes from session to session), *instrumental* (outcomes that activate the learning process), or *ultimate* (outcomes that demonstrate the social or ecological validity of treatment benefits) (Rosen & Proctor, 1981). Outcomes can be characterized at a point along a continuum of impairment (e.g., specific language disorder), functional limitation (e.g., communication difficulties), or disability (e.g., social or learning problems) (Nagi, 1965). At a micro level, an outcome is achieved with the delivery of each treatment stimulus. At a macro level, outcomes can occur long after a regimen of treatment ends, as measured socially, academically, or vocationally (Wilkerson, 1991).

Clinical outcomes are evidence of a clinician's effectiveness (the ability to produce positive outcomes) and value (the ability to produce positive outcomes in the most cost-effective manner). Minifie (1990) states that "the quality of a clinical science is directly related to the ability of its practitioners to produce predictable, efficient, effective, and ecologically sound outcomes with the clinical treatments applied" (p. 239). Why, then, do so little outcome data exist?

The reason rests, in large part, with the multiple dimensions of humanness. Human characteristics, by their nature, add complexity to outcome measurement. Some of the intervening variables that complicate the ability to generalize outcomes research results are age; gender; maturation; left- or right-handedness; intelligence; socioeconomic status; race; ethnicity; education; etiology; type, nature, and severity of disorder; coexisting conditions; and vocational status. Experimental research methods are designed to control for these variables. For example, the use of single-subject experimental designs allows a subject to serve as his or her own control. But single-subject research results are difficult to generalize; an outcome for one may not be an outcome for another. Group design research, on the other hand, calls for subject homogeneity. Group designs must address the ethics of control groups for which treatment (or a favored treatment) is withheld. They must also control for the countless variables that can compromise the study's validity.

Other reasons for the scarcity of outcome data involve time and cost. Outcomes research often is a lengthy and costly proposition. The longitudinal nature of these studies sometimes works at odds with funding, continuing participation of subjects, and administrative support.

From a public policy perspective, however, academic, scientific, and logistic concerns pale to the looming sociopolitical pressures to improve children's access to health care and education. The existing systems are in need of restructuring, and policy makers will not wait for better outcome data to make better policy decisions. In a system of limited resources, outcome data, in whatever shape or form, have been and will be used to make weighty decisions about who receives services, for how much, and from whom.

In this chapter, I will address both the need and the means for collecting clinical outcome data. My perspective will be national in scope and will encompass primarily the viewpoint of policy makers.

Drawing a Profile of Need for Children

Education (and health care) for children is a multibillion-dollar enterprise (Stark, 1992). The extent to which the enterprise has been successful is, however, of deep concern. On the education of children with special needs, Stark (1992) states: "We are well aware of the astronomical costs of these services" (p. 10). But at what return on the investment? Despite the best of intentions and the funding assigned to these special needs programs, many children are not getting the services to which they are entitled as a result of waste, inefficiency, and imbalanced resource allocation. Reform is both necessary and imminent.

In studying the current state of affairs, it is clear that progress has been made; yet the present profile of children's health, development, and educational achievement does not reflect the ultimate outcomes to which our society aspires. Consider, first, some disheartening facts on the status of our children's welfare.

In 1989, nearly 40,000 babies died in the United States before their first birthday (National Health Policy Forum, 1992). Although the U.S. infant mortality rate is at its lowest—9.8 deaths per 1000 live births for that year—it still surpasses that of 21 other industrialized nations. When infant mortality is studied by race, the statistics are even more disturbing. African–American babies are more than twice as likely to die before age one, with a rate of 17.7 deaths per 1000, compared with 8.1 for Caucasian babies. Because prenatal care is associated with good birth outcomes, this statistic is attributed, in large part, to insufficient prenatal care. Between 1980 and 1987, the percentage of women receiving late or no prenatal care was 26% for African–Americans and 17% for Caucasians.

Beyond infant mortality, the health profile of American children has shifted markedly in the past 40 years. Major infectious diseases, such as polio, diphtheria, scarlet fever, pneumonia, measles, and whooping cough, have been virtually eliminated with widespread immunization. Nevertheless, half of the 2 year olds in this country do not receive the necessary immunizations to prevent these diseases. Thus, a program of universal immunization for preschool children recently was instituted.

Several threats to children's health persist and are associated primarily with low socioeconomic status. Mental retardation, learning disorders, emotional and behavioral problems, vision and hearing problems, and speech and language disorders all appear to be more prevalent among children living in poverty, often in inner cities, than among those at higher socioeconomic levels (U.S. Department of Health and Human Services, 1988).

New diseases and syndromes change continually the configuration of the nation's health profile. Consider, for example, children with human immune deficiency virus (HIV), the virus that causes acquired immune deficiency syndrome (AIDS). As of September 1991, the Centers for Disease Control (CDC) reported 3312 cases of AIDS nationwide for children under the age of three. This is a conservative figure. It is estimated that for every child with AIDS, several times more are in various stages of HIV-related involvement (in Seidel, 1991). Typically, most children with HIV have, or will acquire, significant developmental disabilities as a result of intrusion of the virus into the central nervous system. HIV infection has become the major infectious cause of pediatric mental retardation in the United States (Diamond, 1989).

Consider, too, an old problem but new syndrome—shaken baby syndrome. This syndrome describes injuries resulting from care givers shaking young children. Injuries include blindness, spinal cord injury, skeletal injuries, psychological disturbances, mental retardation, cerebral palsy, and brain damage resulting in coma (Keeney, 1992). In addition, when the health profile of U.S. children extends beyond mortality and morbidity data, it includes the emotional, psychological, and learning problems that result from morbidity and add to society's total cost burden (U.S. Department of Health and Human Services, 1988).

A comparable picture emerges in education. A significant "achievement gap" purportedly exists between American students and their counterparts in other industrialized nations (National Education Goals Panel, 1992). Achievement deficiencies, relative to other nations, may be present as early as the first grade. The achievement gap grows as students themselves grow older. Children born at low birthweight because of exposure to toxic substances or poor diets are at risk for maladaptation and experience higher incidences of special education placements, grade retention, and school failure. Fewer than half of preschoolers regularly spend time with their parents in activities such as reading or storytelling, which will enrich their language. Among children aged three to eight, it is the younger ones—those in preschool or kindergarten—who watch the most television.

Although high school dropout rates are declining, the current figures are still highly undesirable. The high school completion rate in 1991 was 85% for 19- to 20-year-olds. Rates for black (80%) and white (89%) students were substantially higher than the rate for Hispanics (61%). The economic consequences of high school dropout are enormous. One half of the heads of households on welfare failed to finish high school. Among the more than 1.1 million persons incarcerated in 1990, at a per-person cost of $22,500 a year, 82% were high school dropouts. Thus, it is much more cost effective to educate young people than to pay for the enormous consequences of their dropping out.

In summary, emotional, psychological, and learning disorders are on the rise among children (U.S. Department of Health and Human Services, 1988). These may be attributed to changing demographics, with increases in minority populations who do not speak English or who are not afforded the same opportunities as other groups; a decrease in mortality (we are saving more lives) and an increase in morbidity (we are seeing more problems as a result); an increase in crime and child abuse; an increase in unintentional injuries such as falls and car accidents; and the erosion of the family as a nurturing unit.

Driven by these data, two national outcome initiatives—one for education, another for health—are underway: America 2000 (U.S. Department of Education, 1991) and Healthy People 2000 (U.S. Department of Health and Human Services, 1990). Both are decade-long projects designed to reach data-based, outcome-oriented goals. America 2000, a long-term strategy to meet national education goals, was adopted by state governors and launched during the Bush administration. The plan attempts to close the achievement gap. The Healthy People 2000 initiative, a national crusade for health promotion and disease prevention launched by the U.S. Public Health Service, involves an enormous effort to meet 300 data-based and outcome-oriented goals. The targets are aimed at creating a healthier society by the year 2000. Characteristic examples of outcome-oriented goals from each national project are listed in Table 1–1.

The nation's health care and education systems are focused overwhelmingly on treatment outcomes. More than ever, substantial outcome data will be needed to make a convincing case for specialized services, including speech-language pathology and audiology services. Health care reforms are moving rapidly toward systems of managed care. Thus, larger but fewer providers will be competing on the basis of quality and cost. Those who cannot provide data supporting predictions about quality (What can be expected as a result of intervention?) and cost (How much will it cost?) will lose to those who can.

What does it cost to remediate a child with a communication disorder? What expenditures can be saved as a result of this remediation? Which remediation methods are the most cost-effective? Can remediation be rendered by or in collaboration with others (e.g., support personnel, families) and achieve the same outcome? How will the child benefit from remediation in his or her functioning at home, in school, and (in the future) on the job? These are the questions of policy makers.

Asking the Basic Question

Measurement of clinical outcomes often begins with a basic question: Does treatment work? Yet the question itself generates considerable debate. Siegal (1987, 1989–1990, 1993), for instance, disputes the value of asking this question. He argues that clinicians know they can change behavior with treatment. Furthermore, he contends that if clinicians were to learn that treatment does not work, they would discount or ignore the results. Siegal (1989–1990) states that

> I [inveigh] against research that asks, "Does therapy work?" I believe that is the wrong question to ask of therapy, but not that no questions should be asked about therapy. I tried to suggest that no clinician worth his salt would ever admit that "therapy" in a

Table 1–1. Examples of Outcome-Oriented Goals from America 2000 and Healthy People 2000

America 2000
By the year 2000, all children in America will start school ready to learn.
By the year 2000, the high school graduation rate will increase to at least 90%.
By the year 2000, American students will leave grades 4, 8, and 12 having demonstrated competency in challenging subject matter, including English, mathematics, science, history, and geography; and every school in America will ensure that all students learn to use their minds well so they may be prepared for responsible citizenship, further learning, and productive employment in our modern economy.
Healthy People 2000
Reduce the prevalence of serious mental retardation in school-age children to no more than 2 per 1000 children. (Baseline: 2.7 per 1000 children aged 10 in 1985–1988)
Increase to at least 80% the proportion of providers of primary care for children who routinely refer or screen infants and children for impairments of vision, hearing, speech, and language and assess other developmental milestones as part of well-child care. (Baseline data unavailable)
Reduce the average age at which children with significant hearing impairment are identified to no more than 12 months. (Baseline: Estimated as 24–30 months in 1988)

Sources: National Education Goals Panel, 1992; U.S. Department of Health and Human Services, 1990.

generic sense doesn't work. A given therapy might not work, or it might not work for a particular client, or at a particular point in the client's development or in view of the client's current family and personal circumstances, etc. That is not to say that clinicians will persist in their "favorite therapies" regardless of the evidence. That would be counterproductive indeed. Rather, research concerning the therapeutic process will be much more informative if it asks questions about that process, and not whether therapy does or does not work. (p. 15)

Thus, Siegal (1993) believes that treatment efficacy research is unlikely to address important questions concerning the underlying nature or the origins of communication disorders. He is increasingly convinced that knowledge about such basic issues is crucial for developing effective treatment regimes.

From a scientific perspective, Siegal's (1993) argument is persuasive. Nevertheless, the fallout of demoting social and political pressures could seriously compromise our professions and the clients whom we serve. Denial of the "Does therapy work?" question most certainly will result in policy development that is arbitrary and flawed at best. The policy maker will not wait for the researcher. Witness Wertz's (1993) defense of the "Does therapy work?" question:

The rationale for not asking appears weak. Knowing that one can change behavior does not demonstrate that one *has* changed behavior (Kent, 1985), that the change is in the right direction, and that the results justify the effort. Moreover, clinicians are very resilient. Negative results do not necessarily dampen enthusiasm or engender disbelief. Most of us are as willing to try something else as we are to "try, try again." Reducing the active uncertainty in what helps and what does not is good for research. It is also good for practice. . . .

"Does therapy work?" is not only a proper question for research, it is also a proper question for challenging or supporting what has become expensive common practice and for supporting or dashing the hopes of sizable populations who seek services. (p. 38)

Both positions have merit. Perhaps we should ask three basic questions: Does therapy work? How does therapy work? and Why does therapy work? These questions, if answered, can best serve the client because they force attention to both the therapeutic process and outcome, as well as the underlying nature of the communication disorder.

Olswang (1993), in formulating basic questions for efficacy research in developmental speech and language disorders, addresses both clinical processes and outcomes and the underlying nature of disorders. She also takes into account the parents' perspective. Parents' questions are these: Is my child impaired? If so, why is my child having these problems? Will treatment improve my child's skills now and in the future? Olswang points out that these questions do not differ from those of the researcher: What is the nature of speech/language acquisition? How can it go awry? Can the organism's naturally occurring acquisition process be accommodated through environmental manipulation? Olswang believes it is not enough to ask "Does therapy work?" We must also ask "How and why does therapy work?" if we are to make convincing statements about treatment outcome.

A Focus on Functional (or Real-World) Outcomes

In the field of rehabilitation, functional outcomes are becoming the primary measure of treatment outcome. If the goal of rehabilitation is to optimize independence and quality of life, a focus on functional outcomes is indeed logical. Yet this focus is somewhat new to the profession of speech-language pathology.

Because many of the frequently used, traditional diagnostic tests measure specific speech and language impairments, the parlance of clinical outcomes often encompasses specific speech and language processes. Specific outcomes, such as enhanced word retrieval, use of action-object utterances, ability to formulate increasingly complex sentences, and ability to follow increasingly complex commands, are found frequently in scientific studies and clinical reports. Today, however, the outcome terminology, perhaps consistent with the World Health Organization's *International Classification of Impairments, Disabilities, and Handicaps* (1980) or Nagi's (1965) conceptualization of the consequences of a disorder, is evolving to a more functional level. Because the term *handicap* has fallen from favor due to implications of negative societal attitudes about individuals with disabilities, the Nagi framework is gaining more favorable attention. This framework provides a solid base from which to articulate a continuum of outcomes at the impairment, functional limitation, and disability stages.

At the impairment stage, it is appropriate to discuss outcomes at the level of specific speech and language deficits. If these deficits (e.g., word-finding difficulties, telegraphic language, and agrammatism) lead to a functional limitation, outcomes are best expressed in functional terms. These include, for example, the ability to communicate basic needs, communication with a familiar partner, and communication with an unfamiliar partner. The third stage, the disability level, creates yet another set of outcomes. This level addresses the consequences of the functional limitation in relation to engaging in socially defined roles and tasks. It focuses, for example, on education, recreation, and employment. Academic achievement and vocational skills are outcomes at this level of disability (or the World Health Organization's level of handicap).

The level of functional limitation is often the point at which policy makers, as well as clients and families, begin to appreciate the positive effects of intervention. Consider the child with a language disorder. Which would be the more relevant outcome: the ability to produce grammatically correct utterances or the ability to use language to communicate immediate needs ("Tie my shoes," "I want a lollipop," "Leave me alone")? It is the functional focus that makes more sense to the client and family as well as the policy maker. It also is the functional focus that looks beyond the ability to master specific (and sometimes isolated) language skills to the ability to learn, work, and develop enduring social relationships.

Nelson (1992) describes changing attitudes toward assessment and intervention. Among these changing attitudes is a focus on functional outcomes. According to Nelson,

> the movement toward measuring communication needs and opportunities as well as processes is accompanied by a clear shift in the kinds of intervention targets that are selected. Intervention targets are not based on the results of formal tests and procedures, but on ethnographic analyses of the child's needs as defined by the important people in his or her life. Functional outcomes and natural consequences are deliberately targeted in intervention. Focus not only on the present, but on preparing children and adolescents for the transitions they will face, from home to school, from early grades to later, and from school to work or post-secondary school that will require new skills and tools. (p. 5)

The shift toward pursuing and measuring functional outcomes is consistent with the speech-language pathologist's changing role. Ferguson (1992) distinguishes the traditional from the emerging role:

> In the traditional role, the medical model defines the parameters of the role played by the speech-language pathologist. We diagnose isolated deficits in a one-to-one setting, and then prescribe developmental tasks to be developed in a treatment room separate from the educational environment of the regular classroom. The IEP [individualized education program] is written to develop isolated skills in this treatment environment. . . .
>
> The emerging role is defined by an educational model. In it we function as a specialist in communication, evaluating student competency in literacy skills (speaking, listening, reading, and writing) in the context of the educational environment (the regular classroom). Rather than work alone, we participate as an active member of a curriculum development team in a collaborative, transdisciplinary role to improve student communication performance. We provide services as a collaborative/consultant or as a team teacher for whole classes or for small groups. (p. 8)

With this emerging role comes the need for better functional outcome measures. But few standardized measures exist currently for the pediatric population. Among the more global measures (measures that span the range of physical, cognitive, communicative, and psychosocial functioning) that include sections on communication are the Pediatric Evaluation of Disability Inventory (Haley, Coster, Ludlow, Haltiwanger, & Andrellos, 1992) and the Wee Functional Independence

Measure (State University of New York at Buffalo, 1991). These are relatively new measures; thus, little information exists regarding their reliability, validity, and sensitivity for children with communication disorders. As the field of functional assessment advances, however, we can expect to see more and better pediatric measures of functional ability in the near future.

An Overview of Methods

At the outset of this chapter, I addressed single-subject and group experimental designs. These are experimental methods designed to yield reliable and valid outcome data. Studies employing these methods must demonstrate that improvement, if it occurs, results from the treatment and not from some unspecified variable (Wertz, 1993). There are, however, other quasi- and nonexperimental methods that can be used to collect outcome data. Although less rigorous than traditional experimental methods, they also can yield useful information. Many researchers, however, will disagree with this position, arguing that efficacy research is the only reliable and valid approach. In fact, the release of outcome data derived from other than experimental methods has received vigorous (and often due) criticism.

In the recent past, for example, the Health Care Financing Administration (HCFA) released mortality data from various hospitals. The data became a kind of report card of quality care for each hospital. Not surprisingly, the action was criticized, for these outcome data did not take into account patient severity, premorbid health status, age, case mix, type of hospital (primary, secondary, tertiary), etc., all of which have a direct impact on mortality rates. Defending this action, however, William Roper, past administrator of HCFA stated that "the perfect should not be the enemy of the good."

This quote exposes the mind-set of many policy makers and is used frequently as a rationalization supporting whatever outcome data exist. Thus, there seems to be little regard for the strict scientific method. Nevertheless, this overview of methods (although showing a clear preference for experimental design) will not discount the practical value of quasi- or nonexperimental methods. Each method can be used to document clinical outcomes. The methods, however, involve varying levels of scientific rigor and, thus, varying levels of confidence about relationships between the process and outcome of care.

Experimental Methods

According to Olswang (1990), *treatment efficacy* is a term open to broad interpretation and involves the use of group or single-subject experimental methods. As mentioned earlier, single-subject designs are those in which a subject serves as his or her own control. One such design (A-B-A design) allows the clinician to begin treatment A, move to treatment B, and then move back to treatment A while measuring behavior across the time continuum to note significant changes. Another suitable design allows the clinician to begin treatment A, withhold treatment, and resume treatment A while measuring behavior across the time continuum. Many such studies must be conducted, however, if behavior-specific results are to be generalized.

Group designs, on the other hand, allow for the study of subject populations, thus permitting the generalization of results. These designs, however, often suffer from problems associated with subject homogeneity, thereby threatening the validity of experimental findings. Group designs typically involve a treatment group and no-treatment (or different-treatment) control group. Behaviors between the groups are compared to note any differences.

Treatment Effectiveness, Efficiency, and Effects: Generating More Research Questions

Experimental methods encompass research that addresses several kinds of questions, which focus more specifically on *treatment effectiveness, treatment efficiency, and treatment effects*. Studies of treatment effectiveness ask whether treatment does or does not work. Treatment efficiency studies ask whether one treatment works better than another. Studies exploring treatment effects ask in what ways treatment alters behavior, specifically examining which aspects of treatment differentially influence which behaviors. Traditionally, clinical researchers have asked effectiveness and efficiency questions.

More and more, researchers are examining treatment effects. According to Olswang (1990), "It is as though after years of wondering *if* our treatments work, we are now examining more critically *why* and *how*. And in reality, isn't the issue of *how* treatment works the most basic?" (p. 100). Studies of treatment effects examine various behavioral outcomes of therapeutic manipulations. Olswang (1990) suggests the use of terminology provided by Rosen and Proctor (1991) to categorize three types of treatment outcome being considered in research on treatment effects: *intermediate, instrumental*, and *ultimate outcomes*.

Intermediate outcomes inform clinicians, from one session to the next, whether treatment is benefiting the client. These studies explore the treatment process. They are designed to answer questions such as What makes a good session? How important is this to the overall goal of treatment (or the ultimate outcome)? How necessary is it for our clients to move through intermediate outcomes? With reference to phonology treatment, Olswang (1990) gives the example of a clinician questioning whether practicing or producing sounds in isolation, syllables, words, and/or phrases is necessary to achieve sound production in conversation.

Instrumental outcomes are those that activate the learning process. These are described as outcomes that, when reached, trigger ultimate outcomes. Once an instrumental outcome is reached, treatment may no longer be necessary because the client will continue to improve on his or her own. The focus is on how long to treat. This kind of research is of particular interest to third-party payers and cost regulators. Again, citing phonology treatment, Olswang (1990) recommends that the clinician question at what level of correct production of the target sound is sufficient to trigger correct production in conversation.

Finally, ultimate outcomes demonstrate the social or ecological validity of treatment benefits. This focus gets at the heart of what is functional. Research designed to study ultimate outcomes explores questions concerning the meaningfulness of treatment. What does it mean to bring about functional communication, and how much direct treatment is necessary? Again, the ultimate outcomes are of prime interest to payers and regulators as well as clients and families: How will this treatment make me a more effective communicator? How will it enhance my ability to learn in school? to get a job?

In summary, treatment effect studies reflect the investigator's interest in determining which components of the treatment seem to be working and how well, or in determining exactly how the treatment affects the client. They are studies of treatment processes and their effect on client behaviors.

Quasi- and Nonexperimental Methods

Most investigators will agree that any inferences made about causal relationships are flawed when the premises of the true experiment are breached (Sechrest & Hannah, 1990). Yet, according to Sechrest and Hannah, causal inferences should not be avoided simply because these inferences may not be as strong as they should be. They cite several reasons why it may not be possible to produce experimental data. Some experiments may not be ethical (e.g., an experiment that withholds treatment); some experiments may be administratively or logistically impossible; some may be too expensive; some may require too much time to complete; some experiments may fail due to loss of subjects. Consequently, studies using quasi- or nonexperimental methods should not be easily dismissed.

These methods include small-area analyses, meta-analysis, case study, group judgment methods, and regression-discontinuity design. Of the less self-explanatory methods, small-area analysis is a technique that uses large administrative databases to obtain population-based measures of utilization and resource allocation (Wennberg, 1990). It is primarily a method of epidemiological investigation. Meta-analysis is essentially a method for reviewing and summarizing clusters of prior studies, irrespective of their research design and methodological differences. The results of studies are statistically combined. This method has the capacity to produce a single estimate of an intervention effect from studies that use different scales to measure the effectiveness of an intervention (Eddy, 1990; Smith & Glass, 1977). Regression-discontinuity design is described as another useful method for determining whether treatment is effective (Trochim, 1990). In its simplest form, it is a pretest-posttest program—comparison group strategy. Regression-discontinuity (RD) is distinguished from other pre-post group designs by the method in which participants are assigned to conditions. Subjects are assigned to program or comparison groups solely on the basis of a cutoff score on a preprogram measure (e.g., this cutoff criterion implies the major advantage of RD design—it is appropriate for targeting a program or treatment to those who need or deserve it).

A Multiple-Attacks Approach

Mosteller (1990) believes that a major approach to outcome evaluation is one of multiple attacks. He bases this on the premise that outcome data from multiple but independent sources, using various methods, are more influential in shaping public policy than outcome data from one study or a collection of studies using the same method. Considering the spectrum of methods available, the concept of multiple attacks has appeal for both the researcher and the clinician.

Historically, we have looked to scientists in the field to conduct experimental research designed to amass outcome data. But what can clinicians do—the vast majority who constitute the field—in efforts to do the same? Over time, the discipline of human communication sciences and disorders has suffered from its increasingly clinical (versus research) orientation. Clinicians are not being grounded in the basic scientific requisites. Siegal (1993) reports that the number of master of arts degree programs requiring original research is shrinking rapidly. Siegal believes this trend will compromise the field's long-standing commitment to research experience as an integral part of professional training. He also believes that future generations of students increasingly will be unfamiliar and uncomfortable with the research process and the interpretation of research methods and results. According to Seigal (1993), "the loss would be profound" (p. 36).

There is optimism that, in the future, clinicians will be grounded in the basic scientific requisites, administrators will support research activities in health care and education settings, and research funding streams will be in rich supply. Until that time, other methods must find their place in the realm of clinical outcome evaluation. Such methods as the clinical case study or group judgments (methods that can more easily be applied by clinicians) will only add to the outcome data available. Thus, the concept of multiple attacks should be supported by both the researcher and the clinician.

Translating Efficacy Data into Practice

The dissemination of treatment efficacy data is too often an overlooked yet critical activity. The best data can exist without practitioners knowing and, thus, without any influence on clinical practice. First, efficacy data should be translated into best practice guidelines. Second, these guidelines should be distributed widely in efforts to change practitioners' ways of doing things and thus reach desired outcomes in a more predictable manner.

Problems with dissemination, however, have become so widespread generally that they became a topic of a conference in 1993 (Darby, 1993). The conference, "Dissemination Strategies for Changing Clinical Behavior," organized by the University of Arkansas Area Health Education Centers, was supported by the U.S. Department of Health and Human Services' Health Resources and Services Administration (HRSA) and Agency for Health Care Policy and Research (AHCPR). William E. Golden, director of general internal medicine at the University of Arkansas for Medical Sciences, states that "you can create beautiful guidelines [based on efficacy data], but if you do not disseminate them, it's kind of like the tree falling in the forest" (Darby, 1993, p. 5).

Supported by research results, conference participants concluded that a multimedia approach to guideline dissemination, aimed at creating a "background of constant exposure" to new information, changed a professional's practice behavior more effectively than two other educational interventions. Similar to a multiple-attacks approach to amassing outcome data, the dissemination approach is a multipronged campaign to influence clinical practice patterns. Efficacy data and practice guidelines should be published in national journals, included in mass mailings, distributed through formation of local education networks (e.g., study groups), presented at continuing education events, summarized in news briefs, incorporated in computer-based treatment programs, and so on.

Audrey Holland (cited in Goldberg, 1993) believes that we must be masters of our fate—for our own professional integrity and for the sake of our clients. To do that, "we must take what we know from efficacy studies, see that the results are translated into practice guidelines, and make sure that those guidelines are widely disseminated and followed" (p. 45). After all, isn't this the right of any individual who seeks speech-language pathology services? Isn't this the right of a child with a language disorder—to expect the best of what exists in clinical practice?

Conclusion

I have constructed a profile of need and presented an overview of the means to collect clinical outcome data. I have reported that little outcome data exist, yet outcome data will be used to set both health care and education policies for the nation's children. I have stated that we must be masters of our own fate. If we do not collect the outcome data, others outside the field will do so with less regard for the rigor of such methods. I have stated a preference for experimental methods, but I have not discounted the usefulness of other quasi- or nonexperimental methods for collecting outcome data. I have supported a multiple-attacks approach to amassing outcome data. Finally, I have emphasized that efficacy data are useless if they are not translated into practice guidelines and disseminated and used widely by the clinical community. It is only until then that we can serve clients in their best interest.

Stark (1992) gives an eloquent epilogue titled, "What's Right for Children":

> What is right for the child is a gentle and sensitive society, a supportive family constellation, and an enriched educational environment. However, contemporary realities force us to look at other issues such as cost effectiveness. We need to examine the effects of early intervention and determine just how early it should be. Could a language learning disability and its concomitant psychosocial consequences have been avoided for thousands (or millions) of children and adults?. . . How can we maximize the use of naturalistic assessment and intervention practices? How can there be effective collaborative management in budget-poor schools? What issues surround the integrity of the family-school relationships? The questions abound and the answers are sometimes elusive. If we are ever to do what is right for children, these questions must be explored. (p. 11)

Clinical outcome investigation begins with scientific inquiry. The clinical question leads to a hypothesis that is accepted or rejected through systematic study. The findings lead to yet other questions that are explored, answered, and generate more questions. Clinical inquiry and its subsequent study form the foundation of any clinical discipline. During a time of cost constraints, the recipient of care depends on the provider of care to submit compelling scientific evidence of the value of clinical services, and thus to meet his or her needs. To this end, we must ask hard questions, such as What is right for the children? Some frank answers may be found in outcome data.

References

Darby, M. (1993). Multi-pronged campaign most effective at disseminating practice guidelines. *Report on Medical Guidelines & Outcomes Research, 4,* 5–7.

Diamond, G. W. (1989). Developmental problems in children with HIV infection. *Mental Retardation, 27,* 213–217.

Eddy, D. M. (1990). The role of meta-analysis. In L. Sechrest, E. Perrin, & J. Bunker (Eds.), *Conference proceedings: Strengthening causal interpretation of nonexperimental data* (pp. 173–176). Rockville, MD: U.S. Department of Health and Human Services, Public Health Service, Agency for Health Care Policy and Research.

Ferguson, M. L. (1992). Changing roles and changing policy. In E. R. Silliman (Ed.), *Special interest division 10 newsletter* (pp. 7–9). Rockville, MD: American Speech-Language-Hearing Association.

Goldberg, B. (1993). Translating data into practice. *ASHA, 35,* 45–47.

Haley, S. M., Coster, W. J., Ludlow, L. H., Haltiwanger, J. T., & Andrellos, P. J. (1992). *Pediatric evaluation of disability inventory,* Version 1.0. Boston, MA: New England Medical Center Hospitals, Inc.

Keeney, S. M. (1992). When children need rehabilitation. *Continuing Care, 11,* 18–34.

Minifie, F. D. (1990). Research in treatment efficacy: Where is the profession? In L. B. Olswang, C. K. Thompson, S. F. Warren, & N. J. Minghetti (Eds.), *Treatment efficacy research in communication disorders* (pp. 239–243). Rockville, MD: American Speech-Language-Hearing Foundation.

Mosteller, F. (1990). Improving research methodology: An overview. In L. Sechrest, E. Perrin, & J. Bunker (Eds.), *Conference proceedings: Strengthening causal interpretation of nonexperimental data* (pp. 221–230). Rockville, MD: U.S. Department of Health and Human Services, Public Health Service, Agency for Health Care Policy and Research.

Nagi, S. Z. (1965). Some conceptual issues in disability and rehabilitation. In M. B. Sussman (Ed.), *Sociology and rehabilitation* (pp. 100–113). Washington, DC: American Sociological Association.

National Education Goals Panel. (1992). *The national education goals report.* Washington, DC: National Education Goals Panel.

National Health Policy Forum. (1992). *Healthy start: Perspectives on the new federal initiative to reduce infant mortality.* Washington, DC: The George Washington University, Issue Brief No. 605.

Nelson, N. W. (1992). Changing attitudes toward assessment and intervention. In E. R. Silliman (Ed.), *Special interest division 10 newsletter* (pp. 3–5). Rockville, MD: American Speech-Language-Hearing Association.

Olswang, L. B. (1993). Issues in treatment efficacy: Developmental speech and language disorders. *ASHA, 35,* 42–44.

Olswang, L. B. (1990). Treatment efficacy: The breadth of research. In L. B. Olswang, C. K. Thompson, S. F. Warren, & N. J. Minghetti (Eds.), *Treatment efficacy research in communication disorders* (pp. 99–103). Rockville, MD: American Speech-Language-Hearing Foundation.

Rosen, A., & Proctor, E. (1981). Distinctions between treatment outcome and their implications for treatment evaluation. *Journal of Consulting and Clinical Psychology, 49,* 418–425.

Sechrest, L., & Hannah, M. (1990). The critical importance of nonexperimental data. In L. Sechrest, E. Perrin, & J. Bunker (Eds.), *Conference proceedings: Strengthening causal interpretation of nonexperimental data* (pp. 1–8). Rockville, MD: U.S. Department of Health and Human Services, Public Health Service, Agency for Health Care Policy and Research.

Seidel, J. F. (1991). The development of a comprehensive pediatric HIV developmental service program. Technical report on developmental disabilities and HIV infection (Report number 7). Silver Spring, MD: American Association of University Affiliated Programs.

Siegal, G. M. (1987). The limits of science in communication disorders. *Journal of Speech and Hearing Disorders, 52,* 306–312.

Siegal, G. M. (1989–1990). Review of "Fragmentation of clinical service and clinical science in communicative Disorders." *Journal of the National Student Speech-Language-Hearing Association, 17,* 15–16.

Siegal, G. M. (1993). Research: A natural bridge. *ASHA, 35,* 36–37.

Smith, L. M., & Glass, G. (1977). Meta-analysis of psychotherapy outcome studies. *American Psychologist, 32,* 752–760.

Stark, J. (1992). What's right for the children. In E. R. Silliman (Ed.), *Special interest division 10 newsletter* (pp. 10–11). Rockville, MD: American Speech-Language-Hearing Association.

State University of New York at Buffalo. (1991). *Functional independence measure for children (WeeFIM),* Version 1.5. Buffalo, NY: State University of New York Research Foundation.

Trochim, W. M. K. (1990). The regression-discontinuity design. In L. Sechrest, E. Perrin, & J. Bunker (Eds.), *Conference proceedings: Strengthening causal interpretation of nonexperimental data* (pp. 119–140). Rockville, MD: U.S. Department of Health and Human Services, Public Health Service, Agency for Health Care Policy and Research.

U.S. Department of Education. (1991). *America 2000: An education strategy—sourcebook.* Washington, DC: U.S. Department of Education.

U.S. Department of Health and Human Services, President's Committee on Mental Retardation. (1988). *Preventing the new morbidity: A guide for state planning for the prevention of mental retardation and related disabilities associated with socioeconomic conditions.* Washington, DC: U.S. Department of Health and Human Services.

U.S. Department of Health and Human Services, Public Health Service. (1990). *Healthy people 2000: National health promotion and disease prevention objectives.* Washington, DC: U.S. Department of Health and Human Services.

Wennberg, J. E. (1990). Small area analysis and the medical care outcome problem. In L. Sechrest, E. Perrin, & J. Bunker (Eds.), *Conference proceedings: Strengthening causal interpretation of nonexperimental data* (pp. 177–206). Rockville, MD: U.S. Department of Health and Human Services, Public Health Service, Agency for Health Care Policy and Research.

Wertz, R. T. (1993). Issues in treatment efficacy: Adult-onset disorders. *ASHA, 35,* 38–39.

Wilkerson, D. (1991, July). *Integrating program evaluation tools and methods with the clinical process.* Paper presented at the annual conference, "Rehabilitation Medicine: Continuous Interdisciplinary Quality Improvement," sponsored by the Buffalo General Hospital and SUNY at Buffalo, NY.

World Health Organization. (1980). *International classification of impairments, disabilities, and handicaps.* Geneva: World Health Organization.

2

The Adaptive Nature of Developmental Immaturity

Implications for Language Acquisition and Language Disabilities

DAVID F. BJORKLUND, PH.D., AND
RICHARD G. SCHWARTZ, PH.D.

Introduction

Developmental psychologists and their intellectual kin have made good livings describing age-related improvements in children's physical, social, cognitive, and language skills. We view ontogenetic development as a steady progression from immature to more mature forms—from embryo through infancy and childhood to reproductive adulthood, old age, and death. From our vantage point, ontogeny is teleological, taking essentially the same course for every biologically intact member of the species. Although there is enough variability in the course of individual development to make life interesting, we know the end state of development and we view preadult periods as preparations for that state. This view of development holds that the young organism is an unfinished form of the adult (a work in progress), needing to acquire or master a set of abilities before achieving completion. From this perspective, immaturity can be seen as a necessary evil, reflecting periods of life that must be endured on the way to reproductive maturity. It would be fully to our species's advantage to skip over or speed through these times of inefficiency, if possible.

This is a wholly reasonable perspective, but it is not the only reasonable perspective of development. Scientists who study that other classic form of development—phylogeny—long ago abandoned a progressive viewpoint, realizing that evolution does not have a plan that must lead to an inevitable conclusion (i.e., *Homo sapiens*). Rather, evolution is blind and more a function of chance or historic contingency than either Newtonian determinism or Divine blueprint (Gould, 1989). As such, evolutionists cannot assume that contemporary functioning is the ineluctable consequence of a developmental past. Current anatomy and behavior may be causally unrelated to phylogenetically earlier anatomy and behavior, each of which may reflect adaptations to particular past environments. There is no reason to assume that the structure or function of evolutionary ancestors were immature or less efficient than the structure or function of extant species.

There are even different forms of ontogeny. Many insects, for example, have evolved a type of ontogeny that is vastly different from our own. Metamorphosing insects often spend long periods of their lives in larval form. A caterpillar is a necessary step on the road to a butterfly, but the former is not simply an incomplete or immature form of the latter. The larvae of many species lead active lives, very different from the lives led by the adult (or imago) forms. Ontogeny is still teleological—butterflies are the inevitable result of caterpillars—but entomologists must recognize the integrity of the various developmental forms and not view one as merely a less effective or inefficient version of the other.

Consequences of Our View of Development

Why question our view of development? Humans (and mammals in general) do not metamorphose, and ontogeny is different from phylogeny because we truly do know the end state. Our view of development as progressing from the immature and inefficient to the mature and efficient cannot be totally wrong, but it may not be totally right, either. We must evaluate our implicitly held assumptions about ontogeny because they affect the type of research questions we ask about development, and they influence how we deal with children's education and remediation. What are some of the consequences of our commonly held and typically unexamined assumptions of development?

Is Faster Better?

When one views early phases of ontogeny as reflecting inefficient functioning, there is the obvious question, asked by developmental scientists, educators, therapists, and parents: "Can we accelerate development?" Perhaps ontogeny is amenable to intervention, to a speeding up of the "normal" rate, thus abbreviating the time children spend as immature and ineffective beings. Some cultures have been more concerned about the acceleration of development than others, with Americans being the twentieth-century champions in fostering the idea that faster is better. One of the reasons for the downfall of traditional Piagetian theory in the United States was persistent evidence that children, who could not spontaneously solve concrete or formal operational tasks, could be trained to do so, often after only a brief period of instruction (Brainerd, 1978). Piaget never seemed to appreciate Americans' fascination with training. Development, for Piaget, was something that occurred through the continual interaction between an active child and his or her environment. It was not something that could be greatly or meaningfully accelerated, and the experiments reporting conservation training in 4-year-olds, for example, reflected less about the nature of development as they did about the ingenuity of the investigator. Piaget referred to training experiments as "The American Question," and this fascination stemmed from a perspective that immature forms of development could and should be overcome by intervention whenever possible.

Our views of development also influence our approaches to education and remediation. If development is seen as a progression from ineffective to more effective forms, then teaching ineffective children the techniques or strategies used by more effective children is an obvious educational objective. With respect to remediation, mentally retarded or learning-impaired children are frequently described as developmentally delayed or as being developmentally disabled. They display skills or attributes characteristic of children younger than themselves. Because these skills represent less mature forms, the remediation attempts, consistent with our understanding of ontogeny, logically focus on providing such children with developmentally more advanced skills.

The Integrity of Immature Forms

We may make different decisions about education or remediation, however, if we viewed different phases of development as having an integrity of their own, much as an entomologist views the caterpillar and the butterfly. Developmental immaturity may provide some benefits of its own to a child who is currently incapable of demonstrating more advanced behaviors. Forcing developmentally more advanced forms of cognition or behavior on such a child may lead to closer approximations to the developmentally appropriate form while not yielding the optimal level of performance for that child. For example, mental strategies of arithmetic or memory are typically associated with enhancements in task performance for the good reason that using such strategies results in more efficient information processing (Harnishfeger & Bjorklund, 1990; Siegler & Jenkins, 1989). Younger children who do not spontaneously use strategies can be trained to do so, sometimes with gains in task performance, but sometimes without (Bjorklund & Harnishfeger, 1987; Bjorklund, Schneider, Cassel, & Ashley, 1994). Mental strategies, although associated with more mature cognition, are mentally expensive in that their execution consumes one's limited mental resources. For the young child, this often results in too few remaining resources to make good use of the strategy, producing no improvement in task performance despite considerably increased effort (Bjorklund, Muir-Broaddus, & Schneider, 1990). Although the results of training experiments demonstrating that children learned the strategy but failed to improve task performance are informative for the psychologist, are such training efforts useful from a pedagogical perspective? Might not there be better ways to enhance eventual performance than simply imposing a mature form of cognition on an immature child? Does such training actually hasten development, or are the effects domain specific and quickly forgotten once training is over?

This is not to take a laissez-faire approach to development, education, or remediation. We firmly believe that children's cognitions are greatly shaped by instruction. Our species's biggest claim to fame is likely our educability (Bruner,

1972).[1] We are the smartest species on Earth, not because we know so much at birth but because we learn so much over an extended childhood. Most of that learning is achieved by an immature organism specially adapted to acquiring the complexities of a human culture (Bjorklund & Green, 1992). Instruction around the world is geared to a child's cognitive level, with parents and other adults working within a child's zone of proximal development (Vgotsky, 1978), which reflects the difference between the level of accomplishment that a child can achieve on his or her own and the level that can be achieved under adult supervision. This zone reaches ever upward throughout development as the child's optimal level of cognitive maturity increases (Fischer & Bidell, 1991). Adult instruction within this zone is most apt to result in cognitive growth, and such instruction is invariably developmentally appropriate.

Similar arguments can be made for remediation. Children who are developmentally delayed or who have specific learning or language deficits can best learn when instruction is within their zones of proximal development. Children who are expected to master skills beyond their abilities may show greater approximation to the adult form, but possibly at an unreasonable expense, much like the expense of using an overly sophisticated memory or learning strategy with a young child.

In this chapter, we will first outline our thinking on the adaptive nature of cognitive immaturity—the idea that young children's cognitive systems may be specially adapted for the tasks they need to learn growing up in human culture. We will present evidence for this position specifically for language acquisition, arguing that infants' and young children's cognitive limitations make the task of acquiring a first or second language easier. We will then discuss the application of these ideas to education, particularly remediation, emphasizing intervention with language-impaired children. The main theme throughout this chapter is that immature cognitive systems should be viewed as having an integrity unto themselves and that instruction and/or intervention is most effective when such integrity is considered.

---

[1]Our species's remarkable educability is chiefly attributable to our possession of language. Although one may argue that language evolved as a consequence of our big brains rather than being their cause, it is inarguable that we would be qualitatively different thinkers and learners without it. The ability of language to displace the speaker and listener from the here and now increases drastically the efficacy of teaching over mimetic instruction (i.e., instruction via imitation; Donald, 1991). Much can be learned by observing another person display some technique and imitating that behavior. In fact, we often equate instructing someone with showing that person how to perform a task. Feedback can be provided, with the target behavior of the novice becoming increasingly like that of the model through practice. In fact, according to social cognitive theory (Bandura, 1989b), it is essentially through this phenomenon of observational learning that most social behaviors and roles are acquired.

But mimetic instruction has serious limitations. It cannot easily escape the immediate environment, cannot explain the caveats associated with the application of any complicated procedure, and is restricted to skills that can be literally shown. With language, both teacher and student can anticipate events in the future relevant to the target behavior and relate the new skill to familiar events of the past. Moreover, the recursive nature of language, the ability to embed ideas within other ideas, makes possible the instruction of complicated skills and procedures that could be mastered only with great difficulty and time, if at all, without it. Language serves not only as a communication system, but also as a representational system, and it may have been its role as a symbol system that, in part, accounted for its rapid evolution in *Homo sapiens* (Bickerton, 1990).

The Adaptive Nature of Cognitive Immaturity

Humans take an inordinately long time to reach maturity. We, as a species, spend proportionally more time as prereproductives than any other primate (Poirier & Smith, 1974). One reason for our prolonged immaturity is the complexity of the world humans must master. It takes time to master the intricacies of human life, even life in hunter-gatherer societies, and the years it takes to reach reproductive age afford the minimal time necessary to be knowledgeable and responsible enough to become a successful adult.

Our physical immaturity is accompanied by cognitive immaturity. We should not be surprised that different systems develop together, but this is not necessary (e.g., sensory systems function at or near adult levels early in childhood). In fact, it might not seem unreasonable for the physically immature child to have mature cognition, producing even faster learning and subsequently a more knowledgeable adult. This is not, of course, the way nature has chosen to work. Given the correlation between physical and mental development, might there be some adaptive value to the intellectual immaturity that accompanies physical immaturity (Bjorklund & Green, 1992; Bjorklund, Gaultney, & Green, 1993)?

The Value of Poor Metacognition

One set of cognitive skills for which immaturity may have an adaptive value for young children has been referred to as metacognition: a person's knowledge of his or her own thought processes. Metacognition has been proposed to influence the efficacy of cognitive functioning and to play an important role in overall cognitive development (Nelson, 1992). Preschool children, in particular, are out of touch with their cognitive abilities. They often think that they never forget things, that garbled verbal messages they send or receive are comprehendible, and that they are generally more competent at a host of cognitive tasks than they actually are (Bjorklund et al., 1993; Flavell & Wellman, 1977; Whitehurst & Sonnenschein, 1985). But in young children, and possibly in older children faced with more difficult tasks, poor metacognition has some advantages.

Following Bandura's ideas about the development of self-efficacy (Bandura, 1982, 1989a), people who *perceive* themselves as effective—who have a sense of positive self-efficacy—tend to be more effective than less positive people. Young children's motor and cognitive performance is consistently below the performance of older children and adults whom they observe and interact with, and, as such, an accurate assessment of their abilities would necessarily yield a low level of perceived self-efficacy. Were children to perceive themselves as ineffective as they actually are, they would begin behaving less effectively, shying away from novel tasks that, as their accurate metacognitive abilities would tell them, were beyond their current competencies.

However, young children rarely make accurate assessments of their performance. Instead they judge their abilities (both before and after performing a task) as being greater than they actually are and believe that they are generally smarter or more competent than an independent observer might judge (Bjorklund et al., 1993; Stipek & MacIver, 1989). Moreover, there is some evidence that whereas metacognitive knowledge and intelligence are positively related for older children

(Schneider, Korkel, & Weinert, 1987), this canonical relationship is not observed for 3- and 4-year-old children, with bright children having somewhat poorer metacognitive abilities (in terms of predicting and evaluating their imitative skills) than less bright children (Bjorklund et al., 1993). As a result, young children continue to attempt new tasks and to persist at old ones, increasing their actual competencies and discovering new skills in the process.

Neural Plasticity

The underdeveloped nervous system of infants and children also has some important adaptive values for cognitive development. For example, the brains of infants and young children are poorly myelinized and process information slowly and inefficiently (Konner, 1991). As a result, little in the way of cognitive processing is automatized, making it difficult for young children to acquire well-established mental habits early in life. The benefit of this lies in the fact that cognitive patterns acquired in infancy would otherwise interfere with later functioning. More so than at any other time in development, the world of infants and young children is very different from the world they will encounter as adults. Some of the lessons learned in infancy and early childhood are just as well forgotten. For example, infantile memories are unavailable to most of us and would be of little interest if we could retrieve them (other than at a New Age cocktail party or at a convention of psychoanalysts). Much of what is learned in infancy is relevant to that time in life only, and having vivid memories of that time may interfere with or contradict later knowledge needed to function well in later environments. Moreover, without giving credence to Freud's (1953) infantile amnesia theory, many of the experiences of infancy may reflect feelings of helplessness, if not actual trauma, and their retention into childhood would likely be maladaptive and impede the development of a positive sense of control.

This inefficient mental processing is likely the factor most responsible for the substantial degree of cognitive and behavioral plasticity humans show over the first 2 or 3 years of life. Babies suffering from malnutrition or reared in stultifying institutions or war-torn lands do show signs of their abuse and neglect, but, given proper stimulation, they can learn new ways of responding (Clark & Hanisee, 1982; Kagan & Klein, 1973; Skeels, 1966). Because of the inefficiency of early cognitive processing, the effects of early deprivation can be ameliorated. If children were born with more mature brains, or if development proceeded more rapidly than it does, the mental, social, and emotional flexibility of young children would be lost. This behavioral and cognitive flexibility is perhaps our species's greatest adaptive advantage, and it is afforded by the prolonged period of mental (and thus brain) inefficiency. Such plasticity declines with age, however (Jacobson, 1963; Lerner, 1984; McCall, 1981; Scott, 1968). As children's brains become more adultlike, they acquire and retain better the knowledge and mental operations they need for effective adult functioning.

Immaturity and Language Acquisition

Although there is strong evidence of early neural plasticity, there is a concomitant lack of uniformity in the young brain or, perhaps, in the genetic program that directs its development in interaction with the environment. In particular, infants and young children seem uniquely prepared for the acquisition of some species-typical skills, the most important of which, for our purposes, is language. The idea of a critical period for language acquisition, although not universally accepted, is strongly supported by evidence from a variety of sources (Hurford, 1990; Lenneberg, 1967; Newport, 1991). Simply put, there is an age after which the acquisition of a first and or a second language is substantially less likely. As the brain matures, the declining plasticity limits the capacity of the developing organism to acquire language.

Language Acquisition as an Inductive Process

To understand the role of immaturity in language acquisition, it is informative to consider current views concerning the nature of language acquisition. For several compelling reasons, some linguists and psychologists maintain that the acquisition of language is, at least in part, innately determined. Language acquisition is different from the development of certain other related abilities, such as reading and writing, in that language is acquired in every culture without direct instruction and in a relatively short period of time. Acquisition is often described as an inductive process. The linguistic data provided by the input serve as the basis for the induction of the adult grammar. Many current theoretical and empirical discussions of language acquisition are based on a logical proof that natural languages are not learnable with only positive evidence (Gold, 1967). Despite that, natural languages are learned. Gold suggested that successful learning occurs because at least some aspects of language may be innate, because there may be indirect negative evidence, or because the input may be ordered in some fashion.

There is a widespread belief that this induction process is governed by a set of constraints. These constraints have been described as passive filters that allow only certain paths in the search for the correct grammar in the hypothesis space. Alternatively, these constraints are sometimes viewed as more actively directing the child's search of the input for critical evidence concerning the nature of the grammar. Regardless of their nature, these constraints are postulated to be innate and domain specific. Their content is posited to be the restrictions on the structures, on the meanings of sentences, and on the mapping between the meanings and structures. In a recent article, Crain (1991) lists three hallmarks of the innateness of these constraints: They are unspecified in the input (i.e., in the language a child hears), they are universal, and the aspects of language they govern are early emerging. Because they are negative in scope (i.e., they specify what cannot occur), it is widely, but not universally, accepted that constraints are not directly available to the child in the input. This argument is based on the assumption that negative evidence (i.e., corrections) occurs infrequently in adults' child-directed speech. Certain aspects of languages are universal, and these are potential candidates for innate specification. Finally, those aspects of language that emerge early are potentially innately specified.[2] Although this is a convincing line of argument,

[2]Leonard (1991) argued that earliness is not reliable evidence for innateness because of the substantially slower acquisition evidenced by children with specific language impairments. However, there may be an even more compelling argument. Although language acquisition *(continued on page 24)*

the absence of negative evidence along with the innateness of constraints may not represent the full range of possible explanations for language acquisition.

In part, these underlying assumptions serve to narrow the scope of a complex problem for developmental psycholinguists, allowing formal argumentation and the description of developmental algorithms. However, this general approach ignores several critical issues. First, it is possible that none of the facilitators of acquisition identified by Gold—negative evidence, innate specification, or ordered input—may alone permit a given instance of a natural language to be learnable. Thus, these facilitators may be individually necessary but not individually sufficient conditions for acquisition. Innate constraints, positive and negative aspects of the input, and some ordering of the input may all contribute to acquisition. Finally, except for maturational proposals in which the later emergence of certain aspects of language are attributed to language-specific biological maturation (Borer & Wexler, 1987), the potential impact of development itself on language acquisition has been ignored. The only specific role ascribed to development is a proposal by Pinker (1984) in which he suggests that morphological acquisition involves the construction of array-like paradigms. Immaturity plays a role in that a premature commitment (i.e., filling in all the cells of the array) may be incorrect and irreversible. This is an interesting notion, but it does not begin to cover the developmental changes that occur during the period of language acquisition.

Cognitive Limitations and Early Language Acquisition

In a recent set of experiments with connectionist networks, Elman (1994) has discovered something rather interesting about language learning that is relevant to the central idea of this chapter. Briefly, connectionist networks are computer models usually implemented as software that consist of layers of units (actually mathematical formulas), each connected to all the units on the adjacent levels. The connections have activation weights with initial values that are selected randomly within a predetermined restricted range. The sum of the weights of the connections to a unit determines the activation level of that unit. Each unit has a threshold of firing. The layers include an input layer, an output layer, as well as several intermediate layers, termed *hidden*. The network takes input and produces output of different forms depending on the purpose of the simulation (e.g., input is a verb root and the output is a past-tense form of that verb; the network is given a segment and its output is the next consonant or vowel in the sequence; or, when given the input one word at a time, the network predicts the next word in the sentence). These simulations also involve sets of learning parameters (e.g., rate of learning, momentum) that determine the changes in the connection weights during a learning phase. During the learning phase, the network is provided with feedback on the accuracy of its output. It takes this feedback and

---

is relatively early, children are immersed in language input beginning at birth. Despite the paucity of information regarding the absolute quantity of input, auditory input is certainly frequent and is certainly more abundant than the exposure young children have to orthographic input. Children actually learn to read (a commonly cited example) with relatively little direct instruction and substantially less time of exposure.

adjusts weights to increase the probability of correct output on successive inputs. The network learns to sequence appropriately words in sentences. But more importantly, analyses of the weight patterns of connections reveal that the network extracts structural information about the input—grouping words together in a way that corresponds to grammatical categories (e.g., nouns, verbs), grouping sets of words in a way that corresponds to clause types (main versus embedded), subgrouping words in a way that corresponds to verb types (transitive versus intransitive), and representing hierarchical relationships among words and groups of words. This aspect of the network structure and performance is an important finding because it indicates that it is possible to extract some abstract features of language from distributional characteristics of the input.

The network employed for Elman's simulation was a specific type called a simple recurrent network (Elman, 1990). Such networks have a set of units called context units that receive input from one of the hidden layers and then feed this back up through the network. The effect of this is that these context units learn and retain information about the internal state of the hidden units, much like some type of memory buffer. In this simulation, the network was provided with a set of input sentences involving subject-verb agreement for number and the potential for multiple relative clause embeddings (in which the heads served as either subject or object of the relative clause). The difficulty for the network is that it has to learn both local and long-distance (i.e., discontinuous) subject-verb agreement (e.g., *The zebras who the lion chases find the hiding place*). In this example, there is local agreement between *lion* and *chase*. However, the agreement between *zebras* and *find* is long distance, dependent on the hierarchical structure of the sentence.

An important result of Elman's simulations was the report of initial failures. Even varying a number of network characteristics (e.g., rate of learning), Elman was unsuccessful in his initial simulations when the entire corpus (embedded and simple sentences) was presented to the network in a random order. The network did not learn correct long-distance subject-verb agreement (i.e., the wrong form of the verb was selected by the network). However, following these failures, the simulation was done in five stages, beginning with only simple sentences followed by subsequent stages, with the corpus containing increasing percentages of complex (i.e., embedded) sentences. Under these conditions, the network was correct in selecting grammatically correct forms of verbs (i.e., that agreed with the appropriate subjects) for all of the different sentence types. Although adults do simplify the language they direct to children, it is not clear that they do so to the extent that Elman reconstructed his input. Consequently, the simulation was conducted again in stages, except that this time the context units were manipulated in a way that simulated an initially limited memory (three to four words), with the memory increasing incrementally with each successive stage. In this case, all simple and complex sentences were presented to the network. Although the pattern of learning was somewhat different from the staged input, it was successful. These findings suggest that the limitation in memory may restrict the solution space for the child in the early stages of language acquisition, which in turn makes the task of inducing the grammar easier. Elman suggested that the critical period represents the delay in development of certain adult abilities rather than the loss of certain capacities. In other words, children's immature memory abilities play an adaptive role in language acquisition.

Newport and her colleagues have made a similar proposal, developing the "less is more" hypothesis of language acquisition (Johnson & Newport, 1989; Newport, 1990, 1991). Based on evidence of second-language learning and from the deaf community learning American Sign Language early versus later in life, Newport proposed that infants' and young children's limited cognitive abilities may provide them with a computational advantage for the acquisition of language, with the increased cognitive abilities of the older child and adult paradoxically making language learning more difficult. Newport (1990) argued that developmental limitations in encoding complex stimuli may facilitate certain aspects of language learning: "If children perceive and store only component parts of the complex linguistic stimuli to which they are exposed, while adults more readily perceive and remember the whole complex stimulus, children may be in a better position to locate the components" (p. 24). Consistent with the data of Elman (1994), Newport (1991) proposed that young children's greater facility for language acquisition is due to their "ability to extract only limited pieces of the speech stream, with a gradual increase over maturation and learning in the amount of material to be analyzed; in contrast, the more capable adult extracts more of the input but is then faced with a more difficult problem of analyzing everything all at once" (p. 126).

Thus, the cognitive limitations of infants and young children serve as a filter, yielding an effectively simplified corpus for children to process. It should not be forgotten, however, that adults in all cultures (Fernald, 1992) also play a cooperative role by speaking to young children in *child-directed speech.* Child-directed speech consists of high-pitched voices; short, grammatically simple phrases; exaggerated emphasis; and many questions and repetitions (Bruner, 1983; Gelman & Shatz, 1977). Infants display more responsive behaviors to child-directed speech than to conventional speech (Stern, Spieker, & MacKain, 1982), suggesting that infants condition their parents to use child-directed speech. Such modified language, accompanied with young children's limited information processing abilities, results in children receiving a much reduced body of linguistic evidence from which to extract the phonological, syntactic, and semantic rules of their mother tongue.

In addition to demonstrations of infants' preference for and attention to child-directed versus adult-directed speech (Fernald, 1992), there is some anecdotal evidence that simply being exposed to adult-directed language is not sufficient for language to develop. For example, Dutch children who watched regularly (and frequently preferred) German television often failed to understand the programs and did not achieve appreciable control of German (Snow et al., 1976). In another case, Moskowitz (1978) reported that the hearing child of deaf parents, who was confined to his home because of poor health, learned sign language from his parents but could neither speak nor understand spoken English by the age of 3, despite frequently watching television. Television not only provides no social reaction to children's speech (television cannot answer questions, respond to a child's comments, or repeat a sentence when requested), but its language is also impoverished in that it consists of adult-directed speech and not the modified child-directed speech that children typically receive from adults.

The suggestion from such research is that young children are neurologically prepared to learn language, although they learn best (or perhaps only) via social interaction with adults or older children speaking to them in nonadult ways (i.e., child-directed speech). For example, one such interchange takes the form of a vertical structure, in which a child produces a single-word utterance about a given scene or event and then the adult asks a question, followed by a single-word response, and so on. The net result is that the child produces a multiword utterance (across several turns) with support from the adult. Such a structure illustrates the possibility of producing more than a single word in relation to a single scene or event, and the questions illustrate the grammatical roles of the individual words. Such exchanges have been reported in various forms when children are between 12 and 18 months of age. The problem for children who have language impairments is that they may be as old as 3 years when they are capable of participating in and benefiting from such interactions. Even if their parents engaged them in this type of discourse at 18 months of age, they would not have been able to participate. By the time they have reached a point in their development at which they could participate in and benefit from this discourse structure, parents may no longer attempt to engage children in this way.

Even with the availability of appropriate input, there is still a question of how children use this information. For example, although there may be extensive prosodic information in the stream of speech to which children are exposed, it is not clear whether they perceive these characteristics and recognize their significance. Although young children have early difficulty in producing unstressed elements in words and in phrases, children seem to have some perceptual preference for prosodic versus segmental information (Echols, 1988). This preference changes direction after 5 years of age. Although we certainly do not know this to be true, it may well be the case that the early preference for suprasegmental over segmental information may point the child to phrase structure boundaries. Perhaps because suprasegmental cues are not consistently reliable cues except when they are highly exaggerated or signaling major syntactic boundaries, they are only used by children in the earliest stages of language acquisition.

Newport's and Elman's results suggest that there may be a developmental sequence of language-related aptitudes, beginning with a facility for analyzing gestalt features of input (e.g., prosodic envelope), followed by a period of facility with salient components, followed by facility with details of the entire complex stimulus. Each period may be adaptive to learning certain features of language.

Linguistic Limitations and Language Acquisition

There are some other phenomena in language that represent examples of the adaptive nature of developmental immaturity across language subdomains. In these cases, however, the immaturity that may facilitate development is actually within the same domain. Children's early lexical acquisition is directed, at least in part, by a phenomenon termed *phonological selection* (Schwartz, 1988). Children between approximately 12 and 18 months of age have gaps in their production vocabularies that can be characterized by the phonological characteristics of the adult targets, most notably initial consonants. Although there are commonalties across children, there are also substantial individual differences in the phonological characteristics selected. For example, a child may have an early production vocabulary that includes words beginning with front stops, labiodental fricatives, and nasals, but none beginning with velar stops, alveolar fricatives, and liquids. This limitation appears to be determined, at least in part, by the child's production abilities. Words with phonological characteristics that the child is capable of producing tend to be selected, whereas novel words with characteristics outside of the child's production abilities are excluded in these early vocabularies. In a small number of cases, these limitations also appear to influence the production of early word combinations (e.g., a child whose early two-word utterances may consist only of words that begin with bilabials; Donahue, 1986). This may serve to reduce the scope of early vocabulary acquisition. Consequently, phonological selectivity may also be an early means of organizing an initial lexicon around a set of structural characteristics. Similar to the effect of the imposed memory limitations in Elman's situation, setting constraints on the range of phonological variation in an initial lexicon may facilitate the subsequent acquisition of a phonologically varied lexicon.

A final example concerns the development of speech perception in young children. There is a series of experiments (Werker & Pegg, 1992) that reveal developmental changes in infants' and young children's perceptual performance in the discrimination of some contrasts that are not part of their native language. Specifically, children under 10 months of age can discriminate a variety of nonnative segmental contrasts. Thus, the children have speech perception abilities that are potentially open with respect to language-specific features. Between 10 and 12 months of age, however, some of these contrasts are no longer discriminable for children. Notably, among the contrasts that continue to be discriminated by children acquiring English (e.g., a contrast between a late and apical click in Zulu) are those that are most unlike any English segmental contrast, whereas those native contrasts that children do not seem to discriminate are closer to English contrasts such as a retroflex/dental contrast in Hindi (Best, McRoberts, & Sithole, 1988).

These examples of adaptive immaturity in subdomains of language, in the relationship between a child's linguistic ability at a given point in time and the characteristics of speech directed to the child, and in language-related domains such as memory point to a maturational view of language acquisition. According to such a view, the sequence of acquisition is directly dependent on a child's maturity or immaturity at given points in development. Given the apparently delicate balance of this relationship, attempts to remediate language disorders in children may pose previously unsuspected problems for interventionists.

Implications for Education and Remediation

When viewing children's immature cognitions as having an integrity of their own—as being adaptive to acquiring knowledge and skills appropriate to their developmental competencies—one must seriously question modes of education aimed at instilling in children skills generally thought to be in advance of their years. For example, what may the consequences be of beginning formal education in the crib (Doman, 1984) or of highly structured, academically oriented preschools (Eastman & Barr, 1985; Engelmann & Engelmann, 1981)? Many psychologists and educators have railed against such "pushing" of young children (Ames & Chase, 1981; Elkind, 1987a, 1987b; Gallagher & Coche, 1987; Sigel, 1987; Winn, 1983; Zigler, 1987); but there are surprisingly little data to support either the academic or developmentally appropriate positions. One recent study is an exception. In research by Hirsh-Pasek, Hyson, and Rescorla (Hirsh-Pasek, 1991; Hirsh-Pasek, Hyson, & Rescorla, 1990; Rescorla, Hyson, & Hirsh-Pasek, 1991), middle-class children who attended academically oriented preschools were compared at the end of kindergarten with a matched group of children who attended nonacademically oriented preschools. Hirsh-Pasek et al. reported no long-term intellectual benefits of academically oriented preschools, mixed with some modest negative consequences. Specifically, children who attended academically oriented preschools showed greater test anxiety and more negative attitudes toward school and were judged to be somewhat less creative at the end of kindergarten than children who attended nonacademic preschools. Based on either a conservative interpretation of these findings (there were no intellectual advantages and no substantial disadvantages) or a liberal one (no advantages with some real, albeit modest, disadvantages), a single conclusion is derived: "If early academic orientations offer no clear benefit to children's development and if they can hinder development, there is no defensible reason to encourage the introduction of formal academic instruction and adult-focused learning during the preschool years" (Hirsh-Pasek, 1991, pp. 44–45).

The Limits of Intervention

Viewing children's immature cognitions as potentially adaptive has significant implications for educational remediation. For example, Goodman (1992) has argued that rigorous educational interventions with delayed preschool children are misguided. Politicians, teachers, and parents have understandably embraced the "optimistic spirit of reform" (p. 250), believing that with enough effort on the part of parents and teachers and by beginning intervention early enough, the effects of mental retardation can be minimized or even reversed. Goodman notes, however, that parents and educators rarely examine the possible detrimental effects of rigorous instruction on delayed preschoolers. Might too much instruction too soon hinder children's spontaneity, suppress creativity and imagination, or negatively affect children's self-esteem as a result of recognizing that their abilities fall far below the criterion of performance demanded by a too rigorous curriculum? Goodman answers yes to each of these possibilities and argues that early education of the developmentally delayed is best achieved by respecting children's pace of development and showing indulgence for their immaturity. Goodman argues that for developmentally delayed children, "slow is fast enough" and that "slowing up will give these children, like other children, the opportunity for mastery and discovery, for fulfillment of their own drives while they meet expectations set by adults" (p. 254).

This position may sound too extreme. However, a weaker version may have implications for a wider range of intervention efforts. Specifically, early intervention for children with developmental disabilities may be limited in value if not undertaken with careful consideration of the child's current developmental abilities. For example, Panagos (in this book) argues that speech therapists' use of highly structured sessions stresses the correct production of speech forms, ignores the social foundation of language, and emphasizes only what children do poorly rather than building on on what they do well. An alternative approach would have the clinician focusing, in a playful and socially appropriate fashion, on aspects of a child's language that are "emerging at age level with the goal of generalization from normal to delayed forms" (Panagos, in this volume). Unfortunately, evaluating a child's current abilities and making use of them in clinical settings is often more easily said than done because of the difficulties in documenting a child's abilities based on observed behavior. Similar-appearing performances can reflect different underlying competencies. For example, although young infants exhibit a stepping reflex that seems to be comparable to later first steps, these are different and, in many respects, unrelated behaviors. Similarly, in the course of phonological acquisition, children sometimes produce one or more individual words in a fashion that is much more advanced (sometimes without any errors) than the rest of their developing phonology. Some of these productions, termed *progressive idioms,* regress in accuracy as the word is brought into line with the rest of the child's phonology. One child who was the subject of a diary study produced the word *pretty* accurately at 10 months of age, a time when she did not produce clusters or voiceless stops in other words (Leopold, 1947). Her production of *pretty* gradually regressed to match her production of other words (i.e., *bidi*). When she ultimately produced this word accurately again, she did so within the context of a more-adult-like phonology. It is unlikely that her initially accurate production was produced as an analyzed form, as would be the case in the later accurate production. There is an analogous situation in syntactic development. Early in the course of normal development (e.g., at the two-word utterance level) or as the result of intervention, children's sentences may be based on linear (i.e., surface) rules that specify structure in terms of the sequential relationships of the words in the sentence. The production of more complex, complete sentences is, by necessity, based on structural rules that are specified in terms of hierarchical structure (e.g., the relationship among sentence components such as noun phrases and verb phrases). Consequently, some earlier developing or intervention-trained structures may not be structurally or linguistically comparable to those that occur naturally at subsequent points in development.

These examples illustrate that apparent advances in a child's productions may not always reflect real changes in linguistic competence. Thus, the success of early intervention may sometimes be illusory. If we persist in early intervention that has little real effect, it is possible, as Goodman suggests, that there will be negative emotional effects because of limited outcomes or the child's frustration. Such intervention, however, should be accompanied by appropriate counseling, guidance, and monitoring to ameliorate any negative effects (see Gillette, this volume). The success of such intervention will depend on selecting and maintaining an appropriate set of goals that are consistent with the child's readiness for change (see Panagos, chapter in this book).

Developmental Language Disorders

Among the central issues regarding the adaptive nature of developmental immaturity are the general appropriateness, the specific nature, and the potential efficacy of intervention for children with developmental language disorders. One question is whether, in some general sense, intervention violates the idea that children's apparent immaturity in language is adaptive. At the extreme, this would mean that the language deficits exhibited by these children are appropriate to their level of development.

DEVELOPMENTAL CONSTRAINTS ON LANGUAGE ACQUISITION

We have some sense that there is a developmentally expanding envelope that restricts the range of language acquisition at given points in time. Depending on the perspective, this envelope may represent a set of constraints imposed by language-related abilities in other domains, such as general cognitive abilities. Alternatively, this envelope might represent the current status of the child's abstract linguistic knowledge (i.e., a set of domain-specific constraints). Finally, the constraint envelope may be specified in terms of peripheral, language-related abilities that permit children to segment, parse, identify, and comprehend utterances, and the peripheral production abilities that permit children to plan and execute the production of utterances (e.g., perception, motor speech production, short-term memory, and long-term memory). Children's linguistic abilities at any given point in time may be developmentally adaptive with respect to their cognitive abilities, their linguistic knowledge, and their peripheral abilities.

Children's overall cognitive development, as typically measured by mental age, is often considered to be a limiting factor in language acquisition. Some clinical investigators have gone so far as to claim that a language disorder is present only if a child's language age is below his or her mental age. Such claims depend on how one views the relationship between language and cognition. The assumption underlying the aforementioned position, that some overall measure of linguistic ability cannot exceed an overall measure of cognitive ability, is but one of several possible relationships between language and cognition (Rice, 1983). In an alternative view, linked to the construct of local homologies, certain specific features of language and related features of cognition (e.g., prelinguistic gestural or vocal requests and object manipulation demonstrating tool use) emerge at similar points in development (Bates, 1979; Greenfield, 1991), with executive control assumed to be a more abstract cognitive ability. There is insufficient evidence to support conclusively any one of these competing views of language-cognition relationships. In fact, except possibly for children with severe to profound developmental delays, there appears to be great variability in the relationship between children's overall intellectual abilities and their language abilities. Furthermore, there is direct evidence that so-called cognitive indexing is not always a reliable way to determine whether a language disorder is present and, if it is, whether intervention will have a significant impact. For example, Cole, Dale, and Mills (1990) found no comparative differences in the linguistic gains following a year of intervention made by a group of children with cognitive skills equivalent to their initial language skills and by a group of children with cognitive skills well beyond their initial language skills. This indicates that, at least for children without severe developmental delays, general cognitive abilities do not necessarily constrain the potential effects of language intervention. Even viewed from the perspective of local homologies, there is no evidence to suggest that specific cognitive behaviors must be present prior to the emergence of their corresponding linguistic abilities (e.g., sound combinations and object combinations).

Perhaps, for these children, the general issue of maturity or readiness for change is more specific to the domain of language or to directly related peripheral skills (e.g., memory, perceptual abilities). Language intervention may fail in several obvious ways. A child enrolled in language intervention may evidence no change, may evidence changes that are limited in their application to novel linguistic contexts, or may evidence changes limited to the communicative context of the intervention setting. Intervention may also fail in less obvious ways. Children may appear to exhibit the desired surface behaviors without a change having occurred in the child's underlying linguistic knowledge. Given the availability of appropriate and efficacious intervention approaches, intervention failures may be attributable to immaturity or a lack of readiness to acquire the targeted linguistic structures or rules. In these cases, the problem may lie in a misalignment of the selected intervention targets and the child's maturational readiness.

No less important are failures that may be attributable to the way in which language is taught or facilitated in the course of intervention. Despite widespread belief in cognitively oriented, structurally hierarchical views of language, intervention often relies heavily on behavioral principles. As a result, children may directly learn linear rules (or surface response patterns) for certain syntactic structures rather than the associated structural rules. To illustrate the differences between a linear and a structural rule, consider the following example of question formation. For the sentence *The man is in the room* to be transformed into a question, it must be changed to the form *Is the man in the room?* Two types of rules could be used to accomplish this change. The simplest would involve a surface, or linear, rule that would move the first *is* in the sentence directly to the sentence initial position. In an intervention activity in which the focus is on simple sentences, a child could easily achieve a high level of success by using this linear rule. However, when the focus of intervention expands to include more complex sentences such as *The boy who is sick is in the room,* this rule will not work. It will yield the ungrammatical question, *Is the boy who sick is in the room?* Instead, a structural rule, which moves the *is* in the highest clause (or main clause) in the syntactic tree to the front of the sentence, is needed. This generates the appropriate question form, *Is the boy who is sick in the room?* Given the format in which intervention most often occurs, it is likely that at least some children learn linear rather than structural rules.

Although we have no direct empirical evidence, the typically larger number of children who fail to generalize intervention gains may do so because they have not acquired or learned to apply structural rules in the course of intervention. Some indirect evidence suggesting that linear rule learning is common is found in an intervention study reported by Leonard (1974). Following training with a modeling procedure, the children generalized training on the auxiliary *is* (e.g.,

Lyle is laughing.) to the copula or main verb form (e.g., *Lyle is relaxed.*) and to question inversions (e.g., *Is Lyle laughing? Is Lyle relaxed?*). It is important to note that the underlying structure of a sentence with an auxiliary places the auxiliary in the verb phrase as a component along with the main verb, whereas the underlying structure of a sentence with a simple main verb (such as the verb *to be* in the copula form) places the verb directly under the sentence node as the verb of the sentence. Generalizing a morpheme across syntactic structures is not a surprising outcome of intervention; it suggests that children are aware of the surface similarities of these forms of the verb *to be*. However, the fact that these children so readily achieved this generalization may also indicate a lack of awareness of the distinction between these sentence structures. These children may have learned to use the two forms of the verb *to be* in these sentence types as a single linear response or rule, without any knowledge of the underlying or structural differences. Although this may serve a child well in simple sentences, as language complexity increases, problems may be revealed. Unfortunately, the measures used to assess a child's pretreatment knowledge and even those used to gauge progress in intervention do not typically reveal anything about children's existing linguistic knowledge.

It is also possible that language impairments are developmentally adaptive with respect to the maturational level of language-related peripheral domains, such as auditory perception or memory. Interestingly, despite substantial evidence of peripheral deficits in children identified as language impaired, interventionists often ignore the potential negative impact of such deficits. Consequently, intervention may involve an attempt to establish linguistic abilities that outstrip children's peripheral abilities in one or more of the aforementioned domains. The relatively constrained communicative setting of intervention may make it possible for a child to demonstrate production or comprehension of the linguistic target. However, because little is typically done to address the relevant peripheral limitation, the child leaves these apparent intervention gains behind in the constrained context.

INTERVENTION GOALS

The potential failure of intervention because of a mismatch with the child's level of maturity poses some serious problems. The solution for interventionists is not immediately evident. Some considerations point to approaches that might be taken in deciding whether to intervene and what to target. Olswang and Bain (1991a) have identified three possible views of the general goal of intervention: (1) To remediate the deficit underlying the disorder (i.e., to remove the adaptive basis of the language disorder such as memory abilities consistent with language abilities below a child's chronological age); (2) to alter the disorder by teaching specific linguistic structures directly;[3] or (3) to focus on compensatory strategies that permit the utilization of more complex linguistic structures and communicative devices within the child's current abilities.

---

[3]It is questionable whether children can be taught, in the traditional sense, abstract structural rules. It may be most reasonable to assume that a subset of input can be manipulated to increase the likelihood that a child will induce the target rule.

The first goal is the ideal. However, children who are identified as language impaired at a young age often continue to manifest language deficits later in life, in both oral and written language, in spite of intervention (Weiner, 1985). Furthermore, we cannot be certain that enough is known about the underlying causes of such disorders to determine what warrants to be remediated. Even when such information is available, it is possible that the underlying deficits will not be responsive to remediation, regardless of whether they are specifically linguistic or language-related peripheral abilities.

The second goal, to alter the disorder by teaching specific linguistic structures, seems to contradict the central premise of this chapter. It may be especially contradictory when language development norms are used to choose goals without considering the child's readiness for particular linguistic structures. In many cases, the result may be either no change or superficial changes that are not truly isomorphic with the targeted changes in underlying linguistic knowledge. However, with the application of more sensitive assessment measures and with alternative approaches to assessment, it may be possible to identify specific features of language that are already established in the child's underlying linguistic knowledge but are not yet part of the child's usage. Such features might be more amenable to intervention than those for which the child does not appear to have underlying knowledge. For example, Crain (1991) and others (McDaniel, Cairns, & Hsu, 1990a) have developed creative comprehension tasks involving picture identification and acting out responses that determine children's knowledge of specific syntactic structures. By carefully selecting sentence and picture stimuli, these investigators have been able to document knowledge of linguistic principles governing pronominal reference that is not yet apparent in young children's simple sentences. However, measurement techniques employed in clinical settings are not designed to reveal these more subtle aspects of linguistic behavior. If these experimental procedures were applied clinically, they might uncover linguistic knowledge not evident in children's language production, which would then be reasonable targets for intervention, consistent with the child's readiness for change.

In a similar vein, Olswang and Bain (1991b) described an approach called dynamic assessment, based on Vygotsky's (1978) previously discussed zone of proximal development. Again, the zone of proximal development is the difference between performance on a given task without extraneous cues or support and performance with added cues and support. Dynamic assessment involves identifying zones of proximal development through trial intervention procedures. Dynamic assessment also is designed to identify points of readiness over the course of development and intervention (Palinscar, Klenk, Anderman, Parecki, & Wilson, 1991).

Olswang and Bain (1991a) characterize this second goal as the prospective aim of current early intervention approaches. These approaches can be categorized in terms of their specific functional outcomes. Intervention approaches may facilitate the emergence (i.e., use) of existing knowledge, or they may facilitate the establishment of new linguistic knowledge. Two types of intervention approaches that might be best suited to facilitating of the emergence of existing knowledge have been referred to child initiated, or hybrid (Fey, 1986; Fey, Cleave, Long, &

Hughes, 1993). Milieu teaching (Warren & Kaiser, 1986), joint action routines (Constable, 1986; Snyder-McLean, Salomonson, McLean, & Sack, 1984), discourse structures (Schwartz, Chapman, Terrell, Prelock, & Rowan, 1985), or focused stimulation (Schwartz & Leonard, 1984) are all examples of these types of approaches. Unlike clinician-directed intervention, these procedures, to varying degrees, follow the child's lead while imposing structured exposure to target structures in a relatively natural discourse context. These facilitative methods typically rely on the course of normal development and target structures at or just beyond the child's current production abilities. However, as just noted, current assessments are not sufficiently sensitive to detect changes in linguistic knowledge that are not directly observable. Thus we have little available empirical evidence of enduring intervention-induced changes in underlying linguistic knowledge. It may be more realistic to expect that child-directed and hybrid intervention methods to facilitate the use of linguistic knowledge are already present.

Within the category of clinician-directed procedures (Fey, 1986), some intervention techniques focus more directly on effecting changes in children's underlying linguistic knowledge, such as the principles of pronominal reference addressed by Cairns (McDaniel, Cairns, & Hsu, 1990b). One example is the induction technique described by Connell (1987, 1988). In this approach, efforts are made to demonstrate the contrast between contexts that require the rule and contexts in which a given rule does not apply. Other techniques, such as modeling and imitation (Connell, 1986), may also be employed with the intent of changing a child's knowledge regarding a particular linguistic structure (e.g., subjecthood). However, because of variations across children in the effectiveness of such approaches, it is not clear that this is a clinical option for all children with language impairments.

The third possible goal for intervention—teaching compensatory strategies that permit children to utilize more complex linguistic structures and communicative devices within the envelope of their existing abilities—has only recently become a focus of clinical research. In the case of children with severe disabilities, selecting alternative modes of communication represents an example of intervention directed toward this goal. However, in the case of less severe speech and language disorders, it is not immediately clear how teaching compensatory strategies might be best approached. As noted earlier, one reason for this uncertainty is our current lack of knowledge of the specific deficits underlying such disorders. Thompson and Shapiro (Shapiro & Thompson, in press; Thompson, Shapiro, & Roberts, 1993) have taken this third approach in treating sentence-production disorders in adult aphasics. They first hypothesized a set of underlying deficits and then trained a strategy that allowed patients to circumvent their limitations and to produce *wh*-questions. However, even if such deficits and compensatory strategies could be identified in young children, learning such strategies and how to apply them may require metalinguistic and metacognitive skills that are not yet in their repertoire, unlike adults with language disorders.

Even though compensatory strategies are seldom the direct focus of intervention for childhood language disorders, the functional outcome of many existing procedures may be compensatory in nature. Many, if not all, past efforts at intervention might have established compensatory strategies rather than the second goal, teaching specific linguistic structures. Even if localized linguistic knowledge is changed, the underlying deficit(s) may remain. This could be why many children who have received early intervention continue to have oral and written language disabilities that persist later in their development. The changes resulting from intervention may, in reality, be the result of a compensatory strategy, such as a reliance on the linear rules described earlier.

An alternative is to provide compensatory strategies for the acquisition of linguistic structures rather than for the use of structures that are already known by the child but are not yet used. For example, if children with specific language impairment actually have deficits in perception, as suggested by some investigators (Leonard, McGregor, & Allen, 1992), an alteration in input may represent a compensatory strategy that would permit acquisition of forms that may be otherwise difficult for children to detect (e.g., grammatical morphemes, final consonants). Similarly, some intervention procedures already in use incidentally alter input by increasing the frequency of target structures.

Of the three goals for intervention discussed, teaching compensatory strategies or providing compensation in input may be the most viable option for achieving true success in intervention. Given the persistence of language disorders, it seems apparent that we do not often succeed in curing these disorders. Effective compensation may be the only real option that does not violate the adaptive nature of immaturity of these children's language disorder and should be pursued more vigorously by interventionists.

Conclusion

How we view development affects the way we look at children, the research questions we ask, and how we approach atypical development. Human cognitive development is generally progressive—children get smarter and more skilled over time. But this is not so for all aspects of development, and it does not necessarily mean that early and immature forms of cognition are ineffective and maladaptive relative to later, more mature forms of cognition. By viewing the behaviors of immature children as having an intellectual/linguistic integrity of their own, we achieve a different perspective, seeing immaturity not as a necessary evil but as reflecting an ontogenetic adaptation.

This perspective is perhaps especially easy to appreciate for developmental psycholinguists because of the long-recognized facility of young children for acquiring both a first and second language. Young children have unique language-learning abilities, and recent evidence points to immaturity in information extraction and memory (Elman, 1994; Newport, 1991) as prime contributors to this special gift. The adaptive nature of developmental immaturity poses a set of issues for clinicians and researchers interested in developmental disorders in general and developmental language disorders in particular. Long-standing assumptions regarding the goals, the appropriateness, and the assumed functional outcomes of various approaches to intervention warrant reexamination in light of this perspective.

Acknowledgments

We would like to thank Barbara Bjorklund, William Cassel, and Lewis Shapiro for constructive comments on earlier versions of this manuscript. Preparation of this chapter was supported in part by a PHS grant from NIDCD to Richard G. Schwartz, "Input-Output Relationships in Speech and Language Impairments," DC00583.

References

Ames, L. B., & Chase, J. A. (1981). *Don't push your preschooler.* New York: Harper & Row.

Bandura, A. (1982). Self-efficacy mechanism in human agency. *American Psychologist, 37,* 122–147.

Bandura, A. (1989a). Regulation of cognitive processes through perceived self-efficacy. *Developmental Psychology, 25,* 729–735.

Bandura, A. (1989b). Social cognitive theory. In R. Vasta (Ed.), *Annals of child development* (pp. 1–60). Greenwich, CT: JAI Press.

Bates, E. (1979). *The emergence of symbols: Cognition and communication in infancy.* New York: Academic Press.

Best, C., McRoberts, G., & Sithole, N. (1988). The phonological basis of perceptual loss for non-native contrasts: Maintenance of discrimination among Zulu clicks by English-speaking adults and infants. *Journal of Experimental Psychology: Human Perception and Performance, 14,* 345–360.

Bickerton, D. (1990). *Language and species.* Chicago: Chicago University Press.

Bjorklund, D. F., & Harnishfeger, K. K. (1987). Developmental differences in the mental effort requirements for the use of an organizational strategy in free recall. *Journal of Experimental Child Psychology, 44,* 109–125.

Bjorklund, D. F., Muir-Broaddus, J. E., & Schneider, W. (1990). The role of knowledge in the development of children's strategies. In D. F. Bjorklund (Ed.), *Children's strategies: Contemporary views of cognitive development* (pp. 93–128). Hillsdale, NJ: Erlbaum.

Bjorklund, D. F., & Green, B. L. (1992). The adaptive nature of cognitive immaturity. *American Psychologist, 47,* 46–54.

Bjorklund, D. F., Gaultney, J. F., & Green, B. L. (1993). "I watch, therefore I can do:" The development of meta-imitation over the preschool years and the advantage of optimism in one's imitative skills. In M. L. Howe & R. Pasnak & (Eds.), *Emerging themes in cognitive development* (Vol. 2, pp. 79–102). New York: Springer-Verlag.

Bjorklund, D. F., Schneider, W., Cassel, W. S., & Ashley, E. (1994). Training and extension of a memory strategy: Evidence for utilization deficiencies in the acquisition of an organizational strategy in high- and low-IQ children. *Child Development, 65,* 951–965.

Borer, H., & Wexler, K. (1987). The maturation of syntax. In T. Roeper & E. Williams (Eds.), *Parameter setting* (pp. 123–172). Dordrecht, Holland: Reidel.

Brainerd, C. J. (1978). *Piaget's theory of intelligence.* Englewood Cliffs, NJ: Prentice Hall.

Bruner, J. S. (1972). The nature and uses of immaturity. *American Psychologist, 27,* 687–708.

Bruner, J. S. (1983). *Child's talk: Learning to use language.* New York: W. W. Norton.

Clark, E. A., & Hanisse, J. (1982). Intellectual and adaptive performance of Asian children in adoptive American settings. *Developmental Psychology, 18,* 595–599.

Cole, K., Dale, P., & Mills, P. (1990). Defining language delay in young children by cognitive referencing: Are we saying more than we know? *Applied Psycholinguistics, 11,* 291–302.

Connell, P. (1986). Teaching subjecthood to language-disordered children. *Journal of Speech and Hearing Research, 29,* 481–492.

Connell, P. (1987). Teaching language rules as solutions to language problems: A baseball analogy. *Language, Speech, and Hearing Services in the Schools, 18,* 194–205.

Connell, P. (1988). Facilitating generalization through induction teaching. In L. McReynolds & J. Spradlin (Eds.), *Generalization strategies in speech and language pathology* (pp. 44–62). Toronto: B. C. Decker.

Constable, C. (1986). The application of scripts in the organization of language intervention contexts. In K. Nelson (Ed.), *Event knowledge: Structure and function in development* (pp. 205–230). Hillsdale, NJ: Erlbaum.

Crain, S. (1991). Language acquisition in the absence of experience. *Behavior and Brain Sciences, 14,* 597–650.

Doman, G. (1984). *How to multiply your baby's intelligence.* Garden City, NY: Doubleday.

Donahue, M. (1986). Phonological constraints on the emergence of two-word utterances. *Journal of Child Language, 13,* 209–218.

Donald, M. (1991). *Origins of the modern mind: Three changes in the evolution of culture and cognition.* Cambridge, MA: Harvard University Press.

Eastman, O., & Barr, J. L. (1985). *Your child is smarter than you think.* New York: Morrow & Co.

Echols, C. (1988). The role of stress, position, and intonation in the representation and identification of early words. *Papers and Reports on Child Language Development, 27,* 39–46.

Elkind, D. (1987a). Early childhood education on its own terms. In S. L. Kagan & E. E. Zigler (Eds.), *Early schooling: The national debate* (pp. 98–115). New Haven, CT: Yale University Press.

Elkind, D. (1987b). *The miseducation of children: Superkids at risk.* New York: Knopf.

Elman, J. (1990). Finding structure in time. *Cognitive Science, 14,* 179–211.

Elman, J. (1994). Implicit learning in neural networks: The importance of starting small. In C. Umilta & M. Moscovitch (Eds.), *Attention and performance XV: Conscious and nonconscious information processing* (pp. 861–888). Cambridge, MA: MIT Press.

Engelmann, S., & Engelmann, T. (1981). *Give your child a superior mind.* New York: Cornerstone.

Fernald, A. (1992). Human maternal vocalizations to infants as biologically relevant signals: An evolutionary perspective. In J. H. Barkow, L. Cosmides, & J. Tooby (Eds.), *The adapted mind: Evolutionary psychology and the generation of culture* (pp. 391–428). New York: Oxford University Press.

Fey, M. (1986). *Language intervention with young children.* Austin, TX: Pro-ed.

Fey, M., Cleave, P., Long, S., & Hughes, D. (1993). Two approaches to the facilitation of grammar in children with language impairment: An experimental evaluation. *Journal of Speech and Hearing Research, 36,* 141–157.

Fischer, K. W., & Bidell, T. (1991). Constraining nativist inferences about cognition. In S. Carey & R. Gelman (Eds.), *The epigenesis of mind: Essays on biology and cognition* (pp. 199–236). Hillsdale, NJ: Erlbaum.

Flavell, J., & Wellman, H. (1977). Metamemory. In R. V. Kail, Jr., & J. W. Hagen (Eds.), *Perspectives on the development of memory and cognition* (pp. 3–33). Hillsdale, NJ: Erlbaum.

Freud, S. (1953). Three essays on the theory of sexuality. In J. Strachy (Ed. and Trans.), *The standard edition of the complete psychological works of Sigmund Freud* (Vol. 7, pp. 125–145). London: Hogarth Press. (Original work published 1905).

Gallagher, J. M., & Coche, J. (1987). Hothousing: The clinical and educational concerns over pressuring young children. *Early Childhood Research Quarterly, 2,* 203–210.

Gelman, R., & Shatz, M. (1977). Appropriate speech adjustments: The operation of conversational constraints on talk to 2-year-olds. In M. Lewis & L. Rosenblum (Eds.), *Interaction, conversation, and the development of language* (pp. 27–61). New York: Academic Press.

Gold, E. (1967). Language identification in the limit. *Information and Control, 16,* 447–474.

Goodman, J. F. (1992). *When slow is fast enough: Educating the delayed preschool child.* New York: Guilford.

Gould, S. J. (1989). *Wonderful life: The Burgess Shale and the nature of history.* New York: W. W. Norton.

Greenfield, P. M. (1991). Language, tools, and brain. *Behavioral and Brain Science, 14,* 531–595.

Harnishfeger, K. K., & Bjorklund, D. F. (1990). Children's strategies: A brief history. In D. F. Bjorklund (Ed.), *Children's strategies: Contemporary views of cognitive development* (pp. 1–22). Hillsdale, NJ: Erlbaum.

Hirsh-Pasek, K., Hyson, M. C., & Rescorla, L. (1990). Academic environments in preschool: Do they pressure or challenge young children? *Early Education and Development, 1,* 401–423.

Hirsh-Pasek, K. (1991). Pressure or challenge in preschool? How academic environments affect children. In L. Rescorla, M. C. Hyson, & K. Hirsh-Pasek (Eds.), *Academic instruction in early childhood: Challenge or pressure.* New Directions for Child Development, Vol. 53 (pp. 39–46). New York: Jossey-Bass.

Hurford, J. R. (1990). The evolution of the critical period for language acquisition. *Cognition, 40,* 150–201.

Jacobson, M. (1969). Development of specific neuronal connections. *Science, 163,* 543–547.

Johnson, J. S., & Newport, E. L. (1989). Critical period effects in second language learning: The influence of instructional state on the acquisition of English as a second language. *Cognitive Psychology, 21,* 60–99.

Kagan, J., & Klein, R. E. (1973). Cross-cultural perspectives on early development. *American Psychologist, 28,* 947–961.

Konner, M. (1991). Universals of behavioral development in relation to brain myelinization. In K. R. Gibson & A. C. Petersen (Eds.), *Brain maturation and cognitive development: Comparative and cross-cultural perspectives* (pp. 181–224). New York: Aldine de Gruyter.

Lenneberg, E. H. (1967). *Biological foundations of language.* New York: Wiley.

Leonard, L. (1974). A preliminary view of generalization in language training. *Journal of Speech and Hearing Disorders, 39,* 429–436.

Leonard, L. (1991). Early emergence as a diagnostic for innateness. *Behavior and Brain Sciences, 14,* 625–626.

Leonard, L., McGregor, K., & Allen, G. (1992). Grammatical morphology and speech perception in children with specific language impairment. *Journal of Speech and Hearing Research, 35,* 1076–1085.

Leopold, W. (1947). *Speech development of a bilingual child, Volume 2. Sound learning in the first two years.* Chicago: Northwestern University Press.

Lerner, R. M. (1984). *On the nature of human plasticity.* New York: Cambridge University Press.

McCall, R. B. (1981). Nature-nurture and the two realms of development: A proposed integration with respect to mental development. *Child Development, 52,* 1–12.

McDaniel, D., Cairns, H., & Hsu, J. (1990a). Binding principles in the grammars of young children. *Language Acquisition, 1,* 121–138.

McDaniel, D., Cairns, H., & Hsu, J. (1990b). Control principles in the grammars of young children. *Language Acquisition, 1,* 297–336.

Moskowitz, B. A. (1978). The acquisition of language. *Scientific American, 239,* 92–108.

Nelson, T. O. (1992). *Metacognition: Core readings.* Boston, MA: Allyn and Bacon.

Newport, E. L. (1990). Maturational constraints on language learning. *Cognitive Science, 14,* 11–28.

Newport, E. L. (1991). Constraining concepts of the critical period for language. In S. Carey & R. Gelman (Eds.), *The epigenesis of mind: Essays on biology and cognition* (pp. 111–130). Hillsdale, NJ: Erlbaum.

Olswang, L., & Bain, B. (1991a). Intervention issues for toddlers with specific language impairments. *Topics in Language Disorders, 11,* 69–86.

Olswang, L., & Bain, B. (1991b). When to recommend intervention. *Language Speech and Hearing Services in Schools, 22,* 255–263.

Palinscar, A. S., Klenk, L., Anderman, E., Parecki, A., & Wilson, A. (1991). Exploring zones of proximal development of literacy acquisition with young children identified as learning disabled. *Exceptionality Education Canada, 1,* 105–125.

Pinker, S. (1984). *Language learnability and language development.* Cambridge, MA: Harvard University Press.

Poirier, F. E., & Smith, E. O. (1974). Socializing functions of primate play. *American Zoologist, 14,* 275–287.

Rescorla, L., Hyson, M. C., & Hirsh-Pasek, K. (Eds.). (1991). *Academic instruction in early childhood: Challenge or pressure.* New Directions for Child Development, Vol. 53. New York: Jossey-Bass.

Rice, M. (1983). Contemporary accounts of the cognition/language relationship: Implication for speech-language clinicians. *Journal of Speech and Hearing Disorders, 48,* 347–359.

Schneider, W., Korkel, J., & Weinert, F. E. (1987). The effects of intelligence, self-concept, and attributional style on metamemory and memory behavior. *International Journal of Behavioral Development, 10,* 281–299.

Schwartz, R., & Leonard, L. (1984). Words, objects, and actions in early lexical acquisition. *Journal of Speech and Hearing Research, 27,* 119–127.

Schwartz, R., Chapman, K., Terrell, B., Prelock, P., & Rowan, L. (1985). Facilitating word combination in language-impaired children through discourse structure. *Journal of Speech and Hearing Disorders, 50,* 31–39.

Schwartz, R. G. (1988). Phonological factors in early lexical acquisition. In M. Smith & J. Locke (Eds.), *The emergent lexicon* (pp. 185–222). New York: Academic Press.

Scott, J. P. (1968). *Early experience and the organization of behavior.* Belmont, CA: Brooks/Cole.

Shapiro, L. P., & Thompson, C. K. (in press). The use of linguistic theory as a framework for treatment studies in aphasia. *Clinical Aphasiology.*

Siegler, R. S., & Jenkins, E. (1989). *How children discover strategies.* Hillsdale, NJ: Erlbaum.

Sigel, I. E. (1987). Does hothousing rob children of their childhood? *Early Childhood Research Quarterly, 2,* 211–225.

Skeels, H. M. (1966). Adult status of children with contrasting early life experiences. *Monograph of the Society for Research in Child Development, 31* (Serial No. 105).

Snow, C. E., Arlman-Rupp, A., Hassing, Y., Jobse, J., Joosten, J., & Vorster, J. (1976). *Journal of Psycholinguistic Research, 5,* 1–20.

Snyder-McLean, L., Salomonson, B., McLean, J., & Sack, S. (1984). Structuring joint action routines: A strategy for facilitating communication and language development in the classroom. *Seminars in Speech and Language, 5,* 213–228.

Stern, D. N., Spieker, S., & MacKain, K. (1982). Intonation contours as signals in maternal speech to prelinguistic infants. *Developmental Psychology, 18,* 727–735.

Stipek, D., & MacIver, D. (1989). Developmental change in children's assessment of intellectual competence. *Child Development, 60,* 521–538.

Thompson, C. K., Shapiro, L. P., & Roberts, M. (1993). Treatment of sentence production deficits in aphasia: A linguistic-specific approach. *Aphasiology, 7,* 111–133.

Vygotsky, L. S. (1978). *Mind in society: The development of higher psychological processes.* Cambridge, MA: Harvard University Press.

Warren, S., & Kaiser, A. (1986). Incidental language teaching: A critical review. *Journal of Speech and Hearing Disorders, 51,* 191–199.

Weiner, P. (1985). The value of follow-up studies. *Topics in Language Disorders, 39,* 202–212.

Werker, J., & Pegg, J. (1992). Infant speech perception and phonological acquisition. In C. Ferguson, L. Menn, & C. Stoel-Gammon (Eds.), *Phonological development: Models, research, implications* (pp. 285–312). Timonium, MD: York Press.

Whitehurst, G. J., & Sonnenschein, S. (1985). The development of communication: A functional analysis. In G. J. Whitehurst (Ed.), *Annals of child development* (Vol. 2, pp. 1–48). Greenwich, CT: JAI Press.

Winn, M. (1983). *Children without childhood.* New York: Penguin.

Zigler, E. (1987). Formal schooling for 4-year-olds? No. In S. L. Kagan & E. Zigler (Eds.), *Early schooling: The national debate* (pp. 27–44). New Haven, CT: Yale University Press.

3

Speech Therapy Discourse
The Input to Learning

JOHN M. PANAGOS

Introduction

When addressing the issue of childhood language disorders, the practicing speech-language pathologist ultimately is confronted with treatment considerations. Regardless of the theoretical foundations employed or the various explanations of language disorders discussed, a clinical treatment perspective is necessary. In keeping with the focus on adaptability and the potential for using compensatory strategies as a viable intervention option,[1] this chapter discusses the role of therapy discourse and how it affects language intervention.

Over the last several years, a number of researchers have published on the topic of speech therapy discourse. In this work, *therapy* is a cover term for techniques, procedures, and intervention strategies incorporated in clinical lessons. The research to date has been descriptive in methodology and directed toward the goal of establishing an independent body of observations about therapy discourse free of prescriptive bias. In these studies, ordinary clinician-child therapy sessions are audio- or videotaped, transcribed verbatim, and analyzed for discourse features. The transcriptions include contextual notes accompanying the verbal material. Speakers' conversational moves are recorded so that the exchange context can be examined. These examinations of the therapeutic context are essential if we are to understand how therapeutic interactions affect treatment considerations. Simply put, if you wish to be an expert in therapeutic intervention, then you should study it in fine detail to develop a descriptive basis for your therapy manipulations.

In this chapter, therapy discourse will be discussed by focusing on three interactive dimensions: the verbal structuring of discourse, the nonverbal structuring of discourse, and the role of perspective taking in intervention. Attention to these

[1] I wish to thank Anna Vlahos for her assistance with this manuscript and Dana Kovarsky, Karen Bobkoff Katz, Penny Griffith, Patty Prelock, and Dani Ripich for their research ideas. Special thanks to Dana, who helped me talk out some of the points about social control and structured therapy.

three dimensions will create a greater understanding of therapy discourse; greater understanding will assist clinicians in monitoring and manipulating their own perspectives and the discourse features of therapy to increase effectiveness in working with childhood language disorders.

Verbal Components

Prutting, Bagshaw, Goldstein, Juskowitz, and Umen (1978) noted that prior work analyzing speech therapy interaction had the purpose of establishing norms for the number of correct responses clinicians should elicit during therapy. However, the clinician might use an analysis of therapy interaction as a self-supervisory tool. Drawing from the theories of Grice, Hymes, Keenan, Searle, and others, Prutting and her colleagues (1978) recommended the following approach:

> In addition to descriptions of procedural techniques, it is necessary to describe the discourse between clinician and child. A description of conversational interaction enhances our understanding of the remediation milieu. At present there are no research accounts regarding how children with delayed language and clinicians communicate with one another in the clinical setting. (p. 124)

Thus our approach should study speech therapy for the sake of studying speech therapy (i.e., it should be basic research).

From 60 audiotapes mailed to working clinicians around the United States, Prutting and her colleagues selected eight lessons for orthographic transcription and speech act analysis. Children with delayed language development between the ages of five and eight were recorded with their clinicians during 20-minute language remediation sessions. Clinicians produced 65% of the speech acts, whereas the children produced 35%. The clinicians made many more requests, many fewer responses, and about an equal number of statements. The clinicians responded to the children's requests less often, either ignoring them or evading them. As to subtypes of speech acts, the clinicians produced the following: requests for verbal information (43%), affirmative-negative (18%), qualification (8%), completion (8%), and imitation (2%). The clinicians never requested permission or responded with polite forms. Clinician statements included description (36%), explanations (26%), and statements of intention (22%). For the most part, the children's speech act frequencies were the reciprocals of the clinician's. As to discourse topics, the adults and children, while making requests, responses, and statements, stayed on topic, occasionally allowing for some subtopics to be introduced. In general, "the findings demonstrated that clinicians were occupying more of the communicative space than the children" (Prutting et al., 1978, p. 134).

The implicit argument in the article of Prutting et al. (1978) is that speech therapy interaction is abstract social interaction subjectable to formal discourse analysis. Clinician-child interaction entails continuous discourse referenced to conversational topics, tasks, and contexts. There is evidence of a speaker-listener relationship, discourse sequences, maxims of agreement, and speech act usage. Speech acts are abstracted away from surface forms, and the listener is required to interpret social messages using the speaking context as a frame of reference. Clinician-child discourse can be compared to mother-child and child-child discourse, yet it is somewhat unique because of the imbalance of power, evasion of requests, and quiz-question sequences. Clinician-child discourse in these ways can also be compared to teacher-pupil discourse.

Becker and Silverstein (1984) replicated the Prutting et al. study while considering factors of variability between samples. Inter- and intrajudge reliability was high, and the proportions of speech acts were virtually the same. There was "a typical pattern of interaction between clinicians and children in treatment settings across geographical areas, personalities and clinical education" (p. 105). Again, clinicians assumed a "dominant role" as manifested in the high density of therapy requests. Prutting (1984, p. 106), commenting that the coding system tested could lead to further examination of the remedial process, added that "one also needs to consider, in a systematic manner, the actual fabric of communication." For Prutting, this endeavor included the study of social roles, speech acts, and discourse roles.

Related Studies

In her study of six clinician-child dyads, Bobkoff (1982) modified the Prutting et al. taxonomy somewhat (e.g., added filler) and used videotape for data collection. Videotape analysis facilitated consideration of the nonverbal contexts for verbal interaction. Drawing from work on classroom discourse, Bobkoff looked closely at request-response-evaluation sequences as therapy units. Within these sequences, the familiar pattern of clinician request and child response was observed. Some 38% of the speech acts were requests, and 62% were statements. Whereas requests for action, confirmation, and imitation were frequent, there were only six clinician requests for clarification. This observation is related to the fact that very little new information was introduced by the clinicians because they already knew the answers to the questions asked. Additionally, there were no clinician requests for permission to act and only two answers to the clinicians' questions, observations indicating the degree of discourse control maintained by the clinicians. Within the statement category, clinician evaluations accounted for 47% of the speech acts. Viewing target structure presentations within a speech act framework demonstrated that therapy procedures are fragments of conversational discourse.

Ripich, Hambrecht, Panagos, and Prelock (1984) asked whether therapy discourse varies with type of therapy (i.e., articulation versus language). Analysis of speech act usage, topic selection, register selection, and underlying intent provided "a way of further clarifying the kinds of *input of learning* provided by clinicians while administering intervention programs" (p. 18, emphasis added). Six clinicians audiotaped one articulation and one language lesson with the same child. Again clinician dominance was evident. The introduction of discourse topics by the clinicians was frequent (85%). Requests (37%) and statements (60%) also occurred frequently. Only 9% of clinician speech acts were responses to child requests. Some 85% of clinician utterances were tied to therapy tasks and activities, suggesting that request-response-evaluation sequences were the key to continuous discourse. Overall, there were only minor differences between the two types of lessons.

Ripich et al. (1984) distinguished between known-information (68%) and unknown-information (32%) requests. Items (1) and (2) in the following excerpt are from language and articulation lessons, respectively. Both sequences are initiated by yes/no requests.

(1) Clinician: Nancy has what? (Request)
Child: Has a broken arm. (Response)
Clinician: That's a good sentence. (Evaluative) (Statement)
(2) Clinician: This one? (Request)
Child: Soap. (Response)
Clinician: Right, nice s on that one. (Evaluative) (Statement) (p. 24)

Both sequences imply that the clinician knows the answer before asking the question, suggesting that there is an abstract process of social discourse operating across speech acts: "For the language learning child the social and role features of discourse constitute, in part, the content of the remediation session" (p. 25).

Ripich, Hambrecht, and Panagos (1985) conducted a similar study with adult aphasic patients. Audiotape samples of four clinician-client dyads were transcribed and analyzed. Patterns of topic control and discourse sequencing were related to the distribution of speech acts:

> The clinician and client shared an underlying orientation about the therapy process. Clinicians were responsible for making appropriate requests, evaluating the client's responses, and generally controlling the topic. Clients were responsive to clinicians' requests and evaluations and only occasionally controlled the topic. (p. 9)

The overall pattern indicated that the "clients were given few opportunities to interact other than in the learner-client role" (p. 9). On the other hand, there were some style differences among the four clinicians. Two clinicians followed a drill format, with the first producing twice as many statements as requests. A third clinician allowed more conversational talk and rarely evaluated responses. The last clinician used an interview style as in item (3), allowing more conversational talk but with greater evaluation:

(3) Clinician: How long have you worked at this job of sales engineer?
Client: Well combined 25 years.
Clinician: Beautiful! (p. 9)

Ripich et al. (1985) thought that the setting (nursing home versus family home) and age similarity (clinician versus client) might be factors influencing therapy style.

Silliman, Gams-Golub, and Chizzik (1979) followed up on the Prutting et al. (1978) study, asking how clinicians organize sequences and conceptual content. One clinician conducted activity-based lessons with four language-delayed children whose language comprehension and production levels varied on formal tests. The lesson entailed following instructions to bake a cake. The clinician asserted the dominant role, directed attention to the task, and chained speech acts (particularly requests) to simplify alternate choices. Although the clinician held form and function constant (requests-responses-statements), she "progressively scaled her level of question content complexity" (p. 3) to approximate the performance levels of her clients. The distribution of speech acts was similar to other studies. For example, the clinician used a high number of requests even though the activity was intended to be child centered and interactive. When these requests were classified by effectiveness in eliciting an appropriate response, 41% were ineffective. Some ineffective requests occurred because the clinician ignored child requests.

Conversation

Studies conducted in the vein of Prutting et al. (1978) had in common the classification and distribution of speech acts within request-response-statement sequences. Related work brings out how conversation spans several turns within the lesson (Panagos, Katz, Kovarsky, & Prelock, 1988). Panagos and Bliss (1990) hypothesized that the therapy characteristic of continuous discourse observed in earlier studies results in part from the dominant role played by the clinician. The clinician has a plan for therapy and its subordinates tasks designed to elicit correct responses. It is the role responsibility of the therapist to keep the child talking so the lesson moves forward.

Within the flow of conversational discourse are cycles of interactive exchange. Bobkoff (1982, pp. 68–69) pointed out that the frequency of speech acts is less important than how they are distributed in sequences. "Elicitation sequences" are hierarchically organized and topically related units governing dyadic interaction. The clinician begins with a request or multiple requests, as shown in item (4):

(4) Clinician: What happened to her in this one?
Here she's what?
Child: Getting dressed. (p. 100)

The child then has the obligation of providing a response because adjacency pairs have been formed (McTear & King, 1991). The child must answer quickly or the clinician restates or rephrases the request. Successive requests are related to one another by paralinguistic cues and by their initial position in the elicitation sequence. After the child's acceptable response, a statement of evaluation is made by the clinician. Rarely does the clinician fail to complete the sequence without some kind of closing statement or evaluation; the tripartite structure commits the clinician to close the sequence as much as it requires the child to respond. Multiple statements and evaluations are fairly common, as shown in item (5):

(5) Clinician: What's happening in this picture?
Child: He is laying in the hammock.
Clinician: Yea.
He is laying in the hammock.
Good for you. (p. 104)

Discourse sequences have internal structure and are marked off externally by boundary markers: "These markers are characterized as sequentially dependent because they anticipate the beginning of one unit (cataphoric) while acknowledging the completion of another (anaphoric)" (Kovarsky, 1990, p. 30). Kovarsky collected a dialogue sample from the lessons of one clinician working with two 9-year-olds. The clinician produced more utterances in therapy than did the clients and used more boundary markers. The words *okay, oh, so,* and *well* serve this purpose.

Kovarsky (1989a, 1989b) looked at the discourse functions of *okay* more closely. *Okay* served as a marker between tasks, discourse sequences, and speech acts. The clinician used *okay* to regulate the child's actions, accept prior responses, approve a response, and release the child from a prior response. The child used *okay* to signal compliance and self-regulation. Role differences were reflected in the functions observed. The okay's of person regulation, evaluation, and approval were inappropriate for the child to use.

Although the clinician sustains therapy discourse through topic reference, task design, sequencing, and focus on correct responses, there are points of interruption and fallback at which conversational repairs were undertaken (Kovarsky & Panagos, in press; Panagos & Bliss, 1990; Panagos, Bobkoff, & Scott, 1986). Most therapy sequences as shown in item (6) are completed efficiently (Ripich et al., 1984):

(6) Clinician: This one? (Request)
Child: Soap. (Response)
Clinician: Right, nice *s* on that one. (Evaluation) (p. 24)

Others, as shown in item (7), are longer and more complex (Bobkoff, 1982):

(7) Clinician: And what are they doing? (Request)
Child: They are. . . .
Clinician: Walking.
Child: Walking.
Clinician: OK.
You can do the whole sentence for me.
Child: They are walking.
Clinician: Good.
They are walking. (p. 193)

Kovarsky (1989a; Kovarsky & Panagos, in press) examined 106 repair sequences in the two dyads he studied and found that 83 were adult initiated and child or adult completed. In 19 instances, the child initiated and repaired sequences. Within sequences, six types of repairs were identified: giving the child a clue for the correct response; giving the response; repetition; silence; reflection time; and hints. Although repairs can be drawn out, with intricate internal structure, there seem to be a finite number of maneuvers to keep the child on track. Bobkoff (1982) described several in terms of remedial sequences containing nested moves.

Register

Microanalysis teases out discourse features and their interrelationships while defining partially the participant structures of talk. Types of talk can be contrasted with others in the sense of registers used across speaking contexts. Panagos and Fry (1976) documented instances of careful speech (formal register), noting that these instances characterized the majority of sequences within the lesson studied. In item (8), the clinician is working on syntactic clauses with a nine-year-old mentally retarded child. The clinician and child speak slowly and clearly with little intonation and emotion.

(8) Clinician: Good. Do you see a mother who has a baby?
Child: I. see . . Mommy . . .

Clinician: (whispers) who
Child: who . have . a baby.
Clinician: Boy, you're really doing a nice job . . . (laughs) You sound sick, I'm just teasing you.
Child: I not sick. (p.11)

The child is hardly fluent in moving between words. After the response, the clinician suddenly switches to casual speech (informal register), in which prosody and grammatical speech are dramatically different. Speech rate increases, there are laughter and lively changes of tone, and word contractions are used. On tape, when the child protests naturally to teasing, we now hear fluent social speech. Rules for register shifting are reflected in lesson sequences but remain abstract to a large extent.

Panagos and Bliss (1990) proposed that one way to understand therapy discourse is to compare it with other social registers. In Table 3–1, we have several similar adult-child dyads and contexts for investigation. Although it may be easy via videotape to describe and contrast the different kinds of talk, at some point one must ascertain on an abstract plane what roles participants give themselves for the purposes of talk.

How we might distinguish speech therapy talk from similar registers seems largely an empirical problem. The descriptive detail available suggests contrastive features at the several levels of discourse (Crystal, 1981; Kovarsky, 1990; Panagos et al., 1986; Spinelli & Ripich, 1985). Compared to ordinary conversation, therapy talk does not go back and forth and allow for extended turns and expanded content; therapy discourse is highly symmetrical and limits the length of turns and details of content within remedial sequences. However, at the level of social discourse, the degree of control exerted by the clinician is highly asymmetrical. The clinician uses boundary markers and regulatives to control sequences and turns. The clinician takes turns at will, assigns turns to the child,

Table 3–1. Systems of Discourse Sharing Features with Speech Therapy Discourse

Social Roles	*Setting*	*Speech Activity*
Mother-child	Home	Story telling
Sunday school teacher-child	Church	Religious lesson
Librarian-child	Library	Story telling
Doctor-child	Clinic	Examination
Teacher-child	School	School lesson
Peer tutor-child	School	School lesson
Teacher aide-child	School	School lesson
Special ed. teacher-child	Special school	Remedial lesson
Remedial reading teacher-child	School	Remedial lesson
Teacher of the deaf-child	Special school	Speech lesson
Speech therapist-child	Clinic	Therapy lesson
Physical therapist-child	Clinic	Treatment
Psychoanalyst-child	Clinic	Psychotherapy session
Psychologist-child	Laboratory	Sign experiment

and takes turns back whenever he or she wants to. The clinician can interrupt but the child cannot. Known-information questions are clinician requests initiating sequences, attentionals are statements serving to keep the child on task, and statements of praise and correction are acts terminating sequences. The child must stay on task even though it may seem peculiar. The child makes few requests compared to the clinician, and when the child does so, the clinician usually evades them and quickly moves forward with his or her agenda. Even when the child is to tell a story, the clinician, instead of saying *mhmm* or asking true questions to clarify content, may violate the norms of narration by saying, "Tell me more." Accordingly, "the child learns that the clinician values the amount of talk rather than the content" (Spinelli & Ripich, 1985, p. 192).

Nonverbal Components

A popular notion is that some 70% of communication between speakers resides in the domain of nonverbal communication. Panagos et al. (1988) argued that nonverbal components of therapy are associated features of situational context, lesson organization, and remedial sequences. Clinician messages are transmitted in parallel through verbal and nonverbal channels; and across discourse sequences, features are added, deleted, substituted, and clustered within and between channels. As shown in Table 3–2, the clinician uses a wide variety of nonverbal mechanisms to manage social behavior and facilitate correct responses. In each channel, features can be modified to change meaning and signal salience.

An example of parallel communication is found in a paper by Moseley (1978):

HIGH PITCH
LIMITED VARIABILITY
(9) Clinician: Show me with your cars what happened yesterday.
AVERAGE LOUDNESS/FAST TEMPO
PRECISE SPEECH/FALSETTO QUALITY
INSINCERE ATTITUDE. (p. 111)

Moseley looked at vocal channels and separated out assorted prosodic features accompanying grammatical utterance. Following a system developed by the linguist David Crystal, Moseley was able to show that changes in rhythm, pitch, loudness, duration, and tone add information to sentence utterances. Thus the client must process information in several parallel channels to understand messages (Panagos, Griffith, & Ripich, 1985). In other words, the child must process nonverbal and verbal information in the therapy context to recover the underlying social intent of the clinician.

Elements

Bobkoff (1982, pp. 82–94) carried out a provocative analysis of nonverbal components as they co-occur with verbal components. She looked at eye gaze (to child, to material), pointing, holding, manipulating, touching, and leaning (forward and back). On tape, these features are clearly evident and variably linked to phases of the elicitation sequence (Panagos et al., 1988). During the request phase, the clinician leans forward, points to objects, and directs eye gaze to the

Table 3–2. Bodily Devices Used in Clinical Lessons

Physical Mechanism	*Nonverbal Signals*
Body	Orienting, relocating, shifting, tensing
Head	Tilting, turning, lowering, raising
Shoulders	Shrugging, curling, slouching
Torso	Leaning, turning, swaying, rotating
Arms	Raising, reaching, encompassing
Legs	Wiggling, opening, closing, crossing
Feet	Tapping, pointing, lifting
Face	Animating, relaxing, talking
Eyebrows	Lifting one, lifting two
Eyelids	Opening, closing, squinting
Eyes	Gazing, staring, shifting, expanding
Cheeks	Smiling, relaxing, flushing
Jaw	Lowering, protruding, tensing
Lips	Pursing, retracting, opening, closing
Voice	Voicing, modulating, silencing
Pitch	Raising, lowering, maintaining
Loudness	Raising, lowering, maintaining
Quality	Slurring, tensing, relaxing
Hands	Gesturing, signing, holding
Palm	Opening, closing, spreading, rotating
Fingers	Pointing, fisting, counting

child. During the response phase, the clinician holds his or her forward body position, point, and eye gaze. When the child's response is slow or diffident, eye gaze shifts rapidly back and forth between the child and object. After the correct response and during the evaluation phase, the clinician leans back, withdraws the point, folds his or her hands, and shifts his or her eye gaze back to the child. On tape, the children can be seen closely watching the clinician's physical communication. One is reminded of Hans the Clever Horse.

Bobkoff and Panagos (1986) looked at the pointing gesture in greater detail. Point occurred as a feature added to verbal requests. With inadequate responses, multiple points occurred prior to the evaluation statement. Point had different functions analogous to emphatic vocal stress. It was used to hold attention, mark nouns and verbs, and signal forward movement. The example in item (10) illustrates the move-forward function. The now-tell-me segment is a request that helps establish the paradigm for the child to follow:

P

(10) Clinician: Now tell me about this boy.
Child: The boy is watching.
Clinician: Uh hum. (p. 57)

Agenda and Plans

Letts (1985, p. 324) studied audiotapes of therapy sessions to see how speech acts function within lessons. She found that one set of organizing principles accounted for lesson activities. Speech acts were used "(i) to set the activity in motion, (ii) to ensure that it did not break down once in motion, (iii) to elicit individual specific responses from the child, (iv) to give the child feedback regarding these responses, and (v) to give information of a more general nature." Letts developed a hierarchy of structure with as many as four nodes of expansion. Most of this structure is implicit: "To ensure an activity does not break down" is an abstraction the clinician cannot verbalize. It organizes verbal behavior but is nonverbal in nature.

McTear and King (1991, p. 203) examined the transcript of a clinician and child to determine their patterns of communication and miscommunication. Adjacency pairs in which the child's response was obligatory were isolated. The percentage of inadequate responses (invalid, irrelevant, or insufficient) was 24.7; the percentage of no-response tallies was 14.3. Topic introduction was also analyzed. The clinician introduced topics at the initial phase of the lesson, but the child tried to change the subject. Such events caused instances of topic negotiation wherein the clinician yielded momentarily to the child only to reintroduce the remedial topic. It turned out that describing the surface levels of dialogue, such as turn taking, repairs, topic organization, and exchange structure, was relatively easy; but the more important issue was "a discrepancy between the goals of the therapist and the child and that this discrepancy in goals gives rise in miscommunication" (p. 203).

Like Letts (1985), McTear and King (1990) set forth the clinician's "ideal plan for the session." The plan entails several logical components "(a) diagnosis; (b) eliciting talk; (c) talk bounded by the starting and ending points of the lesson; (d) cycles of talk associated with the materials; [and] (e) elicitation sequences" (p. 203). Thus there is a hierarchy of goals the clinician operates within, but the child does not grasp the higher levels:

> At the lower levels, miscommunication is likely to be easier to resolve. In the case examined here, problems seemed to occur not only at the higher levels—the inability of the patient to discern the therapist's more global goals—but also at interactions between the levels, that is, an inability to see how the therapist's individual actions were motivated by higher-level goals (pp. 211–212).

The lack of a shared perspective at an abstract level makes a difference in therapy interaction.

Panagos et al. (1986) argued that a clinical lesson is "a hierarchical arrangement of discourse units adapted conversationally for the purposes of controlling lesson behavior and eliciting correct responses" (p. 217). In so doing, they offered the information shown here as Table 3–3. Within the clinical lesson are three phases, of which the work phase is dominant. Within the work phase is one or more therapy tasks, each with its own opening, middle, and closing phases. Within the tasks are request-response-evaluation sequences. When repairs are made, there is further embedding in the lesson hierarchy. Within and across units are speech acts, register shifts, topics, regulatives, turns, narratives, directions, terms of addressives, greetings, leave taking, etc.

Lesson structures co-occur with nonverbal components of therapy exchange (Panagos et al., 1988, pp. 283–284). In the three lesson phases of Table 3–3, we have moves like the following:

Table 3–3. Discourse Components Underlying Phonology Issues

Discourse Feature	*Description*
Lesson	A hierarchical arrangement of discourse units adapted conversationally for the purpose of controlling lesson behavior and eliciting correct responses.
Opening phase	Greetings, reminders, and announced plans for the ensuring lesson.
Work phase	Middle portion of lesson centering around one or more learning tasks.
Closing phase	Comments, reminders, and salutations closing the lesson.
Task	Procedures integrating thematic content, topics, therapy, materials, time allocations, and remedial sequences.
Opening phase	Instructions, illustrations, and task initiation.
Remedial phase	Work phase of task centering around procedures eliciting correct responses.
Closing phase	Termination of tasks, comments, and announced plans for the next lesson step.
Remedial Sequence	Contingently related speech acts governing the elicitation of correct responses.
Request	Utterance requiring a contingent conversational response.
Response	Utterance contingently related to a previous request.
Evaluation	Utterance which evaluates, corrects, or comments on a foregoing response.

Opening Phase
smiling to greet the child
helping pull off garments
making seating gestures
positioning chairs
looking through the therapy bag

Middle Phase
manipulating materials
maintaining and disengaging eye contact
sitting still to listen
pointing with a pencil
manipulating the child's mouth

Closing Phase
putting materials away
leaning back in chairs
getting up from the table
putting on garments
moving toward the door
waving goodbye

How such moves are interrelated with verbal structure, or what salience they have to children, is unknown.

Building on an account of lesson structure, Panagos et al. (1988, p. 291) offered this summary comment:

> Role intent is expressed through the implementation of "structured therapy", dictating the organization of therapy space, objects, and interpersonal distance. The structure of therapy also requires use of the formal therapy register, adapted conversational discourse for lesson organization (phases, tasks, remedial sequences, turns, repairs, speech acts) subsuming nonverbal features at all levels of interaction.

When we look at the inherent structure of speech therapy, we think about courtroom discourse. The architectural layout, furnishings, colors, decor, roles, modes of dress, ritual sequences, mood, and manners of speaking are seriously prescribed. An authority hierarchy exists from law to judge to attorney to bailiff to defendant. There is an overriding goal to be reached that overrides the structure, and it concerns the disposition of clients. There are rules for language forms (Latin) and registers (formal style). Language use is tied to moving clients through the process to a point of final disposition.

Social Abstractions

Prutting (1984) agreed that discovering patterns of speech act usage helps us describe aspects of speech therapy, but she recognized equally the value of parallel work at other levels of analysis—namely, discourse and social roles. Thus the behaviors of speech therapy are related to "obligations and options of speakers and listeners" and "dimensions of relationships" (p. 49). McTear and King (1990) found that such surface details as turn taking, response contingency, repairs, topic organization, and exchange structure are relatively easy to study but are not sufficient to explain instances of miscommunication. Miscommunication must be understood at a deeper level: "the mental states of the participants as they engage in interaction" (p. 207). As to the clinician's agenda, Damico (1990, p. 85) recognized the need "to determine what underlying motivations or mechanisms" shape the clinician's behavior. As to the appreciation of the client's perspective, Maxwell (1990) noted that "one systematically goes through a process of trying to figure out what a client's behavior means to the client and the people around him or her" (p. 4).

The account developed in Table 3–4 provides us with a principled basis for inferring participant knowledge in speech therapy (Panagos & Bliss, 1990). Knowing how to talk for any social purpose is not just a linguistic matter; it entails abstract knowledge of many aspects of communication—organizational patterns; use of space; social roles; social registers, semiotic modes; communication norms; speech activities; grammar, key or mood; discourse rules; norms of affect; knowledge and beliefs; and moral/ethical codes. At each stage of cognitive development, new knowledge is overlaid on old. The clinician's acquisition of therapy skills involves extending and generalizing knowledge of social communication. The norms for therapy interaction are learned through social modeling and practice and are reinforced by those of the institutional setting (clinic). A

Table 3–4. Preliminary Inventory of Features of Speech Therapy Presupposition

Communication Competence: Organizational patterns (meals); uses of space (house); social roles and registers (kinship); semiotic modes (signs vs. speech); communication norms (don't lie); speech activities (story telling); primary linguistic system (grammar); key (irony, moods); verbal and nonverbal discourse rules (sequences, topics, moves, turns, speech acts, kinesics); joint play (sister-brother); norms of affect ("good touching"); knowledge and beliefs (talk right!); moral behavior (praying).
School Competence: Organizational patterns (lunch); uses of space (seating); social roles and registers (teacher-pupil); semiotic modes (reading, spelling); communication norms (don't interrupt); speech activities (reading group); primary/secondary linguistic systems (writing); key (serious school work); verbal and nonverbal discourse rules (classroom lesson sequences, topics, moves, turns, speech acts, kinesics); joint play (friends); norms of affect (don't touch teacher); knowledge and beliefs (prescriptive grammar); moral behavior (no stealing).
Preservice Competence: Organizational patterns (clinic procedures); uses of space (therapy furniture); social roles and registers (therapist-child); semiotic modes (communication boards); communication norms (respect for supervisor); speech activity (therapy session); primary/secondary linguistic systems (target structures); key (exacting therapy work); verbal and nonverbal discourse rules (managing lesson sequences, topics, moves, turns, speech acts, kinesics); joint play (parallel play); norms of affect (physical management); knowledge and beliefs (behavior modification); moral behavior (code of ethics).

short-hand nomenclature—"target structures," "therapy materials," "appropriate responses," "on-task behavior," etc.—enables clinicians to tag the apparent meanings of therapy exchange. Professional meanings are learned rather formally, whereas social meanings are learned with little or no conscious awareness.

Table 3–4 at the first two levels can be viewed from the child's perspective. Language acquisition and talking with others depend on the acquisition of structures of talk. Normal and delayed children master the foundation of talk before school. The acquisition of social roles and registers in the family context is already underway when first words appear. Later children play mommy, daddy, doctor, and teacher, adapting their speech accordingly. The facility to move between registers of speech accounts for variations of linguistic form. Delayed children evidence role and register shifting even though their utterances are largely unintelligible. Through the use of pointing, eye gaze, facial expression, and vocal prosody, the structures of talk are evident. Once school experiences begin, the child has some basis for interpreting the social rules for communication and learning. The pupil-versus-teacher role is learned quickly. Teachers make requests and pupils answer, a discourse rule associated with the relative differences in social power and status. "The higher status person has more rights and privileges and the lower status person has more obligations" (Spinelli & Ripich, 1985, p. 193).

Clinician Perspective

Damico (1990) conducted a relevant ethnographic study to discover the underlying constructs motivating the speech-language pathologist. Two clinicians were observed at work over a 14-month period. Field notes were made throughout the school year. Of the eight themes identified, prescriptionism was by far the most prevalent motivational factor. As Milroy and Milroy (1985) noted, "prescriptionism is an ideology which requires that there is a 'correct' or 'proper' form of language, imposed from above by authority, and that in all aspects of language usage, this correct form shall be employed" (Damico, 1990, p. 86). Prescriptionism is manifested across the domains of clinical assessment, treatment, and professional communication. In treatment sessions, the drive to correct nonstandard linguistic forms can negate the learning goals of the lesson. Consider item (11):

(11) Child: Ain't nobody that can lift that (points to the materials) without that (points to the pulley).
Clinician: (frowning) There isn't anyone who can lift that (points to the materials) without that (points to the pulley).
Child: (tentatively) There isn't anyone who can lift that without that (no pointing).
Clinician: (smiling) Great Bo! I knew you could get it right! (Damico, 1990, p. 89).

The point of the lesson is to facilitate problem solving applied to the science principles of pulleys and fulcrums. The clinician ignores the child's correct answer and goes on to elicit correct form production. Damico reported that the clinician did not realize that she was correcting grammar until he showed her the transcript. The clinician said, "That's pretty weird."

There is some evidence that clinicians have negative views of clients who do not meet their expectations—pay attention, stay on task, and produce correct responses; rather, they prefer clients who respond appropriately and show signs of improvement (Stech, Curtis, Troesch, & Binnie, 1973). An interesting report by McFarlane, Fujiki, and Brinton (1984) categorized 400 difficult clients according to their learning styles and motivational characteristics. Although they should not divulge the therapy agenda, clinicians need special strategies to manage difficult clients. The tone of the report does not honor the intrinsic worth of clients. Figure 3–1 depicts the four types of difficult clients categorized. The cartoon-like images seem to devalue clients because they do not meet performance expectations.

Panagos and Bliss (1990) developed the concept of role drive to explain the therapist's motivation and behavior. During clinical training, the therapist internalizes the therapist role associated with the tight management of therapy tasks and correction of inappropriate responses (i.e., Role ↔ Task ↔ Correct Responses). The role is self-reinforced when treatment sessions are well managed and yield correct responses. From one clinician to the next, structured therapies have more positive social value than child-centered play therapies. In fact, "the scripts of speech therapy lessons may serve as social rituals for mutual identification of therapists across the generations" (Panagos & Bliss, 1990, p. 24). Some years ago, before the clinician was called a speech-language pathologist, he or she was called a speech correctionist.

Table 3–5 (from Panagos and Bliss, 1990) illustrates a clinician's drive to reach goals. The intent is to teach the target structure *can*, and the persistence to get correct responses is apparent. On the one hand, there is some useful syntactic learning going on in the sense of classical notions of auxiliary forms. There are also hints about the use of polite forms such as *may* versus *please*. On the other

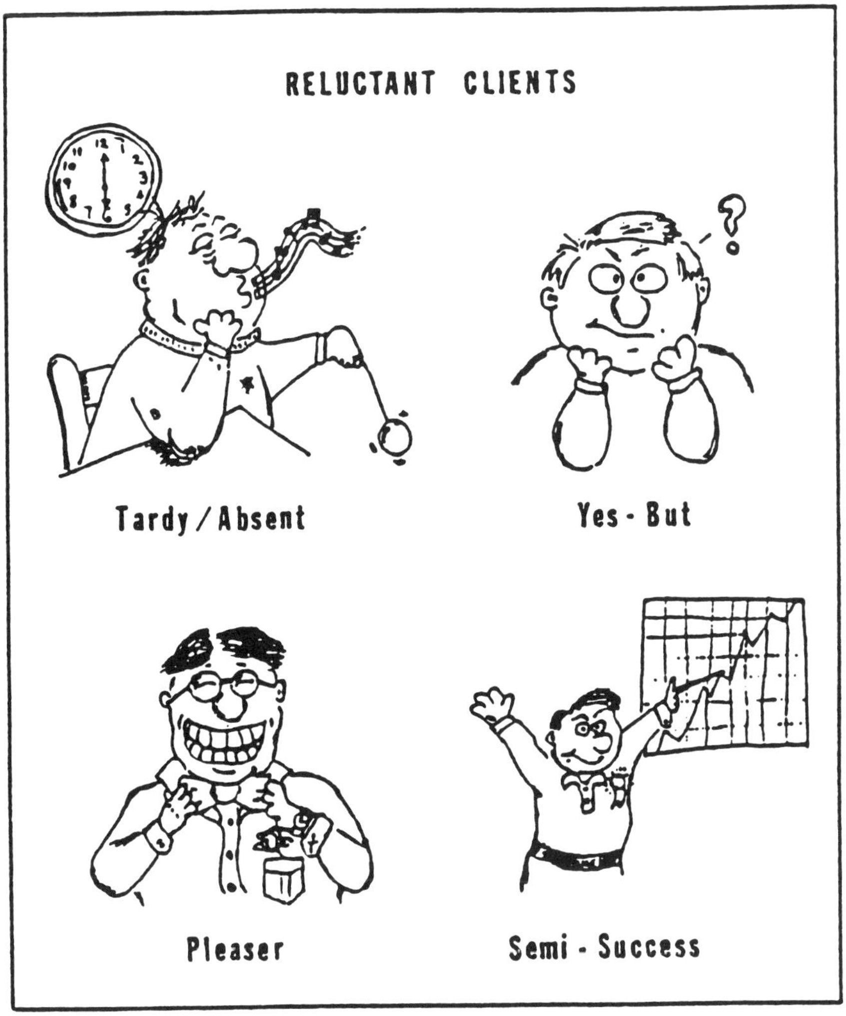

Figure 3–1. Four types of difficult speech therapy clients. Source: *Coping with Communicative Handicaps: Resource for the Practicing Clinician,* by S. C. McFarlane, M. Fujiki, and B. Brinton, 1984, San Diego: College-Hill Press. Copyright 1982. Reprinted by permission.

hand, the push to elicit correct responses creates ambiguities and anomalies of discourse meaning. In item (12), we have ambiguity. English yes/no questions are double signaled through auxiliary preposing and rising intonation.

(12) Clinician: Can you ask?
Child: Give me (reaches to grab cereal).
Clinician: You have to ask, not tell. Say, "Can I have some cereal?"
Child: Have cereal?
Clinician: Good try. Look, Mark. Say—"Can I have?"
Child: Can I have?
Clinician: Yes, you most certainly CAN. (p. 25)

Table 3–5. Therapy Transcript Illustrating Role-Communication Factors

Speaker	*Transcribed Interaction*
Clinician:	Mark, I want you to ask for things, not grab them. Listen and watch—Mark, can I have the cereal?
Child:	(He gives her the cereal.)
Clinician:	Thank you very much. You can give me the cereal, can't you?
Child:	(Nods yes.)
Clinician:	Would you like some? (He nods yes.) Can you ask?
Child:	Give me. (Reaches for the cereal.)
Clinician:	You have to ask, not tell. Say, "Can I have some cereal?"
Child:	Have cereal?
Clinician:	Good try. Look, Mark. Say, "Can I have?"
Child:	Can I have?
Clinician:	Yes, you most certainly can. Since you ask, you can have. (She gives him the cereal, but the lid is on too tight for the client to open up the jar.)
Child:	(He starts to gnaw on the lid. He then throws the jar across the room.)
Clinician:	Mark, do you need help?
Child:	(He hands her the jar but she doesn't take it.) Open.
Clinician:	Oh, you want me to open. Can you ask?
Child:	Please, open.
Clinician:	Say, "Can you open?"
Child:	Can you open, please?
Clinician:	Yes, I can open. You asked me so nicely. (She opens the cereal and gives it to Mark.) Can you pass the milk, please? (He passes her the milk.) Thank you! You can pass. Would you like some milk?
Child:	Can I have some milk, please?
Clinician:	Yes, you can. You can have the milk. You asked, so you can have. (She gives him the milk, which he pours.) Can you pass me those spoons? (He does so, and she thanks him.) Thank you for passing me the spoons. You can pass. (She pulls out a spoon and hands him a broken one. He starts to eat his cereal, balancing the cereal precariously on the side of his spoon.) Hey, that's a neat treat, Mark, but there's got to be an easier way. Mark, what's wrong with that spoon?
Child:	Broken.
Clinician:	Can you fix it?
Child:	No, fix it please! (Hands her the spoon.)
Clinician:	You can ask. I know you can.
Child:	Can you help me, please?
Clinician:	Yes, Mark, I can. (She fixes the spoon, and they eat.)

The clinician says *good try* when intonation is changed but without the production of *can*. Likewise, the child's last response is approved even though an ungrammatical sequence is produced.

Another example is found in item (13). Note that earlier the clinician insisted on Mark's being polite, but later when he is polite, saying *please,* he makes an error because he does not use *can*. The drive to keep the child talking gives neither the child nor the clinician time to observe the nuances of form and meaning.

(13) Clinician: Mark, I want you to ask for things, not grab them.

——

Child: Can I have some milk, please?

——

Clinician: Oh, you want me to open. Can you ask?
Child: Please, open.
Clinician: Say—CAN you open?

Child Perspective

Little is known about how children perceive speech therapy. We surmise that they generalize the social roles and registers of family and classroom experience. Chubrich (1978) had been a client in speech therapy and later became a speech-language pathologist. His recollections of therapy are interesting:

> Going from the classroom to therapy was a little like walking into the twilight zone. The mirrors, tongue depressors, and exercises of therapy had no counterparts outside of therapy. . . . My therapist, like many clinicians, equated her procedures with her goals. Therapy became a succession of contrived tasks that had little to do with reality. The behaviors I acquired could be likened to an elaborate set of parlor tricks. (p. 71)

Through social modeling and conditioning, children in therapy learn the client role. Once the diagnosis is made, the clinician asserts his or her role and status as the professional therapist, while the child's role and status are diminished (McTear & King, 1991; Spinelli & Ripich, 1985). The prescriptionist stance, emphasizing correct or proper language, teaches the child that the clinician is the "error connector" (Kovarsky & Maxwell, 1992). Damico's (1990) notes from the school playground recorded this exchange: "Two girls run up to B (clinician) and one says, 'Lady, you her teacher?' The other child looks up, smiles broadly and says, 'That's her, she helps me talk right, like her'" (p. 77). In this vein, Ripich (1982; see Spinelli & Ripich, 1985, p. 188) interviewed children enrolled in speech therapy and asked them to compare teacher and therapist expectations. The interaction is shown in item (14):

(14) Ripich: What's the most important thing your teacher in your class wants you to do?
Child: Be quiet and listen.
Ripich: How about your speech teacher? What's the most important thing she wants you to do?
Child: Oh, she wants me to talk.

The clinician's goal to keep the child talking is reflected in therapy discourse (Crystal, 1981, p. 200; Spinelli & Ripich, 1985, pp. 192–193) and seems necessary to enable the clinician to correct linguistic errors.

The work phase of therapy formats the context in which the child perceives and learns the client role. Prelock (1990) set up an experimental therapy task directing clinical subjects to at times produce incorrect responses. The aim was to establish a linguistic contrast between words with and without final consonant deletion. Prelock found that some of the subjects refused to respond incorrectly, as seen in item (15):

(15) Child: (selects apple with frown)
Clinician: You picked an apple with a frown, so you need to say the word the wrong way.
Child: I don't want to do that one.
Clinician: You don't want to do that one? You want to do a right one . . . you have a sad one.
Child: No, no, no, no. I have a happy one. (hides the apple with a frown & finds one with a smile) (p.15)

The child is the error maker who must try to make correct responses, not try to make incorrect responses.

Kovarsky and Maxwell (1992) discussed the way the therapist and child set up mutual expectations. The diagnosis establishes the fact of the child's linguistic incompetence, and the child internalizes the clinician's expectations. The child's role is of an error maker. When Kovarsky's two clients looked at videotapes of their therapy sessions, they sat passively except for a few instances when the clinician made negative evaluations: "The children's comments mirrored the evaluative stance taken by the clinician on the videotape . . . [and] the clinician's role was to help [them] correct [their] mistakes"' (Kovarsky & Maxwell, 1992, p. 81).

Kovarsky (1989a) reported additional details about the interviews. He spoke with the clinician, grandparents, parents, and teachers. Carol, the clinician, believed that for years to come the children would have language and literacy problems and would need to develop compensatory strategies. Her long- and short-term goals focused on problem solving and decoding and encoding speech and written material. Word categorization, spelling, and analyzing sound-letter correspondences were the learning activities selected. In contrast, the children believed that classroom difficulties had placed them in therapy, and the activities of therapy focused on writing, reading, performing experiments, and answering questions. They also believed the following: Grandparents give presents to kids, and parents care about feelings. Teachers assign work, and the clinician helps you feel less scared about writing. To make children do things, coaches blow their whistles, and Carol points her pencil (observed on videotape). Whereas parents do not take talking seriously, Carol does. She cares a lot about talking.

Smith-Lewis (1993; reviewed by Blackstone, 1993, p. 6) compared home and school interactions for 10 middle-school children of culturally diverse backgrounds. The children had received augmentative communication services for at least 3 or 4 years. Smith-Lewis wondered how family and school perceived the children. She reported that

> when asked to describe each child, school personnel used medical diagnostic terms. One got no sense of the child's personality. Families gave a psychosocial perspective and told

about the child's likes/dislikes and certain personality traits (e.g., he's stubborn). When videotapes of the children's interaction at home were shown to their speech-language pathologist, they were surprised by the children's communication competence (Blackstone, 1993, p. 6).

Role Interpretation

A study by Ripich (1982; see also Ripich & Panagos, 1985) is noteworthy for its breadth and general findings. School children enrolled in articulation therapy were asked to role-play speech therapist and client. Role-play methodology was viewed as a means of determining the children's social perceptions of therapy. Work in developmental psychology suggested that children are adept at role-playing prior to school, and in peer teaching situations they readily assume the roles of teacher and pupil. The therapy children slipped into their roles without coaching. The excerpt in item (16) shows one exchange.

(16) Clinician: Okay, let's say a good *sh* sound.
Child: /S/ (Clinician looks in the child's mouth).
Clinician: Okay, say *shutter*.
Child: Shutter. (Ripich, 1982, p. 69)

The videotaped sessions were analyzed for various discourse features. The familiar patterns of therapy discourse were observed. Ninety percent of the children's utterances were associated with instructional activities, whereas nonstructural utterances occurred only occasionally at lesson transition points. Speech act distribution paralleled that of Prutting et al. (1978). The clinicians made 91% of the requests and 100% of the evaluations. As to request-response-evaluation sequences, 100% were tied to the instructional context. Topic introduction at 61% was controlled by the clinician, typically within instructional tasks or while shifting to new tasks. For an analysis of management schemes, the clinicians frequently controlled tasks and materials and ignored requests. All of the clients displayed compliance to clinician requests. The clinicians even displayed some physical control to force compliance. One client did not respond to the command to write the word pen. The clinician pushed his arm down to the paper and said loudly, "Write pen!" The Ripich study indicated clearly that children do not perceive speech therapy activities merely as drill and correction; rather, they view therapy holistically as an inclusive pattern of social behavior.

Ripich (1982) also interviewed her subjects after the role-played lesson. One girl was asked about her therapy experiences. Her comments are seen in item (17):

(17) Ripich: What do you usually do in therapy?
Child: Well, I'm supposed to make the bad *r* sounds and Mrs. Marks is supposed to make the good *r* sounds.
Ripich: Don't you ever make good *r* sounds?
Child: No! I'm supposed to make the bad *r's*. (p. 90)

Ripich (1982, pp. 90–91) concluded that "it is conceivable that we identify children as speech and language impaired, tell them they need our help in order to speak better, and create a social contract that says they are supposed to make mistakes so that we can correct them."

Discussion

Our account of therapy discourse is based on the view that description and explanation are equally important and must be considered together as research proceeds. The goal of achieving descriptive adequacy is approachable with continued work (Panagos et al., 1986). Verbal and nonverbal features can be reliably coded from videotape and incorporated into working typologies. Observations can be made across types of therapy, disorders, and clinical settings. A challenge is to sort out the mass of information generated by videotape. For example, although transcribing clinician and client utterances is relatively easy, coding eye-gaze behaviors requires exacting control of recording conditions and reliable tape analysis. Yet such descriptions may produce enough detail to present a clear picture of therapy, apart from a priori stances. That is, the input to learning can be established independent of prevailing clinical notions.

Explaining patterns of therapy discourse is more challenging. Description can lead to inferences about mental states and motivations, and interview and questionnaire studies can tap attitudes and strategies. Triangulation (Kovarsky & Maxwell, 1992)—the comparison of the social perspectives of therapy participants—is one formal method of validating claims. Kovarsky (1989a) used this method when he showed videotapes to clinicians, teachers, children, and parents. Probe questions—asking clients to compare the therapist to other professionals—build on the videotape and interview data. The ethnographer becomes totally immersed in the therapy process to sort out the levels of participant knowledge (i.e., "thick analysis"; Kovarsky & Maxwell, 1992, p. 76). Perhaps 15 to 20 studies are needed.

A logical first step toward explanation is to determine why therapy is so often highly structured and adult centered. Structured therapy is widely promulgated in the field of communication disorders, although I know of no critical evaluation of the arguments for the position. The claim is made that the child has already failed to acquire adequate language in the unstructured home environment and there is no use duplicating that experience in clinical sessions (Letts, 1985, p. 330). It follows that the child needs a structured experience in which there is an opportunity to practice linguistic forms for evaluation and feedback from the clinician. It turns out that support for the child-needs-structure position is found in the research literature. Intervention studies (Hoffman, Norris, & Monjure, 1990; Panagos & Griffith, 1981; Yoder, Kaiser, Alpert, & Fischer, 1993) invariably show that structured therapies produce learning and generalization effects compared to control conditions. Generalization of learning is the pivotal standard against which therapy outcomes are measured.

As tidy as the case for structured therapy appears to be, there is one to be made for a social learning theory: The therapy experience for the child is not just about linguistic learning but also about social relationships and expectations (Kovarsky & Maxwell, 1992; Kovarsky, 1989a; Ripich & Panagos, 1985). At home, family relationships are familiar and center around the use of language to negotiate social roles and standards of conduct. How clearly the child talks is less important than how language is used for socialization and interaction. When the child moves outside the home and encounters doctors, coaches, teachers, and therapists, new role relations and expectations are mapped onto the family (kinship) system. The structures of talk take on new purposes, such as taking talk seriously and speaking clearly. According to this social learning theory, therapy works not because of degree of structure but because the child is placed in a situation in which the negotiated relationship centers around clear speech. Expectations have changed. Although structured therapies are known to promote linguistic learning, differences between types of therapy, if any, are rarely obtained, probably because structured therapies are so similar in the first place (Bobkoff Katz, 1990; Ripich et al., 1984; Panagos & Griffith, 1981). Linguistic generalization is so common that one wonders under what conditions it would not occur. Generalization to nontherapy social contexts remains clinically problematic but is seldom evaluated in treatment studies (Ripich & Panagos, 1985).

The related issue of how heavily structured therapies affect the cognitive abilities of linguistically vulnerable children is a serious one. That structured therapies have side-effects is never studied (Panagos et al., 1986). Many examples can be cited. Children taught to repeat linguistic structures sometimes become echolalic, dysfluent, inattentive, and disruptive—behaviors viewed by the clinician as further confirmation of the child's communication disorders. Some clients develop a labored, monotone vocal pattern in response to therapy demands. Weird generalizations such as placing the article *the* before the main verb or adding the voiceless *th* to all words with fricatives are not uncommon. We have already mentioned the negative impact of structured therapy on the client's self-esteem when the role of error maker is accepted.

It is interesting to note that therapy can be highly structured without the distinguishing feature of speech correction. The clinician can model linguistic targets, expand or expatiate the child's utterances, make comments of genuine interest, and ask true-information questions when the child's meanings are unclear. The clinician can focus playfully on only those forms which are emerging at the age level with the goal of generalization from normal to delayed forms. Nonverbal materials can be arranged carefully to increase the likelihood of the use of target forms. Pointing, leaning, object manipulation, and eye gaze can focus attention on the referential materials. Tallies of the spontaneous use of target structures can be kept to ensure clinical accountability. However, in spite of all of these possible ways of reducing the negative impact of speech correction, aggressive therapies are preferred. The child is put in the position of error maker, with the attendant risks of language confusion and lowered self-esteem.

Why then is structured therapy so universally appealing to clinicians? Why does it occur that even when more child-centered lessons are set up, the clinician takes back the control (Letts, 1985; Silliman et al., 1979)? Why wouldn't child-centered therapy be more interesting, novel, fun, and even humanizing? Why does the clinician invest so much time and energy in controlling every small detail of linguistic performance? The answer seems to be that the clinician needs the structure, not the client (Panagos & Bliss, 1990). The structure says, "I'm professional, well organized, efficient, and accountable. I don't waste time; I keep the child on task and chart the number of correct responses. When the child fails, it's because he or she has a communication disorder. When I fail, it's because I didn't structure the task correctly. Getting down to work means getting down to structure."

Why aren't there more investigations of clinician-child discourse? My view is that discourse analysis lifts therapy out of the realm of techniques, procedures, and strategies and equalizes the role relationship of therapist and client. Whereas prescriptive therapies can be learned by example, even by rote, understanding therapy as social interaction requires reflective thinking and strategic action. Just as there is heavy social control of clients, there is heavy social control of novice clinicians in university clinics. Before insight can be developed, the young clinician is coached to master structured therapies to win the supervisor's approval. When clinician and child become social partners in therapy, the clinician loses status and gains obligations to interact adaptively. Ironically, traditional therapies project failure onto the client when the client has virtually no control of therapy exchange. Scientific analysis of speech therapy points the spotlight at the clinician as much as it does the child.

I once supervised a preschool language program. We had individual therapy followed by structured group therapy followed by child-centered play therapy. At the end of the day, we critiqued our sessions. The five student clinicians inevitably wanted to talk about the problems in the play therapy session. The boys got crazy, marching around the room, chanting, falling down, rolling on the floor, even throwing a few things around. One young woman insisted that we were not getting anything done. I explained that this is often the way boys play and use language when they are growing up. The more I explained the rationale for natural interaction, the more she protested. Finally she said, "I was raised in a strict Catholic family and we just weren't permitted to act that way!" This intrigued me and caused me to think that the issue of structured therapy has deep roots that we need to understand much better than we do now.

References

Becker, L. B., & Silverstein, J. E. (1984). Clinical-child discourse: A replication study. *Journal of Speech and Hearing Disorders, 49,* 104–105.

Bobkoff, K. (1982). *Analysis of the verbal and nonverbal components of clinician-client interaction.* Unpublished doctoral dissertation, Kent State University, OH.

Bobkoff Katz, K. (1990). Clinical decision making as an ethnographic process. *Journal of Childhood Communication Disorders, 13*(1), 93–99.

Bobkoff, K., & Panagos, J. M. (1986). The "point" of language intervention lessons. *Child Language Teaching and Therapy, 2,*(1), 50–62.

Chubrich, R. E. (1978). Session obsession: A former client looks at therapy. *Journal of the National Student Speech and Hearing Association, 6,* 70–78.

Crystal, D. (1981). *Clinical linguistics.* New York: Springer-Verlag.

Damico, J. S. (1990). Prescriptionism as a motivating mechanism: An ethnographic study in the public schools. *Journal of Childhood Communication Disorders, 13*(1), 85–92.

Hoffman, P. R., Norris, J. A., & Monjure, J. (1990). Comparison of process targeting and whole language treatments for phonologically delayed preschool children. *Language, Speech and Hearing Services in Schools, 21,* 102–109.

Kovarsky, D. (1989a). *An ethnography of communication in child language therapy.* Unpublished doctoral dissertation, University of Texas, Austin.

Kovarsky, D. (1989b). On the occurrence of okay in therapy. *Child Language Teaching and Therapy, 5*(2), 137–145.

Kovarsky, D. (1990). Discourse markers in adult-controlled therapy: Implications for child centered intervention. *Journal of Childhood Communication Disorders, 13*(1), 29–41.

Kovarsky, D., & Maxwell, M. M. (1992). Ethnography and the clinical setting: Communicative expectancies in clinical discourse. *Topics in Language Disorders, 12*(3), 76–84.

Kovarsky, D., & Panagos, J. M. (in press). *Repair strategies in child language therapy.*

Letts, C. (1985). Linguistic interaction in the clinic: How do therapists do therapy? *Child Language Teaching and Therapy, 1,* 321–331.

Maxwell, M. M. (1990). The authenticity of ethnographic research. *Journal of Childhood Communication Disorders, 13*(1), 1–12.

McFarlane, S. C., Fujiki, M., & Brinton, B. (1984). *Coping with communication handicaps: Resources for the practicing clinician.* San Diego: College-Hill Press.

McTear, M. F., & King, F. (1991). Miscommunication in clinical contexts: The speech therapy interview. In N. Coupland, H. Giles, & J. M. Weimann (Eds.), *Miscommunication and problematic talk.* London: Sage

Milroy, J., & Milroy, L. (1985). *Authority in language: Investigating language prescriptionism and standardism.* London: Routledge & Kegan Paul.

Moseley, M. J. (1978). Analysis and description of clinician's vocal behavior. *Ohio Journal of Speech and Hearing, 13*(2), 105–115.

Panagos, J. M., & Bliss, L. S. (1990). Presuppositions for speech therapy lessons. *Journal of Childhood Communication Disorders, 13*(1), 19–28.

Panagos, J. M., Bobkoff, K., & Scott, C. M. (1986). Discourse analysis of language intervention. *Child Language Teaching and Therapy, 2*(2), 211–229.

Panagos, J. M., & Fry, J. (1976). *Code switching during language therapy communication.* Paper presented at the annual convention of the American Speech-Language-Hearing Association, Houston, TX.

Panagos, J. M., & Griffith, P. L. (1981). Okay, what do educators really know about language intervention? *Topics in Learning Disabilities, 2,* 69–82.

Panagos, J. M., Griffith, P. L., & Ripich, D. N. (1985). Teacher-pupil discourse in classrooms for hearing-impaired children. *The Exceptional Child, 32*(1), 21–29.

Panagos, J. M., Katz, K. B., Kovarsky, D., & Prelock, P. (1988). The nonverbal component of clinical lessons. *Child Language Teaching and Therapy, 4*(3), 278–296.

Prelock, P. A. (1990). A retrospective examination of interactional behaviors viewed as experimentally nonsignificant. *Journal of Childhood Communication Disorders, 13*(1), 13–18.

Prutting, C. A. (1984). A reply to "clinician-child discourse: a replication study." *Journal of Speech and Hearing Disorders, 49,* 106.

Prutting, C. A., Bagshaw, N., Goldstein, H., Juskowitz, S., & Umen, I. (1978). Clinician-child discourse: Some preliminary questions. *Journal of Speech and Hearing Disorders, 43,* 123–139.

Ripich, D. N. (1982). *Children's social perception of speech-language lessons: A sociolinguistic analysis of role-play discourse.* Unpublished doctoral dissertation, Kent State University, OH.

Ripich, D. N., Hambrecht, G., & Panagos, J. M. (1985). Discourse analysis of aphasia therapy. *Aphasia-Apraxia-Agnosia, 3*(4), 9–18.

Ripich, D. N., Hambrecht, G., Panagos, J. M., & Prelock, P. A. (1984). An analysis of articulation and language discourse patterns. *Journal of Childhood Communication Disorders, 7*(2), 17–26.

Ripich, D. N., & Panagos, J. M. (1985). Assessing children's knowledge of sociolinguistic rules for speech therapy lessons. *Journal of Speech and Hearing Disorders, 50,* 335–346.

Siliman, E. R., Gams-Golub, S. E., & Chizzik, S. G. (1979). *Clinician-child discourse: How accommodating is the clinician?* Paper presented at the annual convention of the American Speech-Language-Hearing Association, Atlanta, GA.

Smith-Lewis, M. (1993). Culturally diverse nonspeakers: Home/school interaction (unpublished report). S. Blackstone (Ed.), *Augmentative Communication News, 6,* 6–7.

Spinelli, F. M., & Ripich, D. N. (1985). A comparison of classroom and clinical discourse. In D. N. Ripich & F. M. Spinelli (Eds.), *School discourse problems.* San Diego: College-Hill Press.

Stech, E. L., Curtis, J. W., Troesch, P. L., & Binnie, C. (1973). Reinforcement of speech clinicians: Factor-analytic study. *ASHA, 15,* 287–289.

Yoder, P. J., Kaiser, A. P., Alpert, C., & Fischer, R. (1993). Following the child's lead when teaching nouns to preschoolers with mental retardation. *Journal of Speech and Hearing Research, 36,* 158–167.

4

Clinical Language Teaching

Theories and Principles to Guide Our Responses when Children Miss Our Language Targets[1]

ALICE VIGIL AND ANNE VAN KLEECK

Introduction

In language therapy, we spend a great deal of effort determining our goals, or target behaviors, for a particular child and deciding on procedures that will help the child achieve those goals. A primary agenda in much of our subsequent intervention, then, is to get children to produce the language (or broader communicative) behaviors we have targeted as goals for them. If the child fails to meet our expectations and does not provide the targeted behavior, we are likely to go back to our original thinking in order to figure out what has gone wrong. We must have erred in our thinking, or the child would not be erring by not responding or not responding appropriately. It must be that either the goals we targeted or the procedures we are using are not appropriate. So, we change one, or maybe even both, in an attempt to correct the situation and create a therapeutic context in which the child will be able to produce the correct (i.e., targeted) response.

Although there is nothing wrong with evaluating the appropriateness of either our goals or the procedures we use to achieve them, there are many other possible reasons why children may fail to meet our clinical expectations. The purpose of this chapter is to provide a framework for considering the myriad reasons why children might err in language intervention. Such a framework will enable us to analyze errors and, by determining their cause, use this to enhance our clinical effectiveness.

Dealing with the complexity of children's language and language learning difficulties is a never-ending challenge that may occasionally border on being overwhelming. Why, you might ask, does the clinician need another framework, yet

[1]This chapter is an updated and revised version of an article that appeared in the *National Student Speech-Language-Hearing Association Journal* in 1986 entitled, "What's in an Error? Using Children's Wrong Responses as Language Teaching Opportunities."

another set of factors to think about? In 1973, Marion Blank suggested that educators do not consider errors worthy of thinking about because they are a natural and expected part of normal learning. Likewise, the presence of errors in language therapy is perhaps so obvious that it does not require our explicit attention.

We believe that the clinician who consciously thinks about errors—what causes them and how to respond to them—will be a much more effective language facilitator. Blank reached the same conclusion regarding teaching in general. She stated, "the effectiveness of any teaching program critically hinges on the management of the wrong response" (1973, p. 85). It is time to add to our treatment plans—along with our goals, activities, methods for measuring progress, and plans for generalization—a serious consideration of how we plan to deal with the child's errors.

What Is an Error?

To analyze errors, we must first be able to agree on what they are. This may seem straightforward—the child either produces the target or does not. Yet the theoretically diverse positions concerning how language is acquired, how it is organized in the brain, and how it might break down make the issue of what constitutes an error a source of controversy. The meaning of the term *error* may vary considerably for different people, and some people may argue that it is not a useful term at all when referring to children's attempts to communicate.

Our own conception of the term *error* derives from the analogy that the term *target behavior* suggests. The clinician selects a target and tries to help the child hit that target. The child may take a shot at the target and may either hit or miss the mark. We often refer to hitting the mark we have selected as a correct response and missing the mark as an error.

However, those of us who have engaged in archery practice will understand what it means to learn a new skill and will feel the injustice wrought by considering each failure to hit the bull's eye as an error. Archers know the skills required to engage in the process (aim, strength, timing) and the variety of factors that affect the accuracy of any particular shot (wind, fatigue, attention, vision, tension). Focusing solely on whether a shot hits the mark ignores the entire process involved in archery. It emphasizes the product or result rather than the process. Missing the mark captures our attention because we are more often aware of our target than of the archery process; but missing the mark can also redirect our attention to the often less directly observable processes involved.

In the same way, the term *error* in children's language production tends to focus us on the product rather than the process of children's language learning, potentially promoting rather all-or-nothing thinking. However, it is the product that catches our attention, signals us that something unexpected has occurred, and can thus remind us to consider the potential processes responsible for the behavior.

In this chapter, we will use the term *error* to focus on how behavior that misses the target signals us to examine the myriad processes that may underlie the behavior. We thus move away from thinking of an error as something the child did wrong and toward viewing it more as a catalyst to promote our understanding of the processes that may be affecting a child's language and other communicative behaviors. We will review the theories that shape often different notions of what constitutes viable language intervention targets and how to respond to them. We describe our own theoretical framework and then propose a set of principles to consider in dealing with children's errors that occur as we attempt to facilitate their language development.

Theories that Influence How We Think about Language Learning

Although the development of explicit techniques for dealing with errors is critical to the field of language intervention, the techniques selected will be highly dependent on the clinician's beliefs and assumptions about how child language behavior changes. As Hoffman concluded, "Perhaps the most immediate manner in which teachers vent their theoretical orientation during instruction is through the form of feedback provided to students when they miscue (err)" (cited in Meyer, 1985, p. 8). Because one's response to children's errors is such a potent factor in teaching and such a sensitive indicator of one's treatment assumptions, it is critical that we select a response framework that is compatible with our theory of language development. To do so, we need first to be clear about what theory or theories we espouse.

Theories that influence how we think about language learning focus on one of two things: (1) how language is acquired, and (2) how it might break down. At the most basic level, theories of language acquisition differ in the degree to which they consider that either innate (i.e., biological) factors or the environment play a key role in the process. Chomskyan linguistic theory lies at one extreme (e.g., 1957, 1965, 1981), touting that syntax is an innate skill, the development of which is merely triggered by environmental input. Learning theory (Skinner, 1957) is at the opposite extreme, awarding great importance to environmental antecedents and consequences of a child's behavior in the development process. In between these two extremes are the cognitive/perceptual and social theories that allow for an interaction between the child's innate endowment and the nurturing role of the environment in guiding language development. Figure 4–1 depicts this continuum of theories. Although learning theory has few advocates in the 1990s as a theory of language development, it continues to have great impact on some language intervention strategies. The other theories are all alive and well in various incarnations. We will briefly explain these theories and consider how each affects both the kinds of errors one looks for (i.e., what language domain or domains the theory is focused on) and how one responds to these errors. They are summarized in Table 4–1.

Operant Learning Theory

In Skinner's (1957) operant learning account, language, as all behavior, is explained using the doctrines of behaviorism, which assert that the input from and the reaction of the environment explain all learning. The sequence of events in any learning situation includes an original stimulus (discriminative stimulus), a response to that stimulus, and then an outcome (reinforcing stimulus). Favorable outcomes (positive reinforcers) increase the likelihood that future

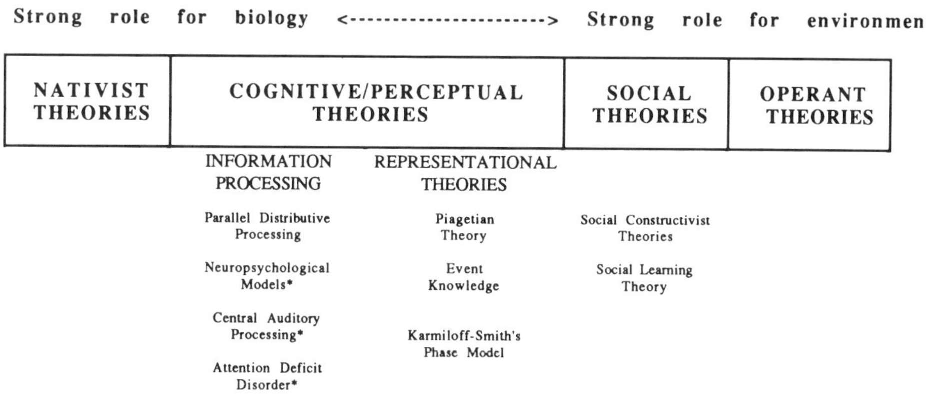

*These theories deal more specifically with breakdowns in cognitive processing that may result in difficulties with learning in general and language learning more specifically.

Figure 4–1. Theories that affect language learning organized along a continuum representing the relative emphasis the theory places on biologic factors (nature) or environmental factors (nurture).

occurrences of the discriminative stimulus will result in the same response, and unfavorable outcomes will decrease that likelihood.

Learning theory applies to all behavior and as such does not focus the clinician's attention on any specific domain of behavior, as long as the behavior is overtly observable and hence measurable. Legitimate targets can be selected from any skill area (syntax, vocabulary, answering questions, etc.) or any problem area interfering with language learning (lack of eye contact, failure to attend, etc.) that can be operationally defined by discrete, observable behavior. The interventionist programs procedures for achieving the desired target by specifying the criteria for mastery, the intervention techniques, and the reinforcements to be utilized.

In learning theory, an error is anything other than the specific response desired following the presentation of a discriminative stimulus. That specific response may be the exact adult form or an acceptable specific approximation that will be gradually shaped to the adult form. Responses to errors are well designated in learning theory. Initially in applying this theory to language intervention, interventionists set up a token economy wherein the child received intrinsically unrewarding but concrete reinforcers (such as plastic chips, blocks, or checkmarks on a paper) that were periodically exchanged for back-up reinforcers, which were extrinsically rewarding for the individual child (such as stickers, little toys, getting to play a favorite game, etc.). Many of the drill-play activities used in direct teaching of language targets include aspects of operant learning theory, attesting to the pervasive impact of this theory on language intervention. Children may win a game piece or turn for an accurate response. Under this system, errors are often responded to by simply withholding a turn, game piece, or token. This clearly indicates to the child that his or her response was not the desired response and that a different response is necessary to win a reinforcer. A somewhat more drastic reaction to an error involves losing a reinforcer that the child has already earned. Many additional techniques for decreasing the strength of

Table 4–1. Summary of Theories

Theory	*Focus*	*Response to Errors*
Operant theory	Environmental antecedents and consequences to any observable behavior	Withhold or withdraw positive reinforcement.
Nativism	Syntax	None, because learning is result of biologic maturation.
Information processing theories		
Parallel distributive processing	All cognitive processing, including syntax and morphology	Supply more input of correct pattern. Provide simple input to beginning learners and learners with too much initial auditory memory capacity.
Neuropsychological models	Attention, memory, sensation, processing speed, spatial skills, auditory and visual processing, executive control of resource allocation	Work with child's processing strengths to Foster development of strategies for learning Help child approach problem differently Make compensatory adjustments to learning environments.
Central auditory processing	Not peripheral hearing impairments, but difficulties with processing auditory information, particularly if signal is degraded or if there is noise	Slow down rate of messages; insert more pauses at phrase boundaries. Decrease background noise and/or improve signal-to-noise ratio (accomplished by seat placement, etc.). Supplement auditory messages with visual and other contextual cues. Teach child to monitor listening and ask for clarification.
Attention deficit or attention deficit hyperactivity disorder	Deficits in attention resulting in inattention and possibly impulsivity, distractibility, and hyperactivity Some believe underlying problem with self-regulation of behavior affecting organizing, planning, monitoring, and evaluating one's own behavior	Inattention: Alert child prior to sending message, or repeat message. Difficulty inhibiting reactions: Reduce extraneous stimuli. Slow processing speed: Reduce length and amount of information, speak more slowly, provide message redundancy, give child longer to respond, or train skill to overlearned level.

Table 4–1. Summary of Theories *(continued)*

Theory	*Focus*	*Response to Errors*
		Difficulty organizing information: Provide supportive organization structure initially and gradually withdraw, model our own organization and planning out loud, mediate problem solving for the child, teach child to recognize own disorganization, and develop plans for responding to it.
Representational theories		
Piagetian theory	Cognitive precursors to symbolic language use Cognitive underpinnings of early semantic relations and later forms expressing time, space, causality	Do not correct errors, but provide environment that encourages child's own active exploration.
Event knowledge	Routine events that constitute earliest mental representations	Provide more experience with the routine. Use a routine more familiar to child
Karmiloff-Smith's phase model	Nature of mental representation changes over time as skill is better learned	Depends on phase of mental representation reached for particular skill
Social theories		
Social constructivist theory	Tutorial skills (mediation, scaffolding) used by adult in teaching child, and how they change as child gains more mastery of that skill	Depends on where skill learning is along the continuum ranging from other-regulation to self-regulation
Social learning theory	Modeling skill for child	Provide correct model.

undesired behavior are specified in operant conditioning technology (see Reese, 1966, for a complete discussion).

Nativism

Chomsky's (1957) well-known view of the language acquisition process, which developed in response to the learning theory view, is that children are born with a special capacity to derive the structural rules of grammar. This innate linguistic knowledge (originally heralded as the language acquisition device, or LAD) consists of a formal system of rules and principles of well-formedness that are universal to all languages. By exposure to a specific language, this universal grammar yields the particular grammar of that language. Language learning is not related to other learning, such as cognition.

Chomsky's theory has changed a great deal since the 1950s, evolving from his generative transformational grammar (1957), which was elaborated in his standard theory (1965), to his current government-binding theory (1981). He now posits that children do not acquire structural rules but rather engage in parameter setting (something akin to on/off switches for all the subsystems of universal grammar that, once they are all set by exposure to a particular language, account for the core grammar of that language).

Although many changes have occurred in Chomsky's thinking, some foundational beliefs remain basically unchanged—that language is innate, that its development is separate from other aspects of development, and that syntax is the central component of language. Chomsky's considerable legacy in linguistics has also spawned additional theories that may differ from his in some critical respects (e.g., the centrality of syntax) but agree with the basic notion that language is innate. Perhaps the most influential of these is the lexical functional grammar (Kaplan & Bresnan, 1982) applied specifically to language acquisition by Steven Pinker (e.g., Pinker, 1984, 1994).

Because they posit that the capacity for language is genetically determined, the ideas of Chomsky and other nativist theorists greatly downplay the role of the environment in language learning. They likewise offer little guidance for how to respond to errors because biological maturation, and not how one responds to the child, determines language development.

Although it offers little in the way of teaching, Chomsky's theory has offered much in terms of providing goals for language intervention. As McLean (1983) noted, "it got us beyond the phoneme as a clinical preoccupation and also allows us to quantify deficits in language through application of syntactic measures" (p. 118). The areas notably lacking in Chomsky's theory—in particular, cognition and some role for environmental facilitation—provided the impetus for many of the later theories of the language acquisition process.

Cognitive/Perceptual Theories

Numerous theories that developed subsequent to Chomsky's notions of innateness have considered language learning not as an entirely unique process but as part of learning in general. These theories divide broadly, although they overlap considerably as well, into those that focus on how the brain processes information and those that consider the nature of mental representation.

INFORMATION PROCESSING THEORIES

These theories focus on some aspect of how the brain attends to, organizes, and stores information. Currently, a plethora of work in cognitive science considers the vast learning potential of the human mind the result of the ability to process many bits of information in parallel or simultaneously. The theories generated from this perspective are often referred to as parallel distributive processing (PDP) or connectionist theories. The other theories considered in this section were developed to explain how different aspects of cognitive or perceptual processing may go awry and result in a language learning disability.

PDP Theories. Traditionally, human information processing was conceived of as occurring in a serial fashion, wherein decisions or operations were performed one at a time, sequentially. Recent work posits parallel processing, wherein multiple decisions or operations may occur simultaneously because networks of processors (called activation nodes) are linked or connected. In this theory, learning involves modifying the strengths of the interconnections between nodes gradually over time as a result of more and more input to the system. As such, the amount of environmental exposure is critical to this model, as is an innate PDP learning mechanism. The system of interconnected nodes learns to detect patterns in the input, and because of this it can produce output that has never occurred in the input based on the similarity of the item to other patterns it has learned.

Rumelhart and McClelland (1986, 1987) conducted pioneering research that applied this model to language acquisition. Using computers programmed to engage in parallel distributive processing, these researchers presented the learning system with over 400 verbs and their past-tense forms. They looked at the machine's "learning" at different points in the input. Furthermore, they attempted to match the input to that which a young language-learning child might receive, so irregular verbs were presented more frequently than regular verbs initially. The computer simulation results exactly mirrored the development of the past tense in normally developing children. The system first used every verb correctly, then passed through a stage of overregularization, and finally correctly produced irregulars.

From Rumelhart and McClelland's work, it is obvious that errors represent one stage in the learning process, a stage that is predicted by a system that is particularly good at detecting patterns and applying them to similar but unfamiliar language forms (so the plural of *mouse* might be produced as *mouses*). These patterns can occur for any aspect of language form (although PDP models may be capable of offering explanations for semantic and pragmatic aspects of language development, we are unaware of any work to date that has done so).

One's response to an error would be to supply numerous examples, over time, of the correct input of the form the child had produced incorrectly. This would act to weaken or lower the weights for the connections between the form produced in error (mouses) and the pattern that had been induced for similar forms (e.g., blouse-blouses, horse-horses, mess-messes). Assuming our input is attended to by the child's learning system, we would expect the child to be sometimes right and sometimes wrong on the form as the connections begin to weaken. The weights on the connections between the activation nodes would continue to be adjusted with each new correct input until eventually only correct output is produced.

More recent work using PDP modeling by Jeff Elman (1993) has different implications for working with children with language disabilities. In a series of brilliantly conceived simulations involving input of both simple and complex sentences, Elman found that learning could occur in two ways. In one study, he first gave input consisting mostly of simple sentences and only later introduced complex sentences. The system was learned eventually in this simulation, although it was unable to learn if both simple and complex sentences were provided equally in the initial input.

Elman did not stop there. He next reasoned that few children would actually receive such developmentally ordered input. How, then, could they learn language? Elman hypothesized that their shorter memory span may actually benefit them in the language learning process. So he gave his computer the equivalent of a shorter memory span (three to four words) that was increased gradually. The input had variable complexity from the outset—some simple and some complex sentences. Initially, the system learned simple sentences only, although this took considerably longer (i.e., much more input) than in the simulation in which only simple input was presented initially. Gradually, however, complex syntax was learned as well. After the initially prolonged stage of learning, subsequent learning proceeded quickly.

Elman's simulations suggest how memory might interact with language input. If memory is too good, learning cannot take place unless only simple input is given initially. This conclusion, if supported in further research, might have implications for a specific type of error encountered in some children with language impairments—the echolalic response. In this case, the child appears to have a good auditory memory span and can repeat language input verbatim, often after a substantial amount of time has elapsed. Echolalic language productions, however, are memorized and not generated by a knowledge of grammar. Elman's research suggests that a therapeutic response to such language would be to offer only simple input until the child provides evidence of understanding the grammar of simple syntax, and then begin to introduce more complex input. The same recommendation would apply to older children (who would presumably have longer memory spans) attempting to learn a second language.

A second implication of Elman's work would be that, for younger children with shorter memory spans, the easiest route to learning might be to provide simple input initially, even though it would not be essential. In this way, the sequential units of language isolated by the child's shorter memory span would be far more likely to contain systematic patterns corresponding to simple sentence grammar, and learning in this stage might proceed more efficiently. This does not offer a way to respond to errors per se but rather suggests that the general nature of our input to language-learning children be kept at a level of simplicity commensurate with (i.e., slightly above) their own budding level of grammatical ability.

Neuropsychological Models. The field of language intervention has a long history of seeking to understand deviant language development through understanding brain-behavior relationships. Early theorists compared the behavior of children with developmental disabilities to that of adults with known neurological lesions and began efforts to map the location of behavior in the brain and to predict the site of neurological impairment in children with abnormal functioning. The early lines of thinking included Werner and Strauss's (1941) exploration of perceptual processing problems, Orton's (1937) theories of hemispheric specialization, and the search by neurologists and educators for neurological soft signs in children with learning problems. More recent research has focused on identifying the relationships between the cerebral hemispheres during information processing, identifying the cognitive processing styles of atypical learners, and understanding the impact of lesions on more plastic, developing brains as opposed to their impact on brains whose functions have become more localized. The brain-behavior relationships of children with language and learning disorders have been explored through analysis of psychometric data, through behavioral tasks such as finger tapping or dichotic listening (which presumably tease apart the functioning of the two cerebral hemispheres), through observation of the activity of the brain with imaging and electrical measurement technology during task performance, and through examination of actual brains of children with disabilities at autopsy.

Neuropsychological models have helped us understand more about the impact of numerous cognitive processes on language learning and language disorders. These models urge us to explore the relationships between performance on language tasks and processes such as attention, memory, sensation, processing speed, spatial skills, auditory and visual processing, and the executive control of resource allocation. Neuropsychological studies that reveal increasingly more subtypes of language and learning disorders illuminate the complexities of brain-behavior relationships and dispel the illusion of simplistic etiologic explanations (Gerber, 1993). The research on cognitive styles urges us to explore the match between our teaching methods and the child's preferred learning avenues.

Research on cognitive processes suggests the need for us to help children develop compensatory strategies for learning or teach them to approach problems differently. We can also attempt to make compensatory adjustments in the learning environment to maximize their success and minimize their frustration. The failure of early attempts to change cognitive processes through direct training (as well as the failure to change children's language by training cognitive processes; see Bloom & Lahey, 1978) has led interventionists to take a more practical and functional approach to clinical teaching.

The more cautious approach focuses on direct teaching of the particular skills a child needs (oral language skills, reading, writing, etc.) while using what is known about the child's cognitive processing strengths and weaknesses to alter *how* the child is taught. When an error arises, it is used as a cue to examine the situation and identify barriers to success. Those barriers are then dealt with directly by making the appropriate modifications in the learning environment or in the instructional methods to work through the child's cognitive processing strengths and to achieve learning. For example, a child who has trouble following oral directions in the classroom might be taught compensatory strategies (such as how to ask the teacher for a repetition), and the environment might be adapted to facilitate success (such as having teachers show the child what to do along with telling him or her). Thus the error is used as a window through which to view the child's processing skills so that a clearer understanding of the child's learning strengths and needs may be obtained.

Central Auditory Processing. Questions about the hearing of children with language disorders have been of great concern since it was first noticed that some children with apparently normal hearing did not learn language normally. Historically these children were sometimes placed in classrooms for children with hearing impairments so that their needs could be met better than in regular classrooms.

More recently, audiologists have been exploring the central auditory processing difficulties of children with apparently normal hearing, using tests originally designed to identify the site of lesion along the auditory pathway in adults with brain trauma. Although imaging technologies have made many of these tests obsolete for confirming lesions of the auditory pathway, many of these tests have been applied in the hopes of identifying the neuroanatomic level of auditory function in children (Keith, 1981). Tallal and her colleagues (e.g., Tallal & Piercy, 1978) have been able to isolate the duration aspect of the acoustic signal as particularly problematic and have identified some language-delayed children who have difficulty processing brief acoustic events.

The debate continues among language researchers regarding whether central auditory processing problems can cause language disabilities (Gerber, 1993). Nevertheless, some children do appear to have particular difficulty with processing auditory information despite having normal peripheral hearing. These difficulties may include problems listening in noisy environments; problems understanding degraded messages; and, in older students, difficulty understanding non-native speakers, hearing or learning the lyrics to songs, or following conversations in a group setting.

Sometimes children are referred for intervention after undergoing auditory testing and receiving a diagnosis of a central auditory processing disorder. A more comprehensive assessment of language and learning needs is then required to plan for communication intervention. If auditory processing problems are found to affect communication and learning, they will affect the way we deal with errors which occur during clinical language teaching. An error may signal the need to slow the message rate, to reduce background noise, to improve the signal-to-noise ratio, or to supplement the auditory message with visual or contextual cues.

For example, we might insert more pauses at phrase boundaries as we speak, seat the child away from a noisy air conditioning vent, demonstrate as well as speak our instructions, or see if the child's frequency modulation (FM) system is working. We might also help the child learn to monitor his or her own listening needs and ask for clarification or accommodation when needed. As with most other information processing theories, this one alerts us to examine how the child is processing our messages and how we can make this processing more successful.

Attention Deficit Disorder or Attention Deficit Hyperactivity Disorder. Another orientation which falls in the category of cognitive processing hypotheses is the notion of deficits in attention. Although the diagnosis of attention deficit (with or without hyperactivity) has become much more frequent in children with and without language disorders in recent years, observers since the time of Strauss and Lehtinen (1947) have noted that children with learning problems often have a constellation of symptoms which include inattention, impulsivity, distractibility, and hyperactivity.

Researchers have offered a variety of theories regarding the underlying difficulty in attention deficit hyperactivity disorder (ADHD), such as problems sustaining focused attention, weak ability to inhibit reactions to competing stimuli, slowed processing speed, and poor regulation of behavior (e.g., Gerber, 1993). Westby and Cutler (in press) describe the pragmatic problems of children diagnosed with ADHD. For example, they have difficulty reading social cues, they may switch topics abruptly, and they have difficulty adapting messages to the listener or to situational nuances. In fact, some of the diagnostic criteria for ADHD are communication problems, such as difficulty awaiting a turn, not listening to what is being said, difficulty following instructions, and interrupting others.

Westby and Cutler suggest that the underlying problem with ADHD may be in the metacognitive skills involved in self-regulation of behavior, such as organizing, planning, monitoring, and evaluating one's own behavior. They point to the dysfluent and incoherent language these children use in language tasks requiring higher levels of organization and to the difficulty they experience in complex problem solving when they cannot rely on external structure and organization. Despite the variety of assumptions regarding the nature of the underlying difficulty, typical treatment for ADHD has involved medication paired with some form of behavioral therapy.

In language therapy, our assumptions regarding the reason for a child's inattentive behavior have major implications for how we deal with the child's errors. If we believe an error is due to inattention, we might either try to prevent such errors in the future by alerting the child prior to requesting a response or we might repeat a request the child did not attend to. If we believe the child's errors are due to difficulty inhibiting reactions to competing stimuli, we might reduce extraneous stimuli as much as possible. We could do this, for example, by having the child look at us when we speak, by removing distracting materials, or by seating the child closer to us or the teacher.

If we believe the child's errors are due to slow processing speed, we might reduce the length or amount of information given at one time, speak more slowly, provide redundancy in our messages, give the child more time to respond, or train skills to an overlearned level so that increased automaticity of skill can reduce the task's processing demand on the child. If we believe a child's error is due to difficulty organizing information, we might (1) provide an organizational structure or scaffolding initially and gradually wean the child to independence in utilizing the structure; (2) talk about our own organization and planning to model or mediate the problem-solving process for the child; or (3) teach the child strategies for recognizing his or her own internal states of confusion or disorganization as a prerequisite to developing a plan for their his or her own behavior or response.

In sum, knowing that ADHD may be affecting a child's responding is only the first step in adapting our responses to meet that child's needs. The important next step is to clarify our own beliefs about the underlying nature of the child's inattention in general or in the moment and adapt our responses so they are consistent with our theoretical assumptions.

REPRESENTATIONAL THEORIES

We are using the label *representational* to consider three theories that have offered insights into the nature of mental representation and how such representation informs us about language development. The most influential of the three is Piaget's theory, which focused broadly on the notion of symbolic function and considered language to be but one manifestation of the capacity to use mental symbols. Katherine Nelson and her colleagues developed the idea of event knowledge, which proposes that routine events themselves, including the language characteristically associated with them, constitute the earliest mental representations of children. Karmiloff-Smith offers ideas similar to Nelson's in her earliest phase of language development, but she goes on to provide a far more refined theory of subsequent phases of representational development.

Piagetian Theory. Although Piaget himself said very little about language development, his work in cognitive development had a great impact on many language development theorists from the 1970s onward. Basically this view proposes that children learn first about the world (cognition) and then learn to convey their ideas through language. The ideas about the world they develop prior to learning language are conveyed through the early semantic relations discussed originally by Bloom (1970) and Brown (1973). Furthermore, to develop "true" language at all, children need first to develop the ability to think symbolically, a hallmark of Piaget's sensorimotor stage of development (which occurs when children are about 18 months old).

The universals needed to develop language are as such cognitive and not specifically linguistic. The system is semantically driven, in that children learn ideas and then learn to convey those ideas linguistically. Syntax is merely the vehicle for transmitting these meanings. Schlesinger (1982) put forth a weaker version of this theory by postulating that children continue to develop concepts by using language throughout the course of development (i.e., cognition does not always necessarily come first).

The focus created by this approach is exemplified in Lois Bloom's pioneering work (1970, 1973), which moved the field of child language from its exclusive focus on syntax to consideration of cognitive and semantic aspects of early language. In language therapy, this theory has created two major types of goals. The first involves developing cognitive precursors to language skills—both prelinguistically and throughout early language development. Prelinguistically, this has involved a focus on Piaget's sensorimotor domains of imitation skills, knowledge of means-end relationships, and the related areas of object permanence (knowing that objects continue to exist when out of sight) and symbolic function (being able to keep in mind nonpresent objects and events). After language development has begun, the clinician continues to teach cognitive concepts, such as those linked to time and space, prior to requiring the child's production of the linguistic forms encoding those concepts.

During the sensorimotor period, children learn about objects—their locations, actions upon them, and that they exist, disappear from view, and come back into view again. Researchers Bloom (1973) and Brown (1973) first noted that when children begin to talk, these sensorimotor cognitive achievements are what they code in language semantically. In their early one- and two-word utterances, they talk about the existence, disappearance, and recurrence of objects as well as actions upon them, their locations, and their salient attributes. Piagetian theory, then, is an indirect catalyst for focusing on semantic relations in choosing language goals for the early stages of language intervention (Bloom & Lahey, 1978; Fey, 1986; MacDonald, 1978).

Regarding responses to errors, Piaget was a pioneer. His famous clinical interview technique was developed to probe the reasoning behind children's errors, and data from this method provide the crux of his theory of cognitive development. Interestingly, although he probed errors for the purpose of assessing a child's intellectual functioning, this theory does not directly advocate using error responses in teaching concepts to children. With this technique you "document a child's unaided development; you don't intervene" (Duckworth, 1979, p. 300). In fact, Piagetian theory views the child as self-pedagogic if the right environmental stimulation is provided. The adult's role is limited to providing the right opportunities for learning to take place spontaneously. The title of Duckworth's 1979 article summed up this stance—"Either We're Too Early and They Can't Learn It or We're Too Late and They Know It Already: The Dilemma of 'Applying Piaget.'" Duckworth stated that this dilemma is false, yet she seemed to agree with it when she concluded that "left to their own rhythm and given the opportunity, children develop the basic frameworks as naturally as walking" (1979, p. 304).

Research that attempts to accelerate the development of cognitive operations discussed by Piaget, such as conservation (the notion that the amount of a substance remains the same even if you change its shape or appearance), has documented the ineffectiveness of attempting to teach this concept to the child who is not yet ready to learn it (e.g., Sigel & Hooper, 1968; Smedslund, 1964). The conclusions of such research seem to be that correcting errors does not help a child learn.

Event Knowledge. Katherine Nelson and her colleagues introduced a concept called *event knowledge,* which views children's knowledge of routine everyday experiences as the initial content of their mental representations and hence as the original foundation for "thinking, talking, and acting" (1986, p. 3). Because it focuses on routines in social contexts as well as the nature of mental representation, her theory actually integrates both cognitive and social theories of language development (see Lucariello, Kyratzis, & Engel, 1986). However, because Nelson says very little about the adult's role in facilitating the child's induction of event knowledge, we have placed her theory with other cognitive theories that deal with the nature of mental representation.

A routine event is any purposeful activity made up of smaller segments of activity and, like the notion of a script (Schank & Abelson, 1977), "it has strong temporally invariant structure, recurs frequently, and has goals, rules and props that are well understood by the participants" (Nelson, 1986, p. 14). For the young child, daily activities of eating, dressing, and bathing constitute such routine events. Grocery shopping, eating in a restaurant, feeding pets, and doing laundry are some further examples. A child is said to understand the event structure when he or she knows the invariant sequence of the events and the roles of the participants.

In responding to children's errors, the notion of event knowledge would have us consider the possibility that the child erred because he or she did not have enough familiarity with the activity or event in which our language targets are embedded. One's response to an error, then, would be to provide opportunities for repetition until the event structure became more familiar to the child. Alternatively, one could try to elicit the target in a routine event known to be more familiar to that particular child.

Karmiloff-Smith's Phase Model. Karmiloff-Smith (1986) proposes an account of children's language development based on phases rather than the global, age-related stages espoused by Piaget. She defines phases as the recurrent cycles of processes that take place again and again as different aspects of the linguistic system develop. This concept is important because it reminds us of the possibility that a child may be at different stages of mental representation, not only broadly for different components of language (e.g., syntax, phonology, morphology) but also for different specific language forms. For example, a child may be able to reflect consciously on a sound that has been in his or her sound repertoire for some time but not be able to do so with a sound recently mastered in speech production. Karmiloff-Smith discusses the nature of the changes in internal representation as the child unconsciously reorganizes mental content to create ever greater cognitive flexibility. So what constitutes an error from this theoretical perspective is completely dependent on the current level of mental representation for that particular language form.

In phase 1, language use is driven by stimuli external to the child. So if a particular form (such as a particular word) is used in different contexts, the child will mentally store two separate representations of that form. For example, *milk* uttered as part of the breakfast routine is mentally stored separately from the *milk* uttered when looking at items in a grocery store. In other words, there is a one-to-one mapping of specific linguistic forms to particular extralinguistic/pragmatic contexts. The goal in using forms is behavioral success in a particular context. Mental procedures run in their entirety. Their components cannot be accessed or operated on separately.

As children move into the second phase, they tend to ignore aspects of external stimuli as they concentrate on gaining control over internal representations. The cognitive reorganization taking place at this juncture involves scanning operations that are sensitive to identical forms that have been paired with different functions. Conversely, the mental operations are also sensitive to identical functions that have been paired with different forms. As the child unconsciously makes these links, a single form becomes pluri-functional (so *milk,* as a single mental entry, can be used to get milk at breakfast and to name the grocery store item) and a single function can be achieved by multiple forms (possession may be signaled by a possessive pronoun or by the final-*s* morpheme).

Karmiloff-Smith posits that for the linguistic content of phase 2, the child is basically impermeable to external correction. This is illustrated in the classic example of the temporarily inexorable overgeneralized past-tense marker, as in *goed* or *wented*. In Karmiloff-Smith's phase 3, the child incorporates into his or her representations the external stimuli that were ignored during phase 2 and is able to make numerous corrections to the system.

In Karmiloff-Smith's view, specific linguistic forms enter the system at different times and hence pass through the phases at different times. The duration of this progression is undoubtedly somewhat different for different forms, depending on their inherent complexity, frequency of usage, and so forth. Therefore, at any given time, a child would have linguistic knowledge at each phase of representation. Thus, what constitutes an error and how one would respond to that error depend on knowing what phase of mental representation had been achieved for the form in question.

In phase 1, an error would consist of not achieving communicative success in a particular pragmatic context. One's response would be to repeat the meaningful routine—because components of more global representations at this point cannot be separately accessed and produced—and to use a virtually identical pragmatic context—because forms are tied to specific contexts at this juncture. Errors in phase 2 are a positive sign that mental reorganization is going on and patterns are being detected by the system. Thus, no reaction to these errors is warranted. Indeed, corrections of mistakenly arrived at patterns (e.g., the child saying "goed") are probably futile because the system at this juncture is not responsive to external feedback. By phase 3, errors of form can be corrected fruitfully. We will discuss this general notion of responding to errors based on the phase of learning later when we present our own theoretical integration of representational and social constructivist theories.

Social Theories

In this section, we will discuss social constructivist theory and social learning theory as explanations for language development. Both theories view social interaction as the basis for language acquisition. Social constructivist theory requires an active, directly participatory role of the adult. "It requires that the adult be a consenting partner, willing to negotiate with the child" (Bruner, 1983, p. 38). In social learning theory, the adult's role is to provide language models for the developing child, a somewhat less demanding role than that posited by social constructivists.

SOCIAL CONSTRUCTIVIST THEORY

Social constructivists consider meaning to be socially created by "the joint intentional actions of minded creatures" (Harré, 1984, p. 8). This philosophical orientation is inherent in the approach to children's psychological development proposed by the Russian psychologist Vygotsky. He claimed that "every function in the child's cultural development appears twice: first, on the social level, and later, on the individual level; first, *between* people (interpsychological), and then *inside* the child (intrapsychological)" (1978, p. 57). Applications of Vygotsky's theory have often focused on the role of adult guidance in fostering various aspects of a child's development, although he clearly acknowledged the realm of the child's internal cognitive restructurings as well.

According to Vygotskian theory, children learn all psychological functioning in social interaction with a more competent, experienced member of their culture. Initially, the adult (or more competent child) provides a great deal of support to ensure the child's successful participation at whatever level he or she is capable of. Over time, the adult gradually relinquishes control of the interaction to the child, who can eventually perform the task independently. Vygotsky refers to this shift as movement from other-regulation to self-regulation or, as mentioned earlier, interpsychological to intrapsychological functioning (Vygotsky, 1978). This process of moving from other-regulation to self-regulation allows for eventual independent problem solving by the child. Bruner refers to this kind of adult support as *scaffolding*. The notion of a "zone of proximal development" is also central to Vygotsky's theory. "It is the distance between the actual developmental level as determined by independent problem solving and the level of potential development as determined through problem solving under adult guidance or in collaboration with more capable peers" (Vygotsky, 1978, p. 86).

In the language development literature, Bruner (e.g., 1966, 1983) has used the term *scaffolding* to refer to the process of adult-guided learning. Adults scaffold the child's language learning of a task by (1) providing simpler talk, sometimes called *motherese;* and by (2) capitalizing on familiar, routine, highly constrained events, which Bruner called *formats*. Formats contain a sequential structure, clearly marked roles and scripts for the accompanying communication. Bruner and his colleagues (e.g., Ninio & Bruner, 1978; Ratner & Bruner, 1978) have focused much research on game formats such as peekaboo, build-and-bash, and object exchange. Others (e.g., Snow & Goldfield, 1981, 1983) have studied book-reading formats.

In responding to errors, Vygotskian theory would remind us to consider the extent to which the child has internalized the skill. That is, the adult's response would differ depending on how much self-regulation the child was currently capable of in executing that skill. Because Vygotskian theory is one that we incorporate into our own theoretical framework for conducting language intervention, we will discuss more specifically how the clinician might respond at different points in the learning process later in this chapter.

SOCIAL LEARNING THEORY

Social learning theory (Bandura, 1977) incorporates some aspects of operant learning theory (such as stimulus, response, and reinforcement), but it also differs in some important ways. First, in social learning theory, learning can and most often does take place through observation rather than overt production of behavior. Furthermore, the child's attention to the modeled event is essential if learning is to occur. In addition to external reinforcement, reinforcement can also be vicarious, as when a child observes another person being rewarded for a behavior, or it can be provided directly by the child (self-reinforcement).

According to this theory, language behavior is learned via a process of abstract modeling, wherein the child abstracts the common attributes of many modeled utterances to "formulate rules for generating behavior with similar structural characteristics" (Bandura, 1977, p. 41). Social learning theory, like operant learning theory, provides no direction in the way of specifying goals for language intervention, because any behavior that can be observed is an appropriate target. The impact of both these theories has been on *how* to teach and not on *what* to teach.

Fey (1986, p. 13) discussed the specific influence of social learning theory on language intervention. He outlined five steps the clinician would take to "motivate the child to attend closely to the target linguistic behavior":

1. Selecting a model with whom the child closely identifies, such as a parent or a peer;
2. Having the model produce numerous examples of target behavior (e.g., subject-verb-object constructions to describe pictures with varying content);
3. Reinforcing the model for correct productions;
4. After the presentation of several uninterrupted models, encouraging the child to "talk just like the model"; and
5. Reinforcing the child for correct productions of the target.

Although Fey's treatment did not directly address how to respond to errors, we can reasonably assume that social learning theory would advocate simply providing the correct model when the child produced the wrong response. In addition, the clinician might use vicarious nonreinforcement by not reinforcing a model who produced the same error.

Our Theoretical Perspective: A Marriage of Representational and Social Constructivist Theories

In discussing how we might explain children's literacy development, Olson (1984) asks, "Do we look into the mental activities of children, an essentially piagetian undertaking, or do we look into the tutorial practices of parents, an essentially durkheimian, vygotskian, or brunerian undertaking?" (p. 185). He goes on to say, "We may note, however, that these two systems are not fully commensurate. They involve different levels of description—the psychological and the social" (p. 185).

It is possible to go a step beyond Olson's important insight that both psychological and social contributions to development are important. One might consider the possibility that these positions (i.e., the social and the psychological) represent different emphases at different points along a developmental continuum. The model shown in Figure 4–2 suggests that social constructivist notions are most explanatory for the initial stages of learning. The behaviors or skills a child is learning are embedded in meaningful activities. Initially, the adult must take major responsibility for the activity's unfolding. Adult input and direct scaffolding are necessary until the child has formed a comprehensive mental representation of the event or activity. Beyond that point, the child can begin the process of internal cognitive reorganizations as his or her mental representations go through the phases outlined by Karmiloff-Smith (1986).

Social transmission, it is suggested, is critical to early stages of learning whereas internal cognitive reorganization is emphasized later. This conceptualization is

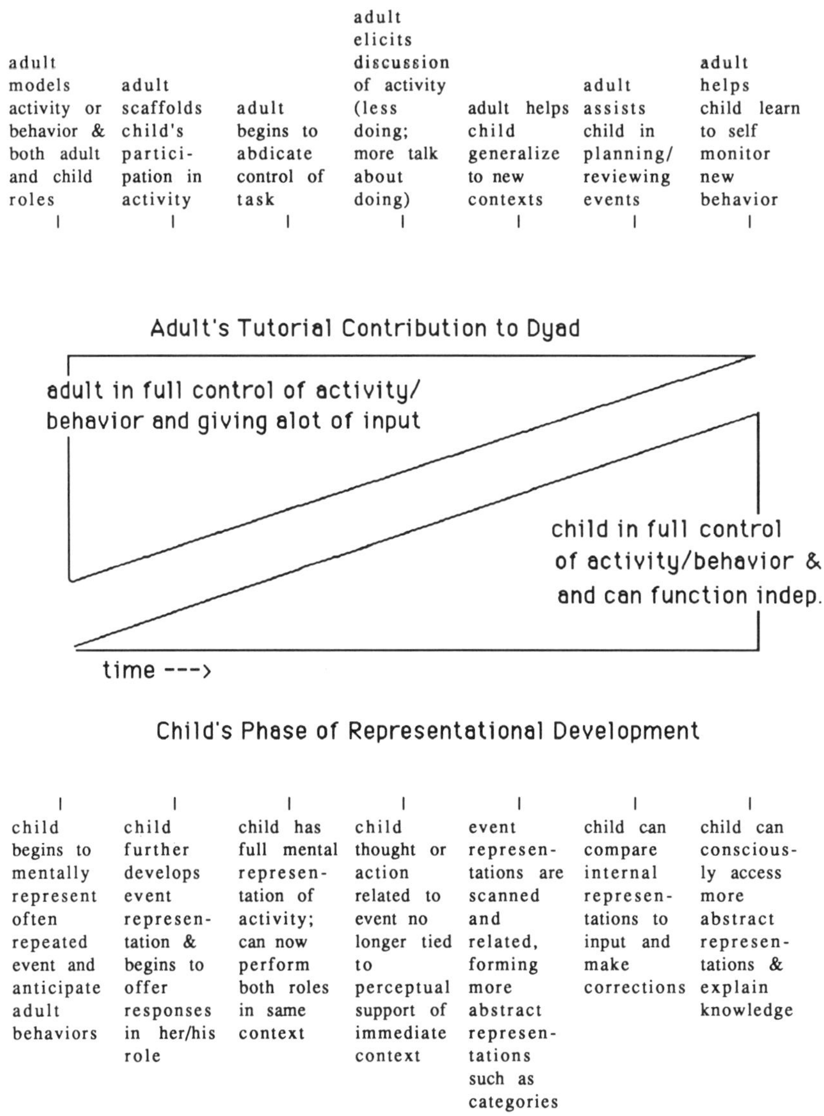

Figure 4–2. Model combining Vygotsky's social constructivism with Karmiloff-Smith's phases of representational development (from van Kleeck, 1994, p. 65).

not entirely new. Vygotsky (1978), as well as both Nelson (1986) and Karmiloff-Smith (1986), imply a progression from socially to cognitively constructed mental representation. The model in Figure 4–2 integrates the social constructivist and cognitivist perspectives far more explicitly.

The general framework suggested by this theoretical integration of the constructivist and cognitivist views allows for consideration of when and to what extent adult intervention is possible in fostering language development. The adult cannot conduct the actual cognitive reorganizations, or the "covert metacognitive processes," as Karmiloff-Smith called them, for the child. However, being aware that any content must hypothetically go through such reorganization would caution adults first to provide the input needed for these covert (what Karmiloff-Smith called metacognitive) processes to work on in the context of a meaningful activity. Then adults must allow the time for mental reorganization to take place covertly before using the language in the earlier input in a more decontextualized context.

The process of passing on a skill or of moving from other-regulation to independent action or self-regulation is presented in Figure 4–2. The role of the adult in the earliest stage of learning involves setting up a positive relationship and enticing the child into attending to the task. At this point, the adult familiarizes the child with the nature of the overall task rather than expecting specific responses. The overall task, like Bruner's formats or Nelson's event structures, is constructed to allow multiple opportunities for the child to produce one or more targeted areas of behavior. The clinician chooses a daily routine or begins to establish a routine activity into which the language goals for the child can be embedded in a pragmatically meaningful manner.

In the second stage, we assume that the child has gained enough familiarity with the event structure of the selected activity that "cognitive space" (i.e., mental energy) is freed to allow the child to begin to participate more actively. The adult's goal then is to increase the child's willingness to participate, to take the risk of trying the new behavior, and to build the child's confidence. "In effect, the child is permitted to do as much as he can spontaneously do; whatever he cannot do is filled in or 'held up' by the mother's scaffolding activity" (Bruner, 1985, p. 85). In practice, this means that the adult responds to the child's less-than-mastery-level response by filling in the response gaps.

In the third stage of learning, the child is so familiar with the event structure of the activity that he or she can initiate segments of the activity and successfully reverse roles with the adult (e.g., the child may begin asking the adult "What's that?" during the book-reading routine). The adult then begins to abdicate naturally some of the responsibility for presenting and structuring the task to the child. In addition, the adult begins to negotiate mutually who will take what roles in the completion of component segments of the activity. The child continues to practice the target behaviors embedded in the activity until they become stabilized and more automatic.

In the final four stages of learning presented in Figure 4–2, the child's complete mental representation undergoes covert reorganization until finally he or she is able to access consciously the knowledge that has been gained. The adult role moves from fostering discussion, to introducing variations of the original activity, to helping with planning and reviewing, and finally to helping the child self-monitor his or her own behavior.

The way in which errors would be responded to at each of these stages of learning will be discussed in the next section.

Responding to Children's Errors

Once our theoretical assumptions about how children learn language are made explicit, the implications for how errors should be responded to become clearer. Some of the key elements of the learning situation include the following:

1. A positive and supportive relationship between the adult and the child;
2. A willingness and skill on the adult's part to guide and fill in for the child as learning occurs while simultaneously giving the child as much control as he or she is capable of handling;
3. Skill at minimizing risk for the child until he or she has achieved some level of competence and confidence in task performance; and
4. A gradual internalization by the child of the adult's thinking out loud about a specific task.

A set of general operating principles for dealing with errors also emerges directly from the theory:

- Principle 1: One's response to an error will depend on the nature of the error, so the clinician must assess why the error occurred.
- Principle 2: One's response to an error will vary depending on the stage the child has reached in the learning process.
- Principle 3: One's response to an error must fit within the perceived role of the participants in the task's event structure.
- Principle 4: In responding to errors, one must have the teaching goal clearly in mind and respond in ways that will facilitate the primary goal.
- Principle 5: Apply these principles when responding to children's correct responses as well as to their errors.

Principle 1

Most teachers realize that a failure to locate the source of a child's error will seriously jeopardize the efficacy of any corrective action taken in response to the error (Meyer, 1985). However, like most other behavior, errors do not stem from a single source. What we have chosen to call skill errors stem from a deficiency in the targeted skill domain. The child makes a mistake because he or she simply does not know how to perform the skill in question. However, deficient skill is only one possible reason for a child's error response. Rather than assume that a lack of knowledge or skill underlies an error, the clinician must also consider other possibilities. We will discuss several types of errors, including (1) skill errors, (2) situationally induced errors, (3) emotionally induced errors, (4) positive errors (those that actually indicate learning or creativity), and (5) errors created by states of the child. In addition, we must consider that multiple sources of error may be operating simultaneously. This is particularly true in the initial stages of learning when newly learned material is still fragile, not automatized, and subject to the effects of any source of stress on the child's system.

Once the nature of the error has been identified, the appropriate response becomes much clearer. The following detailed discussion of several types of errors and their implications for response selection will help illustrate the importance of the first principle.

SKILL ERRORS

The analysis systems we use for identifying types of errors due to skill deficiency will vary with the domain of behavior we are examining—grammar, phonology, pragmatics, math, spelling, etc. Systems also vary in whether they address errors per se or simply categorize behaviors. A variety of category systems has been developed for analyzing language behaviors, and many of those systems utilize a normal developmental model to classify child language behaviors without calling them errors. Bloom and Lahey's (1978) phase levels for categorizing semantic/syntactic relations, Lee's (1974) Developmental Sentence Scoring system for classifying grammatical elements, and Miller's (1981) procedure for assigning sentences to structural stages all fall within this group. When using these systems, errors tend to be viewed as behaviors inappropriate for the child's level of functioning or as unclassifiable behaviors.

Other analysis systems look at particular errors made by children at different stages of development. They simultaneously identify errors by comparing behavior to an adult standard and consider those errors within a normal developmental perspective. Hodson and Paden's (1983) phonological process analysis, Piaget's analysis of sensorimotor and operational thinking as adapted by Uzgiris and Hunt (1975), and Goodman and Burke's (1970) procedure for analyzing reading miscues fall into this group. Finally, classification systems have been developed within a deficiency orientation (primarily by researchers and teachers working with abnormal populations), which analyzes children's errors as evidence for particular skill deficiencies. Feuerstein's (1978, 1980) categories of reasoning deficiencies in adolescents and Lucas's (1980) description of semantic and pragmatic errors in language-disordered children both fall into this group.

Regardless of the system used to analyze skill errors, the collection and analysis of a sample or corpus of errors can provide us with a valuable tool for understanding the child's skill in various domains. It gives us a window into the child's mind. By locating where the breakdown occurs, it becomes possible to identify ways to repair the breakdown. The adult's response to a skill error should assist the child in mastering the skill being targeted. Our model of learning suggests that this is accomplished by the adult's scaffolding the task for the child so he or she can succeed. Specifically, the clinician might ensure the child's subsequent success by selecting from the following clinically viable options:

1. Asking the child for a simpler, more well-established response (making the child's successful participation in the activity more likely);
2. Assisting the child with the task;
3. Breaking the task into smaller steps the clinician knows the child can handle;
4. Shifting to an easier task;
5. Shifting roles and performing the difficult role for the child; or
6. Providing cues and prompts to elicit the target behavior.

Our model requires that the scaffolding be done unobtrusively so that the child perceives the task to be one he or she is capable of performing successfully. In addition, alternating these reactions to errors removes the constant pressure to produce a specific behavior that is typical of much language intervention. Unobtrusive and varied responses should result in a child who is a more self-confident, actively participating learner.

SITUATIONALLY INDUCED ERRORS

There are a number of ways in which the situation the child is placed in can cause errors for a child who might otherwise be able to demonstrate the skill in question. The child may not understand the task, the task may be too complex or presented in an unfamiliar manner, or the child's expectancies may be violated.

Not Understanding the Task. Young children's inability to monitor their own comprehension of a task and consequently seek clarification where they do not understand is well documented (Markman, 1981). Unfortunately, young normal children often learn to indicate (both verbally and nonverbally) that they understand even when they do not. Disordered children are even less likely than normal children to signal when they do not understand (Dollaghan, 1987). This tendency not to signal misunderstanding makes it incumbent on the adult either to verify that the child does indeed understand the task (and not accept the child's verbal or nonverbal assurances as adequate evidence) or to consider lack of understanding as a possible reason for the child's error. Errors due to not understanding the task should be responded to in ways that clarify the task for the child. This may be strategically accomplished by the clinician through

1. Modeling the child's role in the task (with an adult, peer, or puppet serving as a model);
2. Simplifying or repeating the verbal instructions about the task; or
3. Providing visual props to highlight the difficult task elements (e.g., sentence strips of what to say or special hats to signal roles).

Task Too Complex. The effects of task complexity have been shown time and again to affect the child's ability to demonstrate mastery of a particular skill. For example, researchers have often claimed that children are unable to segment sentences into words prior to the early elementary school years (Holden & MacGinitie, 1972; Huttenlocher, 1964; Karpova, 1966). However, the tasks employed in these studies may have been too complex, requiring the child to both repeat an utterance and simultaneously count the words in that utterance. Fox and Routh (1975) designed a simpler method of testing word segmentation abilities by asking the child to say just a little bit of the sentence until the child no longer responded or until all the words had been isolated. With this technique, 5-year-olds achieved near-ceiling scores. These findings suggest that the complexity of the task should always be examined as a potential source of difficulty. Errors may reflect lack of skill with the task rather than lack of underlying knowledge.

Our response to errors caused by task complexity should directly simplify the task to a level appropriate for the child's level of physical, cognitive, linguistic, and metalinguistic sophistication. This usually involves rethinking and redesigning the task.

Task Unfamiliar. Task familiarity is closely related to task complexity. Children may err in the use of a particular skill or structure because they are being asked to demonstrate a language behavior in a context they are not familiar with. For example, whereas Cromer (1971) found that 3- and 4-year-old children were unable to relate events in temporal sequence, Nelson (1986) found that they rarely make temporal sequencing errors as they relate events. Cromer's task required children to order pictures in the correct sequence to depict events young children rarely encounter in day-to-day activities. Nelson examined the language of children as they described familiar events—simply telling about salient activities is a much more familiar task for children. Thus Cromer's sequence errors reflected more a lack of task familiarity than a deficiency in understanding temporal sequence. Nelson and her colleagues (1986) have clearly demonstrated that children's linguistic performance can be greatly enhanced when the task requires that the child describe events that are familiar.

In responding to errors due to lack of task familiarity, the clinician has at least two options to select from:

1. Shifting to a more familiar task; or
2. Repeating the task several times to help the child become familiar with it before expecting extensive participation or production of correct target behaviors.

For example, one child we worked with would never participate in a new task until he had seen it demonstrated on at least three different occasions. This child would not have learned new tasks if we had given up after the first or second demonstration.

Expectancies Violated. A third and related type of situationally induced error is the error caused by violation of the child's expectations. Expectations may be pragmatic, cognitive, or cultural in nature. For example, Donaldson (1978) showed how children's pragmatic expectation that "if they are asked a question twice, they must have answered incorrectly the first time" is partly responsible for their early failure on conservation tasks in which the experimenter makes a transformation and then repeats the same exact question (e.g., "Does this one have the same as this one, or does one of them have more?"). In a similar vein, children's comprehension strategies (Chapman, 1978) often reflect their dependence on contextual expectations in the early stages of language learning. For example, children will often use a probable event strategy when responding to constructions such as passives and temporal adverbials (e.g., "The mother was fed by the baby" and "The boy went swimming after he dried off with a towel"). In turn, they demonstrate understanding of these constructions when probable events are not violated.

The clinician's response to expectancy violation errors might be based on the following response options:

1. Changing the task so that expectancy violations do not occur;
2. Highlighting the trick in the task for the child; or
3. Not responding and allowing the child more time to develop the language skills needed to perform under conditions of expectancy violation.

EMOTIONALLY INDUCED ERRORS

The child's errors may be triggered by a variety of emotional factors, including learned helplessness, a fear of failure, and a power struggle with the clinician. Many language-disordered children have a predominant pattern of offering no response or saying "I don't know" whenever a reply is expected. Although the occasional "I don't know" response may legitimately reflect the child's lack of appropriate skill, if this pattern predominates, it is more likely a reflection of an emotionally induced reaction.

Learned Helplessness. The child demonstrating learned helplessness is conveying a message that "I can do this but I don't want to, because I gain more by your believing I am not able to." It frequently results from the child being placed continuously in the position of the passive responder or recipient of our clinical teaching. Effective responses to errors linked to learned helplessness include

1. Opting for benign neglect by waiting for the child to solve the problem before helping him or her out of an error situation;
2. Putting the child in the role of initiator and controller as frequently as possible;
3. Helping the child save face by avoiding any evaluative or judgmental comments about the child's error;
4. Showing appreciation for the effort the child put into the task; and
5. Expressing encouragement (not praise or coaxing) to help the child appreciate that he or she is doing things not previously done.

Fear of Failure. The message being conveyed by the child afraid of failure is that "Although I have this behavior in my repertoire, I do not believe that it is something I am successful at; therefore, I avoid using it." Bandura (1982) has underscored the importance of the self-perception of efficacy in all human action. Many language-disordered children recognize the distance between the quality of their performance and that of other children. They have encountered many situations in which they could not be successful in the verbal realm. Rather than experience further failure, they avoid difficult situations, even when the expected behavior is within their capability. The child experiencing fear of failure needs many opportunities for success to boost confidence and the sense of efficacy. Confidence during therapy may be built by scaffolding and by providing the support required to perform successfully. A practice of beginning language tasks with a series of successes before attempting difficult material can help desensitize the child to fearful situations. Appropriate behavior in response to errors due to fear of failure includes

1. Avoiding drawing attention to errors;
2. Providing the kinds of support discussed for skill errors; and
3. Shifting to highly motivating tasks that help the child forget himself or herself and his or her fear of failure.

Power Struggle Response. The child who is engaged in the equivalent of a power struggle with the clinician may purposefully offer no response or a wrong response to gain control of the therapy situation. For the child who is rarely given opportunities to control situations, this provides one type of control. The child who is prone to power struggle errors needs opportunities to exercise control in socially acceptable and constructive ways. When intervention is viewed as a process of gradually turning responsibility and control for tasks over to the child, power struggles are usually avoided. The clinician should read power struggle responses as a signal that the therapy relationship needs to be rethought and possibly renegotiated. It is critical that the clinician effectively refuse to participate in power struggles. Thus specific power struggle errors should not be acknowledged. Rather, the clinician should attend to the relationship message the child is intending to send—possibly by giving the child opportunities to have control in constructive ways, such as giving the child choices.

POSITIVE ERRORS

Determining what constitutes an error is critically dependent on how the clinician defines success. If the adult standard is used to define the correct response, then many normal deviations from that standard may be perceived as errors. On the other hand, if a normal developmental sequence is used as a standard or if the child is compared to himself or herself, a variety of positive errors may be identified. These represent improvements relative to the child's system even though it still differs from the adult standard. A frequently encountered type of positive error is an error that represents rule learning. The overgeneralization of the past tense *-ed* to irregular verbs (e.g., *ated*) is one example. Although an error by adult standards, this sort of production may represent a step forward in the mastery of grammar (even if the child previously produced the more acceptable form *ate*). We say that the rote form has been replaced by a rule-governed form. The error resides in the temporary overapplication of the rule prior to figuring out its exceptions.

Another frequently encountered positive error is one that indicates progress toward mastery or a more acceptable approach to a problem. One child who previously ignored all questions not understood suddenly began responding incorrectly to questions he did not understand. Although he persisted in making numerous errors, they represented notable progress in that he was no longer abdicating the conversational responsibility of responding. Another type of positive error is the creative error, wherein the child may create words such as *ballkite* to refer to a frisbee (van Kleeck & Bryant, 1984) to fill in a lexical gap. Responding to positive errors of the sort reflecting the struggle to come to grips with linguistics conventions usually involves (1) recognizing the child's progress and giving no corrective response; or (2) commenting on the child's new rule learning, progress, or creativity (to encourage hypothesis testing and risk taking) while also unobtrusively demonstrating the conventional rule or vocabulary entry the child is seeking.

ERRORS DUE TO TEMPORARY OR PERMANENT STATES OF THE CHILD

Often the child's state or condition or the clinician's disregard of that condition leads to errors even though the child has the capability to respond correctly. The child may err because of fatigue, illness, or a traumatic event that has drained or put additional stress on the system—and thus prohibits responding at higher levels within the zone of proximal development. Long-standing internal states of the child, such as attention deficits, may also interfere with task performance. Habituated response patterns, such as those linked to impulsivity or trial-and-error responding, may also mask the child's knowledge. Additionally, the task may ignore the child's sensory or physical limitations (e.g., a child with limited motor skill may be asked to demonstrate comprehension of *skip* by skipping).

Once the clinician recognizes the nature of the child's error, response options might include

1. Helping the child to control for habituated response patterns (e.g., exploring all choices before answering);
2. Simplifying the task to allow for success and delaying an increase in task difficulty until the child is reasonably prepared;
3. Helping the child to focus attention on the task (e.g., by asking "What did I ask you to do?"); or
4. Devising more appropriate tasks.

An example may clarify how our determination of the nature of the child's error affects the way in which the adult chooses to respond. Assume that the clinician's goal is for the child to understand *where* questions. To the question "Where is the playdoh?" the child answers, "I want playdoh." Consider the following possible reasons for this error and the implications each reason has for responding:

Assumed Source of Error	*Implication for Responding*
Skill error: The child does not understand *where* questions and so responds to the word *playdoh*.	Perform the role for the child: "It's lost. Where is it? Let's look for it. Playdoh, where are you? Are you lost?"
Situationally induced error (expectancy violation): The typical routine when the child enters the room is for him or her to request a toy for play. This time the clinician changes the routine and asks the child where the playdoh is.	Accept the child's request for playdoh. Create a new or different routine for teaching *where* questions.
Emotionally induced error (power struggle): The clinician is holding the playdoh under his or her chair while asking the child to tell its location. The child resists the clinician's quizzing by requesting the playdoh.	Create a context in which the *where* question is pragmatically appropriate (if the clinician obviously knows where it is, there is no genuine need to ask other than to quiz the child).
Positive error: The child typically responds to questions by pointing to an object or using one- to two-word utterances. This was one of the child's first three-word utterances.	Recognize the child's progress and respond to the child's request immediately.
Error due to state of child (inattention): The child was not watching or listening to the clinician and only heard the word *playdoh*.	Get the child's attention first, and then repeat the question.

In summary, once the nature of the child's error has been determined, the adult response should be closely matched to the underlying cause of that error relative to the child's communicative intent. Duchan (1986) described this matching effort as the ultimate fine-tuning of adult responses to child errors. The adult figures out where the child's error likely comes from and then negotiates with the child so the child understands the adult's position and, in turn, the child's position becomes more meaningful.

Principle 2

The adult's response to an error will vary depending on the child's stage in the learning process shown in Figure 4–2. In the first stage, when the adult's goals are to entice the child into a new learning situation and to teach the child a task's event structure, the primary purpose of the adult response to an error must be to increase the likelihood of child participation. The adult response should increase the child's willingness to take risks in learning, the child's willingness to try a new behavior, and the child's confidence in himself or herself as being capable of participating in the communicative exchange. When clinicians forget to make this a primary goal of the early stages of new task or skill learning, they face the consequences of slower learning at best or refusal to participate at worst. Careful attention to the goals of the first stage will help prevent emotionally induced errors at later stages. In fact, whenever emotionally induced errors occur, the clinician should back up and respond as though the child is in the earliest stage of learning. The appropriate responses to errors occurring at the first stage of learning a new task or event structure include

1. Modeling both the adult and the child roles;
2. Giving the child a simpler role to perform; or
3. Assisting the child in his or her role performance.

At the second stage the child is assumed to have learned enough of the event structure so that teaching can focus on the particular skill being targeted. Adult responses to child errors should both sustain the child's motivation to continue and facilitate his or her learning of the target skill. The responses that were described as appropriate for skill errors for Principle 1 can be used at this stage.

In the third stage, the clinician's goals are to shift control of the task to the child. It is at this stage that the skill becomes stabilized and the child learns to perform all of the roles in the event structure. When a child errs at this stage, the adult's response should assist the child to perform successfully and flexibly. Helpful responses include

1. Providing prompts or cues to help the child perform either role; and
2. Giving the child choices of which role to take.

In the next stage, discussions about the event are fostered without the support of the actual ongoing activity. If the child experiences difficulty, some nonlinguistic support may be reintroduced to scaffold the discussion. In the final stages, the adult helps the child generalize the target skills to other contexts, plan tasks, and monitor his or her own errors. The clinician does this by mediating or thinking out loud for the child, by helping the child think of other situations in which the skill can be used, and by helping the child learn ways to adjust to errors in future situations. Clinicians can often achieve error monitoring by helping the child see the value of errors. The focus shifts from correct responding to identifying errors. The child is rewarded for learning to spot his or her own errors, and then ways to handle them are discussed. Dollaghan and Kasten's (1986) comprehension monitoring program is a good example of how error monitoring at this final stage can be taught to school-age children. Hohmann, Banet, and Weikart (1979) provide a good explanation of how to develop "planfulness" in preschoolers, and Feuerstein's (1980) instrumental enrichment program describes ways to teach all of the stages 4, 5, 6, and 7 goals to adolescents. Some appropriate responses to children's errors in the final stage of learning a particular skill include

1. Discussing the nature of the error and ways to identify and deal with similar errors in the future;
2. Shifting the task to one of searching for errors or intentionally making and correcting errors; and
3. Thinking of other situations in which similar errors could occur.

It is important to remember that the stages of learning apply to any age child and any skill area. Clinicians too often quit teaching a young child a skill before the final stage is reached and then do not understand why the child has failed to generalize the target skill. Another important thing to remember is that individual children progress through these stages of learning at different rates depending on the skill being taught, the characteristics of a specific child, and how adaptable the clinician is to error responses. One child might learn a relatively simple skill through the final stage within a single teaching session, whereas another child might require months to reach the same level of mastery.

Principle 3

Each task or activity the clinician sets up has its own event structure. That structure includes the episodes within the event, the roles the participants can play, and the language that is appropriate for each role. The clinician's response to an error must fit within the role the clinician is playing in the event. If either participant's language does not match the expectations for the roles played, the pragmatics of the situation are violated and interaction breaks down. For example, in playing store, the roles might include a shopper and a clerk. Both participants have expectations of what clerks and shoppers say and do. If the child omits a grammatical marker (e.g., "Do you have some apple?") while requesting to purchase an item and the clinician responds by having the child repeat the request correctly (e.g., "Say *apples*"), the clinician has shifted from the clerk role to a teacher role. The event structure then has been changed substantially. The creative clinician will find ways to simplify tasks and scaffold events for the child that leave the event structure intact and thus preserve the credibility of the situation, prevent disruption of the interaction, and maintain the child's trust.

Principle 4

Careful specification of the treatment target is essential so that critical errors can be dealt with and noncritical errors can be ignored. Without a clear awareness of the goal, clinicians are prone to distract themselves and children by attending to irrelevant errors. The following poem was written by an 8-year-old first learning to write poetry:

My *snowfack*
My snowflace is wight
My snowflace is dright.
No snowflace is alice.

The goal of the lesson was to use rhyme in the context of creating a poem. This child achieved this goal despite the misspelling of *snowflake, white, bright,* and *alike.* Drawing the child's attention to the noncritical errors in the poem would most likely serve to discourage future creative efforts. The noncritical errors can serve a useful diagnostic function for the clinician, however. From them we learn that this child has mastered the silent *e* rule and has learned to capitalize the first word in a sentence. He has also learned that *ight* signifies the *ite* sound. However, he is confused about when *c* sounds like *s* and when *c* sounds like *k,* is inconsistent with punctuation, and still reverses the letters *b* and *d.* Not allowing this diagnostic information to interfere with the clinician's response to the child's performance requires a clear specification of the treatment goal.

Principle 5

This final principle is simply a caveat to highlight the intimacy of the relationship between responding to errors and the essence of all teaching. The guidelines clinicians utilize for treating correct responses closely resemble the principles that guide our responses to errors:

1. Clinicians analyze correct responses to determine the nature of the child's performance (e.g., chance versus rule learning).
2. Clinicians' responses vary with the child's stage of learning. (How quickly one moves the child to higher levels within the zone of proximal development depends on the child's current stage in the task-learning process.)
3. Clinicians' treatments of correct responses fit within the perceived roles of the task and the event structure. (When clinicians forget this principle—for example, by praising good talking during conversational exchanges—the communicative interaction is disrupted.)
4. Clinicians avoid attention to irrelevant correct responses because they can distract the child and the clinician as seriously as can attention to irrelevant errors.

There are, of course, additional considerations one needs to include in developing a plan for dealing with correct responses. Several roles adults play in facilitating learning when a child is proceeding successfully are described by Lucariello and her colleagues (1986). These roles and responses are included here as extensions of those just listed because they fit within our model of how learning occurs.

5. Clinicians extend the child's response behavior by widening the range of appropriate situations, the variety of communicative functions, or the language form the behavior is used for.
6. Clinicians act as a "communicative ratchet" (Bruner's term, 1978) by helping the child continue using the target construction and preventing backsliding, thus creating a firm base for the next learning step.
7. Clinicians act as catalysts to help the child find opportunities to use, apply, and draw on the new behavior.

Conclusion

In this chapter, we have argued that how clinicians choose to deal with children's error responses is determined by the explicit and implicit assumptions they hold about how language learning occurs. Because clinicians' responses to errors directly reflect those theoretical assumptions held, it is critical that individual clinicians spend time clarifying their theoretical assumptions about language learning. We have outlined our assumptions about the language-learning process and have explored the implications of these assumptions for our strategic responding to errors.

We believe strongly that further consideration of the role of errors in language intervention is warranted. Each clinician must incorporate strategies for dealing with errors in those plans developed for each treatment goal. Clinicians must clarify the various types of errors that may occur and identify techniques to be used for responding to each error type. Careful attention should also be paid to procedures for dealing with correct responses and moving the child to higher levels of language functioning. Of no less importance, any decisions clinicians make about how to respond to errors should be checked for compatibility with theoretical assumptions about how children learn language.

We suggest that individual clinicians work back through our proposed treatment of errors and apply, where appropriate, various aspects of Principles 1 through 5 to at least one challenging case in their current clinical loads. We believe that a functional appreciation of what Principles 1 through 5 might bring to the clinical enterprise can only be extracted out of dedicated efforts to use those treatment measures discussed in our own day-to-day clinical contexts. For many of us already engaged in the consistent collection and updating of language samples, we might soon begin to see that error sampling and analysis represent a natural and critical extension of language sampling and analysis—with little additional work required.

References

Bandura, A. (1977). *Social language theory*. Englewood Cliffs, NJ: Prentice Hall.

Bandura, A. (1982). Self-efficacy mechanism in human agency. *American Psychologist, 37*, 122–147.

Blank, M. (1973). *Teaching learning in the pre-school*. Columbus, OH: Charles Merrill.

Bloom, L. (1970). *Language development: Form and function in emerging grammars*. Cambridge, MA: Harvard University Press.

Bloom, L. (1973). *One word at a time: The use of single-word utterances before syntax*. The Hague: Mouton.

Bloom, L., & Lahey, M. (1978). *Language development and language disorders*. New York: Wiley.

Brown, R. (1973). *A first language: The early stages.* Cambridge, MA: Harvard University Press.

Bruner, J. (1966). On cognitive growth. In J. Bruner, R. Olver, & P. Greenfield (Eds.), *Studies in cognitive growth* (pp. 1–29). New York: Wiley.

Bruner, J. (1978). The role of dialogue in language acquisition. In A. Sinclair, R. Jarvella, & W. Levelt (Eds.), *The child's conception of language* (pp. 241–256). New York: Springer-Verlag.

Bruner, J. (1983). *Child's talk: Learning to use language.* New York: W. W. Norton.

Bruner, J. (1985). Vygotsky: A historical and conceptual perspective. In J. Wertsch (Ed.), *Culture, communication, and cognition: Vygotskian perspectives* (pp. 21–34). Cambridge, MA: Cambridge University Press.

Chapman, R. (1978). Comprehension strategies in children. In J. Kavanagh & W. Strange (Eds.), *Speech and language in the laboratory, school, and clinic* (pp. 308–327). Cambridge, MA: MIT Press.

Chomsky, N. (1957). *Syntactic structures.* The Hague: Mouton.

Chomsky, N. (1965). *Aspects of a theory of syntax.* Cambridge, MA: The MIT Press.

Chomsky, N. (1981). *Lectures on government and binding.* Dordrecht, Netherlands: Foris.

Cromer, R. (1971). The development of the ability to decenter in time. *British Journal of Psychology, 62,* 353–365.

Dollaghan, C. (1987). Comprehension monitoring in normal and language-impaired children. *Topics in Language Disorders, 7*(2), 45–60.

Dollaghan, C., & Kasten, N. (1986). A comprehension monitoring program for language-impaired children. *Journal of Speech and Hearing Disorders, 51,* 264–271.

Donaldson, M. (1978). *Children's minds.* New York: W. W. Norton.

Duchan, J. (1986). Language intervention through sensemaking and fine tuning. In R. Schiefelbusch (Ed.), *Language competence: Assessment and intervention* (pp. 187–212). San Diego, CA: College-Hill Press.

Duckworth, E. (1979). Either we're too early and they can't learn it or we're too late and they know it already: The dilemma of "applying Piaget." *Harvard Educational Review, 49,* 297–312.

Elman, J. (1993). Learning and development in neural networks: The importance of starting small. *Cognition, 48,* 71–99.

Feuerstein, R. (1978). *The dynamic assessment of retarded performers: The learning potential assessment device, theory, instruments and techniques.* Baltimore: University Park Press.

Feuerstein, R. (1980). *Instrumental enrichment: An intervention program for cognitive modifiability.* Baltimore: University Park Press.

Fey, M. (1986). *Language intervention with young children.* San Diego: College-Hill Press.

Fox, B., & Routh, D. (1975). Analyzing spoken language into words, syllables, and phonemes: A developmental study. *Journal of Psycholinguistic Research, 4,* 331–342.

Gerber, A. (1993). *Language-related learning disabilities: Their nature and treatment.* Baltimore: Paul Brookes Publishing Co.

Goodman, Y., & Burke, C. (1970). *Reading miscue inventory.* New York: Macmillan.

Harré, R. (1984). *Personal being.* Cambridge, MA: Harvard University Press.

Hodson, B., & Paden, E. (1983). *Targeting intelligible speech.* San Diego, CA: College-Hill Press.

Hohmann, M., Banet, B., & Weikart, D. (1979). *Young children in action.* Ypsilanti, MI: The High/Scope Press.

Holden, M., & Macginitie, W. (1972). Children's conceptions of word boundaries in speech and print. *Journal of Educational Psychology, 63,* 551–557.

Huttenlocher, J. (1964). Children's language: Word-phrase relationship. *Science, 143,* 264–265.

Kaplan, R., & Bresnan, J. (1982). Lexical–functional grammar: A formal system for grammatical representation. In J. Bresnan (Ed.), *The mental representation of grammatical relations.* Cambridge, MA: MIT Press.

Karmiloff-Smith, A. (1986). From metaprocesses to conscious access: Evidence from children's metalinguistic and repair data. *Cognition, 23,* 95–147.

Karpova, S. (1966). Abstract of Soviet studies of child language. In F. Smith & G. A. Miller (Eds.), *The genesis of language* (pp. 363–386). Cambridge, MA: MIT Press.

Keith, R. W. (Ed). (1981). *Central auditory and language disorders in children.* San Diego: College-Hill Press.

Lee, L. (1974). *Developmental sentence analysis.* Evanston, IL: Northwestern University Press.

Lucariello, J., Kyratzis, A., & Engel, S. (1986). Event representations, context, and language. In K. Nelson (Ed.), *Event knowledge: Structure and function in development* (pp. 137–159). Hillsdale, NJ: Erlbaum.

Lucas, E. (1980). *Semantic and pragmatic language disorders.* Rockville, MD: Aspen Systems.

MacDonald, J. (1978). *Environmental language inventory.* Columbus, OH: Charles E. Merrill.

Markman, E. (1981). Comprehension monitoring. In W. P. Dickson (Ed.), *Children's oral communication skills* (pp. 61–84). New York: Academic Press.

McLean, J. (1983). Historical perspectives on the content of child language programs. In J. Miller, D. Yoder, & R. Schiefelbusch (Eds.), *Contemporary issues in language intervention* (ASHA Reports 12, pp. 115–126). Rockville, MD: American Speech-Language-Hearing Association.

Meyer, L. (1985). *Strategies for correcting students wrong responses.* Technical report no. 354. Champaign, IL: Center for the Study of Reading, University of Illinois at Urbana–Champaign.

Miller, J. (1981). *Assessing language production in children: Experimental procedures.* Baltimore: University Park Press.

Nelson, K. (1986). *Event knowledge: Structure and function in development.* Hillsdale, NJ: Erlbaum.

Ninio, A., & Bruner, J. (1978). The achievements and antecedents of labeling. *Journal of Child Language, 5,* 1–15.

Olson, D. (1984). "See! Jumping!" Some oral antecedents of literacy. In H. Goelman, A. Oberg, & F. Smith (Eds.), *Awakening to literacy* (pp. 185–192). Portsmouth, NH: Heinemann.

Orton, S. T. (1937). *Reading, writing and speech problems in children.* New York: W. W. Norton.

Pinker, S. (1984). *Language learnability and language development.* Cambridge, MA: Harvard University Press.

Pinker, S. (1994). *The language instinct.* New York: William Morrow and Company.

Ratner, N., & Bruner, J. (1978). Games social exchange, and the acquisition of language. *Journal of Child Language, 5,* 391–402.

Reese, E. (1966). *The analysis of human operant behavior.* Dubuque, IA: William C. Brown.

Rumelhart, D. & McClelland, J. (1986). On learning the past tense of English verbs. In D. Rumelhart, J. McClelland, & the PDP Research Group (Eds.), *Parallel distributed processing: Explorations in the microstructure of cognition.* (Vol. 2, pp. 216–271). Cambridge, MA: Bradford Books.

Rumelhart, D. & McClelland, J. (1987). Learning the past tenses of English verbs: Implicit rules or parallel distributed processing? In B. Mac Whinney (Ed.), *Mechanisms of language acquisition* (pp. 195–248). Hillsdale, NJ: Erlbaum.

Schank, R., & Abelson, R. (1977). *Scripts, plans, goals, and understanding.* Hillsdale, NJ: Erlbaum.

Schlesinger, I. M. (1982). *Steps to language: Toward a theory of native language acquisition.* Hillsdale, NJ: Erlbaum.

Sigel, J., & Hooper, F. (Eds.). (1968). *Logical thinking in children: Research based on Piaget's theory.* New York: Holt, Rinehart & Winston.

Skinner, B. F. (1957). *Verbal behavior.* New York: Appleton-Century-Crofts.

Smedslund, J. (1964). Concrete reasoning: A study of intellectual development. *Monographs of the Society for Research in Child Development, 29,* 3–29.

Snow, C., & Goldfield, B. (1981). Building stories: The emergence of information structures from conversation. In D. Tannen (Ed.), *Analyzing discourse: Text and talk* (pp. 127–141). Georgetown University Round Table on Language and Linguistics, Georgetown University Press.

Snow, C., & Goldfield, B. (1983). Turn the page please: Situation-specific language acquisition. *Journal of Child Language, 10,* 551–569.

Strauss, A., & Lehtinen, L. (1947). *Psychopathology and education of the brain-injured child.* New York: Grune & Stratton.

Tallal, P., & Piercy, M. (1978). Defects of auditory perception in children with developmental aphasia. In M. Wyke (Ed.), *Developmental dysphasia* (pp. 63–84). New York: Academic Press.

Uzgiris, I., & Hunt, J. McV. (1975). *Assessment in infancy: Ordinal scales of psychological development.* Chicago: University of Illinois Press.

Van Kleeck, A. (1994). Metalinguistic development. In G. Wallach & K. Butler (Eds.), *Language learning disabilities in school-age children and adolescents* (pp. 53–98). New York: Merrill.

Van Kleeck, A., & Bryant, D. (1984, November). *Learning that language is arbitrary: Evidence from early lexical changes.* Paper presented at the Annual Convention of the American Speech-Language-Hearing Association, San Francisco.

Van Kleeck, A., & Richardson, A. (1986). What's in an error? Using children's wrong responses as language teaching opportunities. *National Student Speech-Language-Hearing Association Journal, 14*(1), 25–50.

Vygotsky, L. S. (1978). Mind in society: The development of higher psychological processes. In M. Cole, J. Scribner, V. John Steiner, & E. Souberman (Eds.), *Culture and thought: A psychological introduction* (compilation). Cambridge, MA: Harvard University Press.

Werner, H., & Strauss, A. (1941). Pathology of the figure-ground relationship in the child. *Journal of Abnormal Social Psychology, 36,* 236–248.

Westby, C., & Cutler, S. (in press). Language and ADHD: Understanding the bases and treatment of self-regulatory deficits. *Topics in Language Disorders.*

5

Linguistic and Cognitive Aspects of Specific Language Impairment

ALAN G. KAMHI, PH.D.

Introduction

An adequate discussion of linguistic and cognitive perspectives of childhood language disorders is beyond the scope of a single chapter. Such a discussion is manageable, however, if one restricts the focus to a select group of language-disordered children. Because I have spent most of my professional career studying and writing about children with a specific language impairment (SLI), I will restrict the focus of this chapter to these children. The existence of a "pure" or uncontaminated group of language-disordered children continues to intrigue theorists and clinical researchers. Children with SLI have significant difficulty acquiring language that cannot be attributed to sensory, emotional, intellectual, neurological, and social-motivational factors. Language disorders that can be directly attributed to one or more of these predisposing peripheral or central impairments are often considered to be the resulting symptoms of more pervasive disorders such as mental retardation, autism, hearing impairment, and frank neurological dysfunction.

Children with SLI acquire language more slowly than their peers and often continue to have difficulty with spoken and written language throughout the developmental period into adulthood. Research involving these children typically has focused on two basic questions: What is the nature of their linguistic deficits, and why should children with normal nonverbal intelligence, intact speech and hearing mechanisms, and supportive language learning environments have difficulty acquiring language?

In the last 5 years or so, there have been a number of attempts to summarize the literature addressing these questions (Bishop, 1992; Casby, 1987; Ellis Weismer, in press; Johnston, 1988; Kamhi, in press; Leonard, 1987). I will draw heavily on these reviews (particularly my own) in addressing these questions. The nature of SLI will be considered in the first part of the chapter. The majority of the chapter is devoted to the research that has attempted to explain SLI.

The Nature of SLI Children's Language Disorder

A central question underlying much of research on SLI children's language abilities is whether these children follow the same course of language development as normally developing children. A related question is whether SLI children's language systems are different from the language systems of normally developing children. Some researchers (e.g., Casby, 1987) refer to these questions as the language delay versus language deviance issue. To address these questions, investigators typically have compared a particular aspect of language functioning in SLI children and language-age–matched normally developing children. Comparable performance of the two groups is taken as evidence that SLI children are following a normal course of development. Such evidence is used to support the delayed-language view.

Johnston (1988) provided a comprehensive review of studies that examined SLI children's language abilities across a number a variety of domains. These domains included (1) syntax (Johnston & Kamhi, 1984; Morehead & Ingram, 1973), (2) grammatical morphology (Johnston & Kamhi, 1984: Johnston & Schery, 1976), (3) relational semantics (Johnston, Kamhi, & McDonald, 1981; Leonard, Steckol, & Schwartz, 1978), (4) lexical semantics (Leonard et al., 1982), (5) narrative discourse (Liles, 1985), and (6) conversational abilities (Brinton, Fujiki, Loeb, & Winkler, 1986; Gallagher & Darton, 1978; Leonard, 1986).

It is possible to review in detail all of the studies that have examined SLI children's language abilities as Johnston and others have done. I feel, however, that such a detailed review would not add anything new to this body of literature. Twenty years of research in this area has eliminated the methodological problems, such as the use of age- or mental age (MA) level matched comparison groups, that plagued earlier studies (e.g., Leonard, 1972; Menyuk, 1964). This research has been thorough in its use of different language assessment procedures and linguistic perspectives. For example, structural (syntactic-semantic) and functional (pragmatic-discourse) linguistic perspectives have been used to characterize SLI children language and communication abilities. Recent attempts to explain SLI children's language learning difficulties using current linguistic theories (e.g., parameter theory and lexical functional grammar) will be discussed in a later section.

Johnston's summary comments (1988) capture the essence of SLI children's language abilities:

> Although further work is needed in each of the areas investigated, there are now sufficient data to make an interim global conclusion. SLI children acquire major grammatical categories and syntactic ordering rules in the same order as normally developing children, albeit more slowly and at a later age. Grammatical morphology also follows the same sequence of development in SLI children, but the acquisition of these forms is markedly protracted. Semantic studies indicate that SLI children follow normal acquisition patterns in most lexical domains and are able to express a variety of relational meanings. Although narrative discourse abilities are clearly delayed, conversational abilities are basically intact. For the most part, SLI children are purposeful and responsive conversationalists, limited only by their relatively poor mastery of grammatical form. (p. 693)

This body of research provides unequivocal support for the delayed-language position. However, as Johnston (1988) notes, the aforementioned studies focused on one linguistic domain at a time. The deviant or disordered aspects of SLI children's language can be captured only by looking across language domains. For example, Johnston and Schery (1976) found that SLI children acquired grammatical morphemes in the same sequence as normally developing children. However, the protracted development of these forms meant that they were being acquired at later mean length of utterance (MLU) stages with more complex sentence structure. The association between syntactic and morphological development in SLI children thus is atypical.

Studies that have examined SLI children's language across domains have revealed a more disordered picture. Johnston and Kamhi (1984) conducted one of the first multidomain studies of SLI children's language. Subjects in the study were 5-year-old SLI children and younger normal-language children matched for MLU. The MLUs ranged from 4.2 to 5.5. Samples of spontaneous language were obtained from each child and evaluated for syntactic, morphological, semantic, and pragmatic knowledge. Although many of the sentence patterns produced by the two groups were similar and both groups showed comparable use of ellipsis, pronominalization, and imperatives, two notable group differences were found. The SLI children made significantly more grammatical morpheme errors and produced significantly fewer sentences with embedded propositions than their language-matched peers.

These findings indicate that SLI children acquire some aspects of language more readily than others. Different acquisition rates lead to asynchronies in development. For example, normally developing children acquire most grammatical morphemes during early stages of language development when sentences are relatively short. In contrast, SLI children will still be acquiring grammatical morphemes at later stages of language development when sentences are much more complex. Thus, even though SLI children acquire various language forms in the normal developmental order, they will produce some utterances that are unlike any of those produced by normally developing children. These different utterances represent the deviant aspect of SLI children's language.

At the beginning of this section, two questions were posed: (1) Do SLI children follow the same course of language development as normally developing children? and (2) Are SLI children's language systems different from the language systems of normally developing children? The literature suggests that the answer to both of these questions is yes.

Explaining SLI

Information processing accounts of cognitive function provide a framework for evaluating the possible causes of language-learning difficulties. Information processing models distinguish between mental representations of information (knowledge states) and the cognitive operations or processes that operate on the mental representations (Bishop, 1992). Consider, for example, the levels of representation and cognitive processes involved in language comprehension and production. With language comprehension, a spoken utterance is initially represented and stored in terms of its auditory or acoustic features. This acoustic representation is converted first into a phonetic representation and then a phonological (phoneme-based) representation. Familiar sequences of sounds are then matched to existing lexical representations stored in long-term memory. Higher level syntactic, semantic, pragmatic knowledge will be combined with knowledge of the meaning of the lexical items to provide the meaning or gist of the utterance (Bishop, 1992; Clark & Clark, 1977).

In contrast to language comprehension, the process of language production starts with the idea or message to be communicated and ends with the actual production (articulation) of the utterance. In between, one must generate a grammatical structure that accurately conveys the idea units (propositions) in the message, determine which words best express the particular propositions, access the phonological sequences associated with each word, and transmit this information to the articulators (Bishop, 1992; Bock, 1982).

An information processing model of language leads naturally to the question of where in the system SLI children break down. For example, are language comprehension difficulties caused by deficient lower level perceptual processes required for encoding linguistic information or higher level conceptual processes involved in constructing meaning? In the same vein, do SLI children produce grammatically simplified utterances because the underlying representation of grammatical structure is deficient or does the problem lie somewhere in the chain of processes involved in converting ideas into speech (Bishop, 1992)? In the following sections, these questions are addressed.

Perceptual Aspects of SLI

Normal language learning and conceptual processing require the effective functioning of a variety of perceptual mechanisms. These mechanisms include not only those that are bound to specific senses, such as vision and audition, but also attentional and memory processes that span the senses. A large body of literature has examined auditory processing abilities in children with SLI. This literature has been reviewed in a number of recent articles and chapters (Bishop, 1992; Casby, 1987; Ellis Weismer, in press; Johnston, 1988; Kamhi, 1993; Leonard, 1987). In brief, the work of Tallal and her colleagues over the past 20 years has shown that compared to age-matched peers, SLI children have difficulty processing information that is represented at a rapid rate. The poor performance of the SLI children on visual tasks suggests that the processing deficit is not specific to auditory input (see Elliot, Hammer, & Scholl, 1989, for an alternative view). The "neural timing deficit," as Tallal (1988, p. 164) referred to it, accurately predicts (1) performance on the nonverbal and verbal serial memory tasks, (2) the pattern and type of speech production and perception errors, (3) the degree of receptive language impairment, and (4) classification of SLI.

Despite the overwhelming evidence suggesting that a timing deficit provides a sufficient explanation for SLI, many remain unconvinced that such a deficit can account for the extent and nature of the SLI (Johnston, 1988; Leonard, 1987; Rees, 1981; Tomblin, 1984). The problem lies not in the data or methodology of the studies but in the bottom-up information-processing or specific-abilities models that provide the theoretical backdrop for most of the studies that evaluate perceptual abilities in SLI children. An assumption that underlies these studies is that there are fundamental perceptual and memory processes that are necessary for, but independent of, language learning (Tomblin, 1984). That is, language usage and learning depends on a set of component auditory perceptual abilities that are arranged in some serial, bottom-up fashion. The perception and processing of sensory information is viewed as passive and unaffected by situational factors, knowledge states, and previous experiences of the individual.

The counterclaim is that perceptual and memory processes do not function independently of knowledge states and other conceptual processes. Several contemporary theories of language processing emphasize the complex interactions that occur among structural mechanisms, cognitive processes, knowledge states, and environmental forces (see Bohannon & Warren-Leubecker, 1988). Piagetian (constructionist) notions that emphasize the active role the child plays in organizing and making sense of the world have become an important component of current accounts of language learning (e.g., Ingram, 1989). There is a rich experimental literature that demonstrates the effects of higher level language abilities on speech perception (Pisoni, 1978; Rees, 1981). In the same vein, short-term memory abilities are known to increase when the individual is able to relate the information to previous knowledge or experiences (e.g., Bransford & Franks, 1971; Chi, 1976; Huttenlocker & Burke, 1976).

There are at least two other significant problems with perceptual explanations of SLI. The first stems from the fact that normally developing children younger than 4;6 cannot perform the Tallal tasks (Tallal, 1976). Four-and-a-half-year-old normal language (NL) children, however, have sophisticated language abilities. By this age, they produce many complex sentence structures and use a wide range of grammatical morphemes (Ingram, 1989; Miller, 1981). Given that young NL children have sophisticated language abilities and cannot perform the processing tasks, one must seriously question what successful performance on Tallal's tasks means for language learning. The perceptual processing abilities of young NL children are apparently sufficient to comprehend and produce sophisticated language forms.

The second problem follows directly. In Leonard's (1987) words, "we cannot lose sight of the fact that, although normal children improve across time in their performance on auditory processing tasks, there has been no serious attempt to explain language development on the basis of developing auditory skills" (p. 22). Leonard's point is that to draw causal connections between perceptual deficiencies and language impairment, there must be some theorizing about how particular developments in auditory skills affect the acquisition of specific linguistic forms and structures. Such theorizing would make specific predictions, for example, about what kinds of perceptual developments precede the acquisition of first words, word combinations, canonical word ordering (SVO), complex sentences, and so forth.

Interestingly, as discussed earlier in this section, since Leonard wrote these words, he has made a serious attempt to relate SLI children's problems with grammatical morphemes to the acoustic characteristics (i.e., low phonetic substance) of these forms. Using Pinker's (1984) learnability theory, Leonard (1989) suggests that SLI children have difficulty acquiring particular grammatical morphemes because these forms have low phonetic substance. Pinker has suggested that grammatical elements that are low in phonetic substance are more difficult to acquire or build into the child's grammar. Low phonetic substance is defined as "monosyllabic consonant segments and unstressed syllables, characterized by shorter duration than adjacent morphemes, and, often, lower fundamental frequency and amplitude" (Leonard, 1989, p. 186). Leonard (p. 187) goes on to show how SLI children have difficulty with grammatical morphemes that meet the low phonetic substance definition and do not have difficulty with grammatical morphemes that do not meet the definition.

Although Leonard (1989, p. 193) finds the low phonetic substance hypothesis attractive, he also recognizes some of its major limitations. One problem is that the definition of low phonetic substance is simplistic because once a certain absolute duration is reached, relative duration may not be important. Another problem is that although low phonetic substance provides a reasonable explanation for protracted acquisition of grammatical morphemes, it does not account for the continued difficulty older SLI children have with these forms. Older SLI children have heard these forms millions of times and can recognize them in reading but still use them inconsistently in their speech (Tomblin, 1990).

In light of these concerns, the most optimistic interpretation of the data is that perceptual limitations account for protracted acquisition of selected language forms, such as grammatical morphemes and structures that depend on grammatical morphemes for their meaning. However, the perceptual deficit does not account for continued problems with these language forms (e.g., through childhood and adolescence), nor does it account for other language problems. The most pessimistic interpretation of the data is to argue that the findings merely establish a strong correlation between rapid perceptual processing and SLI. The relationship between these perceptual skills and language is not unidirectional (i.e., from perception to language) but interactive and reciprocal. That is, a perceptual deficit may cause certain language problems, but the language problems may, in turn, cause certain perceptual problems (Rees, 1981). If the perceptual deficit is secondary to the language impairment, one is left to explain what causes the primary language impairment. Three possibilities will be considered: (1) short-term memory limitations, (2) a specific deficit in the language-learning mechanism (module), and (3) a nonspecific deficit in some aspect of general cognitive functioning.

Short-Term Memory Limitations in SLI Children

Short-term memory refers to a capacity for keeping a limited amount of information in a special active state. Information can be used (stored, transformed, manipulated) only when it is in this active state (Anderson, 1985). Short-term memory deficiencies have been well documented in SLI children (see recent reviews by Ellis-Weismer, in press, and Johnston, 1988). Specific deficits have been found in the use of rehearsal strategies (Kirchner & Klatzky, 1985), scanning speed (Sininger, Klatzky, & Kirchner, 1989), and storage and retrieval processes (Kail & Leonard, 1986).

Gathercole and Baddeley (1989, 1990) have argued that short-term memory plays a significant role in language learning. A central principle of what is referred to as "the working memory approach" is that the temporary storage of information plays an important role in a range of complex cognitive tasks such as learning, comprehension, and reasoning. The model proposed (Baddeley & Hitch, 1974) consists of three main components: an attentional system known as the central executive and two subsidiary slave systems, one for construction of visual images and the other for the temporary storage of phonological information. Phonological representations are assumed to fade within 2 seconds unless kept active in some way (e.g., by rehearsal). The basic claim is that phonological memory limitations affect language learning. Vocabulary and reading are particularly affected by such limitations.

To support these claims, Gathercole and Baddeley (1989) studied the relationship between phonological memory as measured by a nonword repetition task and receptive vocabulary in 4- and 5-year-old normally developing children. They found that children's scores on the nonword repetition task were highly correlated with receptive vocabulary scores, even after nonverbal IQ and age had been taken into account. In a subsequent study, Gathercole and Baddeley (1990) found that 7- and 8-year-old SLI children had more difficulty repeating single nonwords and recalling word lists than younger children of comparable verbal abilities.

These findings are consistent with findings of two studies that my colleagues and I conducted several years ago with SLI children (Kamhi & Catts, 1986; Kamhi, Catts, Mauer, Apel, & Gentry, 1988). In these studies, young school-age SLI children consistently performed more poorly than peers matched for nonverbal IQ in repeating single-syllable nonsense words, three-item strings of single-syllable nonsense words, and multisyllabic nonsense words. These studies also contained a group of reading disabled (RD) children. The SLI children performed comparably to the RD group on the single-word repetition tasks but significantly worse than the RD group on the multisyllabic word repetition task.

Gathercole and Baddeley (1990) suggest that the difficulty SLI children have repeating nonwords is caused by limitations in phonological storage rather than impairments in auditory perceptual processes, articulation rate, phonological encoding processes, and rehearsal processes. They suggest three possible explanations for the phonological memory storage deficit. The first possibility is that the SLI children's acoustic and segmental analysis of phonological events may be "noisy," such that the resulting phonological representations are less discriminable when they are retrieved. The second possibility is that SLI children have less phonological storage capacity, leading to either fewer items being stored or to the same number being stored less richly and redundantly. The third possibility is that the phonological trace decays faster in SLI children than in normally developing children. Gathercole and Baddeley (1990) propose that phonological storage limitations are directly responsible for the vocabulary and comprehension deficits exhibited by SLI children.

Although Gathercole and Baddeley (1990) make a nice case for a phonological storage deficit in SLI children, many researchers do not accept their conclusion that a phonological storage deficit is the primary deficit. Other researchers are not so willing to accept Gathercole and Baddeley's claim that perceptual, encoding, articulatory, and rehearsal limitations have little influence on SLI children's word repetition and language-learning abilities. For example, Tallal clearly would disagree with Gathercole and Baddeley's (1990, p. 356) claim that SLI children's neural timing deficit is caused by limitations in memory storage.

I am not so willing to dismiss the importance of speech production and encoding processes. Kamhi and Catts (1986) suggested that encoding processes, rather than storage or retrieval processes, were particularly taxed by the multisyllabic nonsense word repetition task. We argued that storage and retrieval processes were minimal because immediate repetitions were required. Gathercole and Baddeley (1990, p. 336) point out that phonological representations fade within about 2 seconds. If Gathercole and Baddeley's proposal is correct, SLI children's word repetition performance should deteriorate as the interval between the word presentation and repetition increases. This could be tested easily. I have no argument with Gathercole and Baddeley's claim that SLI children have the ability to encode (i.e., represent accurately) phonological information. But this ability is taxed by tasks that require accurate representations of discrete, sequential phonological information, such as repeating multisyllabic nonwords. Moreover, the ability to encode phonological information does not mean that the phonological representations generated by SLI children have the same quality as those generated by normally developing children. For example, SLI children as well as children with reading disabilities have considerable difficulty with phonological awareness tasks that involve accessing discrete phonological information (Kamhi & Catts, 1986; Kamhi et al., 1988; Wagner & Torgesen, 1987). Poor-quality representations may be "fuzzy" or lack the discrete, sequential phonemic information one must have to perform well on phonological awareness tasks.

Speech production factors may also play some role in SLI children's poorer word repetition performance. Although Gathercole and Baddeley (1990) rule out peripheral articulatory processes, SLI children may have higher level speech programming or planning difficulties that make them less proficient than normally developing children in planning complex phonological sequences (Kamhi et al., 1988). Without recognition data, it is not possible to rule out the influence of such higher level programming processes. Kamhi, Catts, and Mauer (1990) examined novel-word acquisition in reading-disabled children. The paradigm included both production and recognition conditions. In most cases, production difficulties were associated with recognition failures, suggesting that speech production and planning factors contributed minimally to novel-word learning in reading-disabled children. SLI children, however, may not show the same pattern of performance as reading-disabled children.

Conceptual Aspects of SLI

By definition, SLI children exhibit a significant discrepancy between language abilities and nonverbal performance scales of intelligence, such as the Leiter International Performance Scales (Arthur 1952), the Wechsler Intelligence Scale for Children (WISC), and the Columbia Mental Maturity Scale (Burgemeister, Blum, & Lorge, 1972). SLI children's age-level performance on nonverbal intelligence tests initially discouraged investigations of cognitive abilities in areas not tapped by the intelligence tests. The assumption was that SLI children would show age-level performance in other cognitive measures, as long as the verbal component was minimized. The rediscovery of Piaget in the early 1970s led Morehead and Ingram (1973) to speculate that SLI children might have a more general deficit in symbolic representational abilities. This speculation was based on Piaget's view of language development. According to Piaget (e.g., 1952), language emerges as part of a more general symbolic function—a function defined as the ability to represent symbolically an external event or object in its absence.

This view led researchers to look for parallels in the development of language and other symbolic behaviors in normal language (NL) and SLI children. Early studies with NL children (e.g., Bates, Benigni, Bretherton, Camaioni, & Volterra, 1979; Nicolich, 1977) found relationships between developments in language and nonlinguistic symbolic behaviors, such as means-ends relations and symbolic play. Subsequent studies involving SLI children (e.g., Johnston & Ellis Weismer, 1983; Kamhi, 1981; Kamhi, Catts, Koenig, & Lewis, 1984; Roth & Clark, 1987; Savich, 1984; Terrell, Schwartz, Prelock, & Messick, 1984) found that SLI children did not perform as well as NL peers on measures of symbolic play and mental imagery. The SLI children generally performed better than language-age–matched peers on these measures. Other aspects of cognitive functioning with presumed links to language learning also have been examined in SLI children, including hierarchical planning (Cromer, 1983; Ward & Mills, in press; Kamhi, 1991), hypothesis testing (Ellis Weismer, in press; Kamhi, Nelson, Lee, & Gholson, 1985; Nelson, Kamhi, & Apel, 1987), and analogical reasoning (Kamhi, Gentry, Mauer, & Gholson, 1990; Nippold, Erskine, & Freed, 1988).

The same articles that reviewed the perceptually oriented literature have also provided comprehensive reviews of the cognitively oriented literature (Bishop, 1992; Ellis Weismer, in press; Johnston, 1988; Kamhi, in press). A brief summary (adapted from Johnston, 1991b, pp. 76–77) of the major findings from this body of literature is that SLI children

1. Exhibit deficient symbolic, adaptive, and integrative play skills (Roth & Clark, 1987; Terrell et al., 1984)
2. Have difficulty generating, maintaining, and interpreting mental images (Johnston & Ellis Weismer, 1983; Savich, 1984)
3. Can solve mental imagery problems when multiple resources (i.e., alternative strategies) can be used to solve the problems (Kamhi, 1981)
4. Show deficiencies in hierarchical planning (Cromer, 1983; Ward et al., 1991)
5. Have difficulty solving certain complex reasoning problems (Ellis Weismer, in press; Kamhi et al., 1990; Nelson et al., 1987)
6. Use age-appropriate reasoning processes (e.g., hypothesis testing and analogical) to solve problems (Kamhi et al., 1984; Kamhi et al., 1990)
7. Are adept at solving problems that require visual, spatial pattern analyses (e.g., Johnston, 1982; Kamhi, Minor, & Mauer, 1990).

Twenty years of research have shown that SLI children demonstrate particular cognitive strengths and weaknesses. SLI children do not have domain-specific cognitive deficiencies, nor do they have deficits in fundamental reasoning processes. Domain-specific deficits are inconsistent with findings that SLI children can play symbolically, generate mental images, exhibit hierarchical planning, generate hypotheses, and reason analogically. However, compared to their normal language peers, SLI children show deficiencies in each of these areas.

These deficiencies are thought to be caused by some type of cognitive processing inefficiency. Although many researchers have recognized SLI children's cognitive processing inefficiencies (e.g., Ellis Weismer, 1993; Johnston, 1988, 1991; Kamhi, 1993), identifying the specific cognitive limitation that underlies the processing inefficiency has proved to be elusive. This is because any number of factors can cause processing problems, such as basic capacity limitations, perceptual or short-term memory deficits, reduced processing speech, attentional speech motivational factors, metacognitive deficiencies, the language impairment itself, and so forth.

Several authors, most notably Johnston (1988, 1991), have suggested that capacity limitations underlie SLI children's cognitive weaknesses. Current limited capacity models of information processing view changes in capacity as a result of the automaticity of various skills or cognitive operations. The automatization of a particular behavior (e.g., speech production, word recognition) frees up cognitive resources, thereby increasing processing capacity. Johnston (1991b) has suggested that SLI children might be slower that NL peers in automatizing certain skills or operations. Even if this is the case, one is still left to explain why SLI children take longer to automatize (i.e., learn) the particular skill, operation, or knowledge in question. As Ellis Weismer (1993) notes, capacity limitations can be caused by a range of factors. Indeed, each of the factors that might cause inefficient cognitive processing also could cause capacity limitations. This last point raises some questions about causal-based research that attempts to uncover/discover the cause of SLI. Before considering these questions, however, I consider briefly the possibility that SLI children suffer from a specific deficiency in the language-learning module.

Linguistic Aspects of SLI

It may seem curious to consider linguistic interpretations of SLI impairment after reviewing a body of literature that shows that learning and processing problems are not restricted to the linguistic domain. Given, however, that grammatical difficulties are a hallmark of SLI and that some form of grammatical (syntactic) modularity is still a dominant linguistic theory, one must consider the possibility that SLI children have some specific deficiency in the language-learning module. The existence of cognitive deficiencies per se does not rule out the existence of a language-learning module and coexisting deficiencies in such a module.

HIERARCHICAL STRUCTURE DEFICIT

Bishop (1992) provides an excellent review of the literature that addresses the possibility that SLI children have a specific deficiency in the language-learning module. The first possibility Bishop considers is that SLI children have a specific problem in appreciating underlying hierarchical structure. The hierarchical nature of language is well known. Consider the sentence *The leaves on the trees are falling.* Without appreciating the hierarchical structure of this sentence, one would conclude that the trees rather than the leaves are falling. Cromer (1983) used a construction task adapted from Greenfield and Schneider (1977) to determine whether SLI children had a general hierarchical planning deficit.

Unfortunately, there were a number of methodological flaws in the study (see Bishop, 1992; Kamhi, in press). For example, the subjects ranged in age from 9 to 16 years and ranged from having convulsive disorders to being profoundly deaf. The most serious problem with the research is that no attempt was made to link performance on the construction task to language performance.

Bishop (1982, cited in Bishop, 1992) devised a set of items to examine whether SLI children had difficulty processing sentences with hierarchical structure. Test items were a series of sentences and four pictorial response choices. All sentences had the structure "The X in/on/under/behind the Y is Z," where X and Y were nouns and Z was a color term (e.g., "The circle on the star is black."). If a child was using a sequential processing strategy, he or she would choose the picture in which the star was black. Test items were presented in three modalities: spoken, written, and signed. Subjects consisted of nine children with severe receptive language problems. Bishop (1992) notes that performance was poor, but the errors were not random. Subjects tended to attach the adjective Z to the nearest noun, Y. Although these findings support Cromer's hypothesis, Bishop reports that profoundly deaf children showed the same pattern of performance with the same materials. She takes these findings as evidence against the view that SLI children have a primary impairment in the language acquisition (device) module. Bishop argues that SLI children's problems with hierarchical sentences are a "consequence of auditory processing deficits that force children to rely on the visual modality for language learning" (p. 27). She bases this conclusion on the assumption that no one would maintain that deaf children are born without a language acquisition device. Although no one would dispute this assumption, it is unclear how this assumption leads to the conclusion that an auditory processing problem underlies SLI children's problem with hierarchical sentences. Curiously, Bishop does not consider whether other linguistic-based explanations or cognitive ones (which she reviews in later sections of her chapter) can account for difficulties in understanding hierarchical sentences. Some of the alternative linguistic-based explanations are considered next.

DIFFICULTY ASSIGNING GRAMMATICAL FUNCTIONS AND SYNTACTIC-SEMANTIC MAPPING

Van der Lely and Harris (1990) raise the possibility that SLI children have difficulty assigning grammatical functions and integrating syntactic and lexical information. These authors performed two experiments in which they examined comprehension of reversible sentences in 5- to 7-year-old SLI children and normally developing children matched for chronological age (CA) and language age (LA). Children were asked to act out sentences such as *The boy pushes the girl* and *The girl is pushed by the boy.* The SLI children showed significantly poorer comprehension than both control groups. In a second experiment, the same sentences were presented using a picture-pointing task. A single-word vocabulary test was also given to rule out potential differences in word comprehension. The results of the second experiment were consistent with those from the first experiment.

In discussing the findings, Van der Lely and Harris (1990) noted that a particularly striking finding was that a significant proportion of SLI children had difficulty understanding transitive and dative sentences with canonical word order (i.e., simple active sentences). No differences were found between the SLI and LA children on the vocabulary test. Another interesting finding was that for the LA children there was a significant negative correlation between language age and proportion of word-order errors. As language age increased, normal children made fewer word-order errors. This was not the case, however, for SLI children, suggesting that increases in general language age were not related to increases in knowledge of the relationship between grammatical functions and thematic (semantic) roles.

Van der Lely and Harris (1990, p. 112) present a three-part model of sentence processing to explore the implications of their findings. The first process involves parsing or syntactic analysis of the sentence. Such parsing involves identifying and sequencing words, storing these words in short-term memory until the phrase structures are identified, and then assigning grammatical functions (e.g., subject, verb, object) to the words. Another process is required to identify the predicates of the sentence and access the argument structure for each predicate (e.g., the predicate *eat* has two inherent arguments, an agent and a patient/object). A third process is required to integrate the first two processes, thus enabling the appropriate arrangement of thematic roles in relation to grammatical functions.

Van der Lely and Harris (1990) interpret SLI children's frequent word-order errors as evidence of difficulty in assigning grammatical functions and integrating syntactic and lexical information. In both experiments, SLI children had particular difficulty assigning thematic (semantic) roles to syntactic structures. Van der Lely and Harris question whether deficient mapping abilities underlie the SLI children's sentence comprehension problems or whether the mapping problem is secondary to a more basic perceptual problem that affects low-phonetic-substance morphemes, as proposed by Leonard (1989). They argue that a perceptual problem cannot account for the difficulty some SLI children had understanding simple active sentences. Van der Lely and Harris conclude that the fundamental deficit in SLI children is grammatical rather than cognitive-semantic in nature because these children have difficulty figuring out thematic roles from syntactic information but do not have difficulty mapping cognitive or semantic representations to grammatical structure.

FEATURE BLINDNESS

Gopnik (1991, 1992) and Gopnik and Crago (1991) have suggested that the grammatical impairment in SLI is confined to grammatical morphology. They propose that SLI individuals demonstrate a pervasive difficulty in mastering syntactic-semantic features, which they term "feature blindness." Gopnik and Crago's claim is based on data from a large, multigenerational family in which a developmental language impairment recurs over three generations. Of the 30 family members studied, 16 have been diagnosed as SLI. Data from several different studies indicated that the affected family members exhibited morphophonemic errors across different measures of language in spontaneous speech, grammatical judgment tasks, sentence imitation, and writing. Moreover, these errors affected a wide range of features, including number, person, tense, aspect, and gender. These data led Gopnik (1992) to conclude that these individuals with SLI cannot construct general rules that govern morphological development. The deficit is in the underlying grammar rather than merely a performance problem. In recent work, Gopnik (1992, p. 33) attributes the morphophonemic deficiencies to a single gene that interferes with the ability to construct morphological rules in the grammar. Gopnik (1992) does note, however, that SLI individuals can learn appropriate surface forms and the semantic content of these forms by memorizing individual lexical items.

Bishop (1992) raises several questions about the logic of Gopnik's claims. For example, Bishop thinks that Gopnik's dismissal of a perceptual basis for morphological errors is premature (p. 32). Bishop also finds a number of differences in the data reported by Gopnik and those reported by Leonard and his colleagues (e.g., Leonard, Sabbadini, Volterra, & Leonard, 1988). Some of the discrepancies in the data may be a function of test procedures. For example, Gopnik's failure to find deficits in her subjects' comprehension of thematic roles may be due to the use of a comprehension test designed for aphasic adults. Bishop recognizes, however (and I agree), that some of Gopnik's findings reflect genuine differences between her subjects and other SLI individuals. Gopnik's subjects were members of a single extended family with a dominant pattern of genetic transmission of SLI. The severity of the language impairment was probably greater in Gopnik's subjects than in other studies with SLI individuals. The SLI individuals in Gopnik's study may represent a unique subgroup of individuals with SLI and, as such, conclusions about the nature of these individuals' language impairment may not be applicable to the general population of individuals with SLI.

PARAMETER-SETTING PROBLEMS

Parameter-setting theory attempts to account for the generality of the language-learning mechanism (Hyams, 1986). In this theory, it is assumed that certain components of the grammar can be marked or unmarked. The initial value is unmarked. This value or parameter is changed to the marked setting if the evidence from the language input is inconsistent with the initial unmarked setting. Loeb and Leonard (1988) tested the hypothesis that SLI children may be slow in setting the Null Subject parameter. All children start out with this parameter set to [+ uniform], indicating that the language permits sentences lacking an overt subject and that verb morphology is uniform. This setting is appropriate for languages such as Italian but not for English, because overt subjects are required and verb morphology is not uniform (e.g., some verb forms require inflectional endings and others do not [pushed, pushing, push]). Loeb and Leonard examined language samples from eight SLI children. They found no support for a parameter-setting deficit. In a subsequent study, Leonard (1989) also found no support for the theory.

Bishop (1992) notes that despite the inadequacy of parameter-setting theory to explain errors patterns in SLI children, the theory does suggest a different way to think about some of the counterintuitive cross-linguistic differences in Leonard's work. Rather than hindering language learning, a complex morphological system, if it is consistent, may facilitate acquisition. For example, Rom and Leonard (1990) found that Hebrew SLI children were more likely to produce present and past verb inflections and noun plural inflections than English SLI peers. The high frequency of the obligatory nature of morphological information in Hebrew apparently tunes in the child to morphology in general.

EVALUATION OF LINGUISTIC INTERPRETATIONS

Bishop (1992) finds the evidence in support of linguistic explanations of SLI "both logically inadequate to make the point and inconsistent from one study to another" (p. 37). Although she finds linguistic explanations undeniably plausible, she does not think that those advancing linguistic explanations have considered alternative hypotheses. She concludes her evaluation by noting that

> a minimal requirement would be to compare SLI children with younger normal children to demonstrate that language seen in SLI is deviant rather than merely delayed. It would then be necessary to show that SLI children differ also from children with language deficits arising from other causes (e.g. hearing impairment, mental retardation). (p. 37)

Like Bishop, I also find the linguistic claims plausible. I do not find her reasons for dismissing the claims convincing, however. Inconsistency between studies is easily accounted for by the different language tasks used and different linguistic claims evaluated. Alternative explanations for SLI were considered extensively by Gopnik and Leonard, with Gopnik rejecting nonlinguistic explanations and Leonard embracing a perceptual explanation. Van der Lely and Harris (1990), however, failed to consider alternative explanations for their findings.

I found Bishop's "minimal requirement" for the linguistic explanation lacking on two accounts. First, it is unclear how evidence showing language deviance and language differences relative to normal language age and mentally retarded peers would support the linguistic explanation. Language deviances or differences need not reflect deficiencies in the language-learning module. Second, as indicated in the first part of this chapter, a number of studies have documented language deviance in SLI children. Others (e.g., Kamhi & Johnston, 1982) have found language differences between SLI and retarded children. The best reason for rejecting linguistic explanations is the large body of literature indicating that SLI children's deficiencies are not restricted to language. The lack of specificity of the language impairments means that one must consider seriously the possibility that the same processing or capacity limitations that cause various cognitive and conceptual deficits in SLI children also cause these children's various language deficits.

The Pros and Cons of Causal-Based Research

Reading or writing a review of SLI children's perceptual and cognitive strengths and weaknesses (as I did recently; see Kamhi, 1993) is bound to leave one feeling somewhat unsatisfied. This is because no single factor (perceptual, cognitive, or linguistic) or obvious combination of factors can explain the extent and nature of SLI. Failure to find the primary causal factor(s) has led some researchers and clinicians to question the value of continued research and clinical efforts that address causal issues.

Leonard (1987) has made the most compelling arguments to date about the inadequacy of causal research. In the final section of his critical review of causal research, he noted that "accounts of specific language impairment fall short not only because they fail to identify the proper cause of this condition, but also because they assume that the condition is one for which a tangible cause must exist" (p. 30). Although some factors seem to have more explanatory adequacy than others, no factor by itself can explain the extent and nature of SLI children's language impairment. Most researchers or chapter authors end up with an unsatisfying conclusion that SLI is caused by a variety of factors.

Leonard (1987), in contrast, views the cause of SLI children's language limitations as "simply the product of the same types of variations in genetic and environmental factors that lead some children to be clumsy, others to be amusical, and still others to have little insight into their own feelings" (p. 31). Leonard's view draws on Gardner's (1983) theory of multiple intelligences, in which seven different kinds of intelligence are proposed. If the language delay is viewed as normal variation rather than a disorder or deficit, one effectively eliminates the need to search for a cause. In other words, there can be no cause for the disorder if there is no disorder. This view leads Leonard to the logical conclusion that research efforts in search of causal factors will not be high-yield enterprises and seem unjustified.

There is a certain appeal to Leonard's view: By embracing it, we prevent future researchers from expending large amounts of time and resources searching for underlying causes that do not exist. But there are several reasons not to view causally oriented research as fruitless. Johnston (1991a), for example, points out that the claim that most SLI children are normal is not the same as the claim that the condition has no cause. Normal variation in an ability does not mean that the cause of the variation is of no interest. Some researchers are presumably interested in the neurological correlates of exceptional musical ability. The same holds true for language variation. As Johnston notes, even if we agree with Leonard that the primary cause of SLI is variation in genetic and environmental factors, we can still wonder about the causes of these variations. Why do these children have difficulty learning to talk?

Aram (1991) proposes four reasons why it is important to understand why SLI children have difficulty learning language. First, there is the level of science to which we want our profession to aspire. Without explanatory power, she argues, ours is a dead-end science, with the risk that we might become a dead-end profession. Second, there is our clinical responsibility to parents of SLI children. Most parents want to know why their child has a language impairment. Aram asks, "How long can a profession continue to say 'We don't know' to the questions that prompt their consultation (pp. 85 & 86)?" Aram's third reason is that identification of causal factors has major implications for intervention programs. Finally, there is the issue of prevention. Aram argues that only through understanding *why* can we have an impact on preventing specific language impairments. If we act as if causation does not matter, is unknowable, or is simply the inevitable result of a normal distribution, we will be unable to prevent future generations of children from having specific language impairments.

Aram concludes by noting that we do know something about the causes of SLI. Johnston (1991b) makes a similar point in arguing that we should abandon "etiological" jargon because it has connotations of pathology and primary cause, and we should attempt to identify the mental processes and mechanisms that influence success in the language acquisition task.

There have been several other benefits of causally oriented research. For example, based on this body of research, one can reason, as Johnston (1991b) has done, that language learning requires (1) the ability to perceive and produce rapidly presented information; (2) the ability to generate, maintain, and interpret symbols; (3) the ability to organize information hierarchically; and (4) a variety of reasoning processes. Although these claims are by no means earth shattering, they do represent progress. The weakness of the work, according to Johnston, is not in the direction it takes but in its infancy. Johnston finds no fault with the general research strategy in which (1) we compare the performance of SLI and NL children on various linguistic and nonlinguistic tasks, and (2) we make inferences about the mental abilities that are causally linked to language learning based on patterns of performance.

All researchers seem to agree that the basic research strategy needs to be refined. Aram (1991) sees particular promise in using sophisticated neuroimaging techniques, such as magnetic resonance imaging (MRI) and positron emission tomography (PET), to determine whether there are subtle differences in brain morphology and/or activity in SLI children. Another promising avenue of research addresses the genetic bases of SLI (e.g., Lewis, Ekelman, & Aram, 1989; Tomblin, 1989).

Johnston (1991a) suggests three refinements in future research efforts. First, we need to explore more complex patterns of association. Most research, she notes, has primarily tried to link language learning to another single mental ability, such as the symbolic function or perception of rapidly presented events. But simple causation models, as Hubbell (1981) has pointed out, do not adequately capture the complex biologic and environmental interactions that underlie developments in language throughout the developmental period. Future studies need to examine the reciprocal causation effects that occur among maturing perceptual, cognitive, linguistic, and social abilities throughout the developmental period.

Second, we need to figure out how to formalize and operationalize promising mental constructs. For example, there should be other ways to measure hierarchical planning ability than using three-dimensional mobiles. Or, as Johnston notes, there is currently no experimental task to evaluate the construct of "extracting regularities," which has been suggested as a possible weakness in SLI children.

Johnston's third refinement is that we need to break down familiar constructs, such as language, into their component parts. Instead of looking for associations between generic notions such as language-learning ability and other mental functions, we need to look for associations between discrete language subskills and nonverbal competencies. Leonard's (1989) work, in which he suggested a perceptual explanation for SLI children's difficulty with grammatical morphemes, is an example of the kind of research needed.

One area of research that holds particular promise for better understanding language disorders focuses on the various processes involved in language comprehension and production. In the preface to Chapman's (1992) book on language processes, Chapman notes that process approaches to adult language use have long been the norm, whereas child language research has traditionally focused on modeling linguistic competence rather than use. In recent years, researchers have shifted their focus from describing SLI children's linguistic knowledge to showing how SLI children use language. This chapter provides information on the processes SLI children use to understand and produce language.

Conclusion

In this chapter, I have described the linguistic, perceptual, and cognitive abilities of children with SLI. In doing so, I have attempted to answer two basic questions about these children: What is the nature of their linguistic deficits, and why do these children have difficulty learning language? The answer to the first question is considerably more clear cut than the answer to the second question. SLI children's basic deficit is in the grammatical component of language, particularly grammatical morphology. With respect to the issue of language delay versus language deviance, the literature indicates that SLI children follow the same course of language development as normally developing children, but their language systems differ from the language systems of normally developing children. SLI children thus exhibit a delay in acquiring language, but their language systems at any one point in time are deviant because these systems are different from those of normally developing children.

The review of causal-oriented research revealed no clear consensus about why SLI children have difficulty learning language. For some, this lack of consensus is good reason to abandon causal-oriented research and direct efforts in more productive areas, such as devising better intervention programs. Others, however, feel strongly that abandoning causal-based research would be a serious mistake. Yet even the theorists who feel the strongest about continuing causal-based research recognize that refinements are needed in future research efforts. With such refinements, I am optimistic that during the next 20 years we will uncover the specific neurological correlates and cognitive processing limitations that underlie language-learning difficulties in SLI children.

Acknowledgments

Portions of this chapter have been adapted from a recent chapter I wrote, entitled "Children with Specific Language Impairment (Developmental Dysphasia): Perceptual and Cognitive Aspects," which will appear soon in *Linguistic Disorders and Pathologies: An International Handbook,* published by De Gruyter, New York. The book is edited by G. Blanken, J. Ditmann, H. Grimm, J. Marshall, and C. Wallesch.

References

Anderson, J. (1985). *Cognitive psychology and its implications,* 2nd ed. New York: Freeman.

Aram, D. (1991). Specific language impairment as a clinical category. *Language, Speech, and Hearing Services in Schools, 22,* 84–88.

Arthur, G. (1952). *The Arthur adaptation of the Leiter international scale.* Chicago: Stoelting.

Baddeley, A., & Hitch, G. (1974). Working memory. In G. Bower (Ed.), *The psychology of learning and motivation* (Vol. 8, pp. 47–90). New York: Academic Press.

Bates, E., Benigni, L., Bretherton, I., Camaioni, L., & Volterra, V. (1979). *The emergence of symbols.* New York: Academic Press.

Bishop, D. V. M. (1992). The underlying nature of specific language impairment. *Child Psychology and Psychiatry, 33,* 3–66.

Bock, J. (1982). Toward a cognitive psychology of syntax: Information processing contributions to sentence formulation. *Psychological Review, 89,* 1–47.

Bohannon, J., & Warren-Leubecker, A. (1993). Theoretical approaches to language acquisition. In J. Berko Gleason (Ed.), *The development of language* (3rd ed.). Columbus, OH: Merrill.

Bransford, J., & Franks, J. (1971). The abstraction of linguistic ideas. *Cognitive Psychology, 2,* 331–350.

Brinton, B., Fujiki, M., Loeb, D., & Winkler, E. (1986). Development of conversational repair strategies in response to requests for clarification. *Journal of Speech and Hearing Research, 29,* 75–81.

Burgemeister, B., Blum, L., & Lorge, I. (1972). *Columbia mental maturity scale,* 2nd ed. New York: Harcourt Brace Jovanovich.

Casby, M. W. (1987). Competing bases of language impairment in children. *National Student Speech Language Hearing Association Journal, 15,* 120–137.

Chapman, R. (1992). Preface. In R. Chapman (Ed.), *Processes in normal language acquisition and disorders* (ix–x). St. Louis: Mosby.

Chi, M. (1976). Short-term memory limitations in children: Capacity of processing deficits? *Memory and Cognition, 4,* 559–572.

Clark, H., & Clark, E. (1977). *Psychology and language.* New York: Harcourt Brace Jovanovich.

Cromer, R. (1983). Hierarchical planning disability in the drawings and constructions of a special group of severely aphasic children. *Brain and Cognition, 2,* 144–164.

Elliot, L., Hammer, M., & Scholl, M. (1989). Fine-grained auditory discrimination in normal children and children with language-learning problems. *Journal of Speech and Hearing Research, 32,* 112–119.

Ellis Weismer, S. (1991). Hypothesis testing abilities of language impaired children. *Journal of Speech and Hearing Research, 34,* 1329–1338.

Ellis Weismer, S. (1993). Perceptual and cognitive deficits in children with specific language impairment (developmental dysphasia): Implications for diagnosis and intervention. In H. Grimm, & H. Skowronek (Eds.), *Language acquisition problems and reading disorders: Aspects of diagnosis and intervention* (pp. 75–103). New York: de Gruyter.

Gallagher, T., & Darton, B. (1978). Conversational aspects of the speech of language disordered children: Revision behaviors. *Journal of Speech and Hearing Research, 21,* 118–135.

Gardner, H. (1983). *Frames of mind.* New York: Basic Books.

Gathercole, S., & Baddeley, A. (1989). Evaluation of the role of phonological STM in the development of vocabulary in children: A longitudinal study. *Journal of Memory and Language, 28,* 200–213.

Gathercole, S., & Baddeley, A. (1990). Phonological memory deficits in language disordered children: Is there a causal connection? *Journal of Memory and Language, 29,* 336–360.

Gopnik, M. & Crago, M. (1991). Familial aggregation of a developmental language disorder. *Cognition, 39,* 1–50.

Gopnik, M. (1991, June). *Theoretical implications of inherited dysphasia.* Paper presented at the Workshop Cross Linguistic and Cross Population Contributions to the Theory of Acquisition, Jerusalem.

Gopnik, M. (1992). *Linguistic properties of genetic language impairment.* Paper presented at AAAS Meeting.

Greenfield, P., & Schneider, L. (1977). Building a tree structure: The development of hierarchical complexity and interrupted strategies in children's construction activity. *Developmental Psychology, 13,* 200–313.

Hubbell, R. (1981). *Children's language disorders.* Englewood Cliffs, NJ: Prentice Hall.

Huttenlocker, J., & Burke, D. (1976). Why does memory span increase with age? *Cognitive Psychology, 8,* 1–32.

Hyams, N. (1986). *Language acquisition and the theory of parameters.* Dodrecht, Holland: D. Reidel.

Ingram, D. (1989). *First language acquisition: Method, description and explanation.* Cambridge, UK: Cambridge University Press.

Johnston, J., & Schery, T. (1976). The use of grammatical morphemes by children with communication disorders. In D. Morehead & A. Morehead (Eds.), *Normal and deficient child language* (pp. 239–259). Baltimore: University Park Press.

Johnston, J., Kamhi, A., & McDonald, J. (1981). Patterns of predicate use in language impaired children. *Proceedings of the Symposium on Research in Child Language Disorders, 2,* 17–28.

Johnston, J., & Ellis Weismer, S. (1983). Mental rotation abilities in language disordered children. *Journal of Speech and Hearing Research, 26,* 397–403.

Johnston, J., & Kamhi, A. (1984). Syntactic and semantic aspects of the utterances of language-impaired children: The same can be less. *Merrill-Palmer Quarterly, 30,* 65–85.

Johnston, J. (1988). Specific language disorders in the child. In N. Lass, L. McReynolds, J. Northern, & D. Yoder (Eds.), *Handbook of speech-language pathology and audiology* (pp. 685–715). Philadelphia: B. C. Decker, Inc.

Johnston, J. (1991a). The continued relevance of cause: A reply to Leonard's "Specific language impairment as a clinical category." *Language, Speech, and Hearing Services in Schools, 22,* 75–80.

Johnston, J. (1991b). Questions about cognition in children with specific language impairment. In J. Miller (Ed.), *Research on child language disorders: A decade of progress* (pp. 299–309). Austin, TX: Pro-Ed.

Kail, R., & Leonard, L. (1986). Word-finding abilities in language-impaired children. *ASHA Monographs, 25.*

Kamhi, A. (1981). Nonlinguistic symbolic and conceptual abilities of language impaired and normally developing children. *Journal of Speech and Hearing Research, 24,* 446–453.

Kamhi, A., & Johnston, J. (1982). Towards an understanding of retarded children's linguistic deficiencies. *Journal of Speech and Hearing Research, 25,* 435–445.

Kamhi, A., Catts, H., Koenig, L., & Lewis, B. (1984). Hypothesis-testing and nonlinguistic symbolic abilities in language-impaired children. *Journal of Speech and Hearing Disorders, 49,* 169–176.

Kamhi, A., Nelson, L., Lee, R., & Gholson, B. (1985). The ability of language disordered children to use and modify hypotheses in discrimination learning. *Applied Psycholinguistics, 6,* 435–451.

Kamhi, A., & Catts, H. (1986). Toward an understanding of developmental language and reading disorders. *Journal of Speech and Hearing Disorders, 51,* 337–347.

Kamhi, A., Catts, H., Mauer, D., Apel, K., & Gentry, B. (1988). Phonological and spatial processing abilities in language- and reading-impaired children. *Journal of Speech and Hearing Disorders, 53,* 316–327.

Kamhi, A., Gentry, B., Mauer, D., & Gholson, B. (1990). Analogical learning and transfer in language-impaired children. *Journal of Speech and Hearing Disorders, 55,* 140–148.

Kamhi, A., Minor, J., & Mauer, D. (1990). Content analysis and intratest performance profiles on the Columbia and the TONI. *Journal of Speech and Hearing Research, 33,* 375–379.

Kamhi, A., Catts, H., & Mauer, D. (1990). Explaining speech production deficits in poor readers. *Journal of Learning Disabilities, 23,* 632–636.

Kamhi, A. (in press). Specific language impairment: Perceptual and cognitive aspects. In G. Blanken, J. Ditmann, H. Grimm, J. Marshall, & C. Wallesch (Eds.), *Linguistic disorders and pathologies: An international handbook.* New York: De Gruyter.

Kirchner, D., & Klatzky, R. (1985). Verbal rehearsal and memory in language-disordered children. *Journal of Speech and Hearing Research, 28,* 556–565.

Leonard, L. (1972). What is deviant language? *Journal of Speech and Hearing Research, 37,* 427–446.

Leonard, L., Steckol, K., & Schwartz, R. (1978). Semantic relations and utterance lengths in child language. In F. Peng, & P. von Raffler Engel (Eds.), *Language acquisition and developmental kinesics* (pp. 93–105). Tokyo: University Tokyo.

Leonard, L., Schwartz, R., Chapman, K., Rowan, L., Prelock, P., Terrell, B., Weiss, A., & Messick, C. (1982). Early lexical acquisition in children with specific language impairment. *Journal of Speech and Hearing Research, 25,* 554–563.

Leonard, L. (1986). Conversational replies of children with specific language impairment. *Journal of Speech and Hearing Research, 29,* 114–119.

Leonard, L. (1987). Is specific language impairment a useful construct? In S. Rosenberg (Ed.), *Advances in applied psycholinguistics* (Vol. 1, pp. 1–39). New York: Cambridge University Press.

Leonard, L., Sabbadini, L., Volterra, V., & Leonard, J. (1988). Some influences on the grammar of English- and Italian-speaking children with specific language impairment. *Applied Psycholinguistics, 9,* 39–57.

Leonard, L. (1989). Language learnability and specific language impairment in children. *Applied Psycholinguistics, 10,* 179–202.

Lewis, B., Erelman, B., & Aram, D. (1989). A familial study of seven phonological disorders. *Journal of Speech and Hearing Research, 32,* 713–724.

Lieb, O., & Leonard, L. (1988). Specific language impairment and parameter theory. *Clinical Linguistics and Phonetics, 2,* 317–327.

Liles, B. (1985). Cohesion in the narratives of normal and language disordered children. *Journal of Speech and Hearing Research, 28,* 123–133.

Menyuk, P. (1964). Comparison of grammar of children with functionally deviant and normal speech. *Journal of Speech and Hearing Research, 7,* 109–121.

Miller, J. (1981). *Assessing language production in children.* Baltimore: University Park Press.

Morehead, D., & Ingram, D. (1973). The development of base syntax in normal and linguistically deviant children. *Journal of Speech and Hearing Research, 16,* 330–352.

Nelson, L., Kamhi, A., & Apel, K. (1987). Cognitive strengths and weaknesses in language impaired children: One more look. *Journal of Speech and Hearing Disorders, 52,* 36–43.

Nicolich, L. (1977). Beyond sensorimotor intelligence: Assessment of symbolic maturity through analysis of pretend play. *Merrill-Palmer Quarterly, 23,* 89–99.

Nippold, M., Erskine, B., & Freed, D. (1988). Proportional and analogical reasoning in normal and language-impaired children. *Journal of Speech and Hearing Disorders, 53,* 440–449.

Piaget, J. (1952). *The origins of intelligence of children* (M. Cook, trans.). New York: International Universities Press.

Pinker, S. (1984). *Language learnability and language development.* Cambridge, MA: Harvard University Press.

Pisoni, D. (1978). Speech perception. In W. Kates (Ed.), *Handbook of learning and cognitive processes* (Vol. 6, pp. 171–203). Hillsdale, NJ, Erlbaum.

Rees, N. (1981). Saying more than we know: Is auditory processing disorder a meaningful concept? In R. Keith (Ed.), *Central auditory and language disorders in children* (pp. 94–102). San Diego: College-Hill Press.

Rom, A., & Leonard, L. (1990). Interpreting deficits in grammatical morphology in specifically language-impaired children: Preliminary evidence from Hebrew. *Clinical Linguistics and Phonetics, 4,* 93–105.

Roth, F., & Clark, D. (1987). Symbolic play and social participation abilities of language-impaired and normally-developing children. *Journal of Speech and Hearing Disorders, 52,* 17–29.

Savich, P. (1984). Anticipatory imagery in normal and language disabled children. *Journal of Speech and Hearing Research, 27,* 494–501.

Sininger, Y. Klatzky, R., & Kirchner, D. (1989). Memory scanning speed in language disordered children. *Journal of Speech and Hearing Research, 32,* 289–306.

Tallal, P. (1976). Rapid auditory processing in normal and disordered language development. *Journal of Speech and Hearing Research, 19,* 561–579.

Tallal, P. (1988). Developmental language disorders. In J. Kavanagh & T. Truss, Jr. (Eds.), *Learning disabilities: Proceedings of the national conference* (pp. 181–272). Parkton, MD: York Press.

Terrell, B., Schwartz, R., Prelock, P., & Messick, C. (1984). Symbolic play in normal and language disordered children. *Journal of Speech and Hearing Research, 27,* 424–429.

Tomblin, J. (1984). Specific abilities approach: An evaluation and alternative method. In W. Perkins (Ed.), *Language handicaps in children* (pp. 27–41). New York: Thieme-Stratton.

Tomblin, J. (1989). Familial concentration of developmental language impairment. *Journal of Speech and Hearing Research, 54,* 287–295.

Tomblin, J. (1990). *Language cognition and social characteristics of young adults with histories of developmental language disorder.* Paper presented at the Symposium for Research on Child Language Disorders, Madison, WI.

Van der Lely, H., & Harris, M. (1990). Comprehension of reversible sentences in specifically language-impaired children. *Journal of Speech and Hearing Disorders, 55,* 101–117.

Wagner, R., & Torgesen, J. (1987). The nature of phonological processing and its causal role in the acquisition of reading skills. *Psychological Bulletin, 101,* 192–212.

Ward, M., Mills, E., & Kamhi, A. (in press). Hierarchical planning abilities with specific language impairment. *Journal of Speech and Hearing Research.*

Part II
Practices and Populations

6

Children with Developmental Language Disorders

Outcomes, Persistence, and Change

ANTHONY S. BASHIR, PH.D., AND
ANN Z. STROMINGER, SC.D.

Introduction

Language serves many different functions and purposes in a person's life, and its development continues from infancy into adulthood. Because language comprehension, production, and use are fundamental to social interaction and academic success, children with developmental language disorders are at risk for problems in social relations and school learning (Bashir, Wiig, & Abrams, 1987). This chapter addresses issues related to the continuous vulnerability of children with developmental language disorders, especially during the school years.

A number of terms are used to designate these individuals, including *childhood or developmental aphasia* (Eisenson, 1972; Proceedings, 1962), *children with language disorders* (Berry, 1969), and *specific language impairment* (Lahey, 1988). The term *children with developmental language disorders* will be used in this chapter, which states that the personal, academic, and social vulnerability of children with developmental language disorders results from the life-long need to acquire language, to learn and interact with language, and to apply accrued knowledge of language to other related learning tasks, such as reading and writing.

The Language Continuum: Contributions to Understanding Natural History

Basing her work on that of Myklebust (1954, 1960), Johnson developed a perspective that language processes and functions are best understood along a continuum of developing cognitive and linguistic abilities (1968). Johnson (1991) argued that the initial aspects of the continuum begin with the child's development of symbolic representations of the world. It was this evolving cognitive system—this inner language—that would form the basis for the development of understanding and expression.

The language continuum begins with oral language comprehension and expression and develops through reading and writing. Johnson noted that this specific continuum is similar to the language arts curriculum of schools. In the language continuum, emphasis is placed on the reciprocal relationships between the components of language and the ways in which development in one aspect of language facilitates development in other aspects of language. The interrelatedness of language development and reading thus becomes clearer (Catts, 1989a; Dickinson & McCabe, 1991; Stanovich, 1986).

Although there were challenges to the notion of a hierarchy of language functions in that it was too simple and linear, the earlier work of Johnson and Myklebust formed the basis for understanding the complexity of language learning, both developmentally and academically. Their work also provided a model for understanding why children with preschool developmental language disorders often evidence persistent problems in language learning and school achievement. For example, the speech-language clinician treats a child with a developmental language disorder and, seeing the child achieve therapy goals, discharges the child from therapy. Within a year or two the child is, once again, brought to the clinician's attention; the parents now note that the child is having difficulty participating in school, understanding the teacher, and learning to read and write. What might explain this "new" set of problems? Part of the answers can be found in the language continuum and its relation to the natural history of developmental language disorders.

Follow-Up and Longitudinal Studies of Preschool Children with Speech and Language Problems

Concerns for the late sequelae of early childhood language disorders were first expressed in the late nineteenth century (Weiner, 1985), yet systematic follow-up studies did not begin until the mid-1960s (de Ajuriaguerra et al., 1976). In the 1960s and early 1970s, longitudinal studies of children with developmental language disorders included illustrative case histories (Berry, 1969; McGinnis, 1963; Ward & McCartney, 1976; Weiner, 1974) or personal accounts by mothers of children with language disorders (Clarke, 1973; Kastein & Trace, 1966). Without exception, these accounts are of children with severe and often multiple handicaps, yet they provide remarkable insights into the ways in which the lives of these children were affected. Along with extensive clinical descriptions of developmental language disorders (Berry, 1969; Eisenson, 1972; Johnson & Myklebust, 1967; Myklebust, 1954), these case studies demonstrated that developmental language disorders were heterogeneous and occurred across different clinical groups. From these cases it was clear that language disorders persist in time and have consequences throughout the life of the individual. Generalizations based on clinical reports and descriptions would have to await systematic documentation and research within carefully defined populations.

Early Studies: The 1960s and 1970s

By 1968, children with developmental language disorders were included in the definition of learning disabilities written by the National Advisory Committee on

Handicapped Children (1968); this definition was incorporated into Public Law (P.L.) 94-142. The association of language disorders with learning disabilities postulated by Johnson and Myklebust was documented by the mid-1970s (Denckla, 1977; Mattis, French, & Rapin, 1975). Recent studies further elucidate the close association between language development, language disorders, and dyslexia (Catts, 1989a; Scarborough, 1990).

A number of different follow-up study designs are used. Some follow a group of children from preschool into the school years (e.g., Rissman, Curtiss, & Tallal, 1990; Scarborough & Dobrich, 1990; Tallal, 1988), whereas others use a follow-up format and assess the child's language and academic performance at a later age (e.g., Aram, Ekelman, & Nation, 1984; Aram & Nation, 1980; Catts, 1991; Garvey & Gordon, 1973; Hall & Tomblin, 1978; Strominger & Bashir, 1977; Wolpaw, Nation, & Aram, 1976). Direct comparison of study results is difficult because various criteria are used for subject inclusion. In addition, there are different descriptions of subjects provided; there is little uniformity in the measurements used to determine current status; there are different lengths of time between diagnosis and follow-up; and different designs are used (i.e., prospective and retrospective). There are reviews that summarize the research on preschool children with language disorders and their academic performance (Aram & Hall, 1989; Bashir et al., 1987; Maxwell & Wallach, 1984; Tallal, 1988; Weiner, 1985).

Early studies relied on the use of surveys with heterogeneous groups of children with communication disorders. Beagley and Wrenn (1970) followed 192 normally hearing children all with delayed speech, whereas Morley (1965) was interested in the developmental outcomes of 162 children with speech delay. In both of these studies, the vast majority of children improved, but residual concerns for articulation status persisted in 20% to 27% of the children. The children studied represented different clinical syndromes, including those with and without neurological problems as well as with and without hearing impairment.

Griffiths (1969) surveyed 24 children who had attended a special school for children with severely delayed language; follow-up occurred over a period of from 1 to nearly 8 years. Of her original group, only 5% were without problems in latter childhood, whereas the majority continued to evidence problems in language social and emotional development and school learning. The persistence of problems in language development and the difficulty in educational progress were also reported by Garvey and Gordon (1973) in their follow-up study of 58 children. Sheridan and Peckham (1975), reporting on a follow-up at 11 years of 215 children with marked speech defects recorded at 7 years, indicated that a large proportion of the 11-year-olds, regardless of their speech outcomes, had reading difficulties; unfortunately, developmental language status was not available. Weiner's (1972) follow-up of seven dysphasic boys noted persistence of language comprehension problems and reduced auditory processing abilities, in spite of normal nonverbal intelligence.

In 1976, a report of the work of de Ajuriaguerra and his colleagues became available, in which 17 children with dysphasia (from an original group of 40 children) were followed 2 years after their initial assessments. Although all children were found to have improved their communication abilities, the effects of early language disruption on later development were seen as pervasive: "Dysphasia is not merely reducible to an obstruction in the development of the language, but rather seems to be a special kind of disorganization of language spanning its entire development" (p. 384). This work shows the importance of studying developmental language disorders within a longitudinal perspective. The study results brought together for the first time the idea of the convergence of different domains of development (linguistic, cognitive, academic, social, and emotional) in the natural history of language disorders.

Studies of the late 1970s, while stressing the growth and development of children with developmental language disorders over the follow-up period, began to document the differential outcomes for these children. Wolpaw et al. (1976) reported follow-up findings from a study of 30 children diagnosed between 3 and 7 years and followed again between 9 and 11 years using the same assessment scales. Included within the study were children who were both retarded and nonretarded. Of the nonretarded group, however, 43% continued to demonstrate language problems. Although there was variation in the type of presenting language problems on follow-up and although all children evidenced growth in language, there was persistence of comprehension deficits with variations in severity. This indicated that underlying problems in language development may persist over time and change in degree and type of problem.

Strominger and Bashir (1977), in a 9-year follow-up study, examined cognitive, linguistic, and academic outcomes for a group of 40 children diagnosed as language disordered before 5 years of age. They were interested in whether a continuum of language-learning failure might be evident in these children. Consistent with the findings of Evans and Bangs (1972), they found that no child was without residual deficits. Only two children were reported to be at or above grade expectations on oral reading, reading comprehension, and written language. These two children continued to experience problems with sound sequencing and spelling as well as naming retrieval problems. Of the remaining 38 children, all performed below grade level on both read and written language assessments. Clearly, preschool children with language disorders were vulnerable to problems in their subsequent development of reading and writing. These findings proved consistent with those of the Collaborative Perinatal Project (Lassman, Fisch, Vetter, & LaBenz, 1980). Those children who evidenced problems on the 3-year speech and language protocol were two to three times more likely to fail on the written communication section of the 8-year protocol. Early failure in language acquisition was implicated in later problems with reading and writing.

Outcomes for children with speech disorders were different from outcomes for children with developmental language disorders. Using data that is part of a comprehensive follow-up of children with language or articulation disorders, Hall and Tomblin (1978) reported outcomes for 18 language-impaired and 18 articulation-impaired children, followed for both communication and educational outcomes 13 to 20 years after initial assessment. Differences were noted between the two groups in persistence, associated educational problems, and negative postsecondary education outcomes. Young adults with histories of language impairment evidenced persistence of language problems in 9 of the 18 individuals followed, whereas only one of those in the articulation group showed such impairments. Educational differences were noted across grades; those with language impairment achieved below those with articulation problems. Fewer young adults with language impairment were involved in postsecondary pursuits. Differential outcomes for those with phonological problems and those with phonological and language problems were supported in a study of individuals with a history of early phonological disorders (Lewis & Freebairn, 1992). Similarly, differences in psychological status for those with speech disorders only and those with speech and/or language disorders are well documented (Baker & Cantwell, 1982, 1987). By the late 1970s, it was clear that sequelae associated with developmental language disorders included problems in learning to read and write as well as differences in psychological adjustment and later life pursuits.

Later Studies: The 1980s and 1990s

The studies conducted in the 1980s and 1990s clarified outcome data and allowed for the isolation of factors that can predict risk variables and influence school learning and placement. After following a group of 63 children with developmental language disorders 4 to 5 years after initial diagnosis, Aram and Nation (1980) reported that approximately 40% of these preschoolers continued to present with speech and language problems and approximately 40% with learning problems. They reported a moderate correlation between preschool levels of language and later class placement in the elementary grades. For example, 40% of the children were not yet placed in regular classroom settings and performed below age and grade expectations in reading and arithmetic. Both the language arts and basic arithmetic pose a problem for these children; to date there have been no extensive studies of mathematics in children with developmental language disorders. A disconcerting finding to the authors was that preschool therapy did not relate to later speech, language, and academic abilities. As with Strominger's data (1983), the receipt of therapy did not seem to alter persistence of language and academic learning problems for some children. As noted by Aram and Nation, we needed to work in the area of differential effects of early language intervention on subsequent language and academic learning.

Further appreciation of the complex of variables that must be considered in studying outcomes is evident in the retrospective 15-year follow-up study of King, Jones, and Lasky (1982). Working from clinical records and interviews, King and her associates followed a group of 50 individuals whose length of time in therapy varied considerably from less than 6 months to more than 5 years. Length of therapy was on the average greater for those with language disorder/delayed speech than those with articulation problems. As was true with Hall and Tomblin, persistence of communication concerns was greater among those with language problems than those with only articulation problems. The findings indicate that concerns for reading were present in all communication-disordered groups (i.e., 46% of those with language disorders and articulation deficits, but only 17% of those with articulation problems alone). Math concerns were reported only for the articulation group. Academic achievement by the group as a whole was better than had been reported by Griffiths (1969). Although tutoring was needed in 52% of the cases, 76% of the group had received average grades or better.

In a follow-up study of 20 preschool children with language disorders into adolescence, Aram and Nation (1980) noted that with the exception of five young adults, the remaining 15 required some special education. Early IQ scores were strongly related to later IQ, class placement, language, and academic achievement. Of the early measures, the Letter International Scale was found to be the best single predictor of later language and reading achievement. Using the Northwestern Syntax Screen Test, Aram and Nation found that the Expressive subtest was a significant predictor of language outcomes in adolescence. In addition to these predictive measures, their study revealed that social and behavioral consequences needed to be addressed to understand the natural history of developmental language disorders. Preschool language disorders were known to have a general effect on other aspects of development (Howlin & Rutter, 1987).

Some children who demonstrate problematic language development do seem to achieve age-appropriate levels on follow-up. Across studies, there is wide variation in the reported recovery figures, ranging from 7% in the Stark et al. (1984) study to 50% in Aram and Nation (1980). Bishop and Edmundson (1987) noted that the child's age at time of diagnosis and follow-up as well as his or her intellectual level influence predictions of recovery from early development problems. Bishop and Edmundson (1987) reported that 37% of their 87 language-impaired children demonstrated normal language development by age 5½. Aram and Nation (1980) noted that nonverbal intelligence as measured by the Leiter was an important predictor of outcome. Status of language comprehension in the preschool years also is another major predictive factor, as is range and severity of language impairment. However, even children who seemingly resolve developmental problems are not free from later educational challenges (Scarborough, 1991; Stark et al., 1984). It may be that different components of language predict future status in different ways and to different degrees.

Persistent language deficits are not only evident at the beginning of schooling but can emerge from time to time during the middle, junior, and high school years. Because language learning continues through adolescence, additional language problems may not be evident until then (Ehren & Lenz, 1989). In fact, the learning of language forms, meanings, and uses continues into late childhood and adolescence (Menyuk, 1983; Simon, 1985). These later attainments of language are critical for socialization, content learning, and reading and writing (Wiig & Semel, 1984).

Some of the later-appearing language problems include delays in the learning of grammatical morphology (Johnston & Schery, 1976; Wiig & Fleischman, 1980), differences in syntactic abilities as seen in both comprehension and production (Menyuk & Flood, 1981; Wallach, 1985; Wiig & Semel, 1973, 1974), problems in the development of figurative language (Lee & Kamhi, 1990), word retrieval deficits (German, 1979, 1982; Rubin, Berstein, & Katz, 1989; Wolf, 1982), problems in the development of oral and written narratives (Garnett, 1986; Montague, Maddus, & Dereshiwsky, 1990; Nodine, Barenbawn, & Newcomber, 1985; Roth & Speckman, 1986; Scott, 1989; Westby, 1985), and difficulties in text comprehension (Conte, 1993; Westby, 1989).

Finally, clinical experience and research findings suggest that persistent problems with later language learning do not exist apart from other problems in cognitive development, including nonverbal abilities (Johnston, 1994). As noted for individuals with learning disabilities, children with language disorders also experience loss of effective and efficient learning of strategies, difficulty in the integration of subskills, problems in activation of what is learned, and changes in problem-solving approaches (Meltzer, 1990; Swanson, 1987; Torgesen & Licht, 1983). Because of the effects of language on cognitive development during the school years, persistent problems with growth and generalization of learned material pose serious obstacles for children with language disorders (Johnston, 1988; Kamhi, 1988). Neuropsychological approaches to the study of patterns of cognition and language abilities have integrated perspectives which were previously considered discrete and noncontinuous (Rudel, Holmes, & Pardes, 1988).

A Recapitulation

What can we realistically expect as outcomes for children with preschool developmental speech and language problems? After considering some of the major research findings, we can assert that children with only developmental speech problems experience a better outcome than do those with developmental language problems; this is so in terms of education and psychological adaptation. Second, persistence of language problems into the school years is reported in 40% to 88% of the children. The variance in reports is a function of type, range, and severity of the presenting problem as well as intelligence.

The results of these and other studies (Johnston, 1982) suggest the following: (1) Children with language disorders do show changes in the type and severity of their language problems over time; (2) the order of acquisition of language forms mirrors that of nonaffected children, but the acquisition of language occurs more slowly and over an extended age span; (3) language problems persist for many of these children throughout childhood as well as adolescence and young adult life; and (4) additional language problems may not be apparent until the middle school years, when children are required to understand or produce complex language, develop narratives, understand or create expository texts, or use language for higher order tasks, such as argument and interpretation. The problems can change and manifest differently across time; other domains of development emerge as problematic. This convergence of language acquisition problems, school learning problems, and social development problems is difficult to explain; one way of explaining it is through a demands-capacity model, discussed later in this chapter.

The Persistence of Language Disorders

Summarizing their longitudinal data on lexical, syntactic, and semantic development in four children with expressive language problems who were identified at age 2½, Scarborough and Dobrich (1990) noted that "over the preschool period these children underwent concurrent developmental changes in the severity and breadth of their productive language impairments" (p. 80). As the children developed from 2½ years old to 5 years old, the researchers noted differences with respect to selectivity of the language deficit and pattern of language problems. The progression was from broad to specific aspects of language. The findings are consistent with those about changing patterns of language behavior with increasing age (Aram & Nation, 1975). In summary, language differences persist as children with language disorders continue to develop; severity, range, specificity, and patterns of language differences vary across age and from child to child; and the learning of language can be affected differentially.

It is possible for a child to evidence normal language functions at the time of school entry. This is the case in the subjects reported by Aram and Nation (1975), Bishop and Edmundson, (1987), and Scarborough and Dobrich (1990). However, this does not mean that these children will not have additional problems in learning when application of language knowledge is required. Scarborough and Dobrich (1990) apply the term "illusory recovery" to the fact that some children can appear normal and then go on to experience additional problems.

Differences in later development of children with developmental language disorders can be seen after they pass through a plateau of normal acquisition of selected aspects of language. However, because language can be regarded as a componential system, it is unlikely that equality of development or plateau achievement should be expected across all components. The reemergence of problems would occur consistent with the ability to meet challenges at the next developmental stage of growth and demand.

Consequently, the data suggest that for at least 40% of preschool children with developmental language problems, language differences and a slower rate of language acquisition persist into the early school grades. These occur across the same developmental time span when the child is required to learn to read and write. As a consequence of the time needed for mastery of certain language forms (Johnston, 1982; Johnston & Schery, 1976; Stark et al., 1984), the child with a language disorder continues to need additional time to acquire aspects of language often after peers have accomplished the same task. However, in school the assumption is made that the child has mastered certain language forms and concepts and can use language and knowledge about language for learning to read, write, and participate in classroom activities. The differences between the child's language status and the language required for learning in school can result in recurrent learning difficulties for children with language disorders. This is a major reason why children with language disorders remain academically vulnerable throughout the school years (Bashir, 1987; Bashir & Scavuzzo, 1992; Blank, Rose, & Berlin, 1978; Nelson, 1984, 1994).

Addressing the issue of chronicity, Scarborough (1991) argues that the persistence of problems does not reflect a single factor. Rather she hypothesizes that "the appearance of each symptom is primarily determined by the underlying condition itself which impedes the mastery of each developmental challenge" (p. 218). Although other factors—such as motivation, prior learning and experience, and treatment effects—may all influence eventual outcomes, problems in learning are seen when the developmental or task challenges require some aspect of verbal-cognitive processing. This idea is consistent with the postulates of Wiig and Semel (1976), who argue that cognitive-linguistic interactions are the principal determining factors in late sequelae of early disruption in language learning.

Children with Language Disorders and the School Years

Not all preschool children with language disorders have problems learning when they attend school. Nonetheless, reports indicate that at least 50% to 75% of children with language disorders will evidence persistent academic problems (Aram & Hall, 1989). A reduced rate of learning as well as level of achievement also are reflected in other longitudinal studies (Shaywitz, 1989).

In the work of Tallal and her associates, it is apparent that across the early school grades, children with language disorders achieve, but at a reduced rate and amount when compared to their normal peers (Tallal, 1990). The San Diego Longitudinal Study was developed to study various outcomes for preschool children with language disorders (Rissman et al., 1990; Tallal, 1990). For children with language disorders, types of educational placements changed across the 5 years of the study. At 4 and 5 years of age, the use of special self-contained classes predominated, with approximately 53% of the children placed in a special day class by kindergarten. After the kindergarten period, there was a gradual increase in the use of pull-out service programs and a decline in self-contained class placement. Finally, by 8 years of age, only 23% of the children were in special class placements, whereas 40% were involved in pull-out programs and 37% in regular class placements.

Although an expressive language deficit was used most often to determine school placement in the San Diego Study, it was the child's receptive language abilities as measured at 4 years of age that predicted school placement at age 8 years, especially for those who remain in self-contained classes (Rissman et al., 1990). Again, different aspects of language may predict with differential effectiveness depending on setting requirements and task demands. The data suggest that the children with language disorders become "increasingly differentiated from each other" (p. 56). Achievement in language arts and nonverbal IQ measures also influenced placement in the early elementary grades.

Educational outcomes at the postsecondary level suggest the importance of language abilities in determining success. In a study of the extrinsic and intrinsic factors affecting college success for students with learning disabilities, Vogel and Adelman (1990) note that support services provided to students with learning disabilities were effective in assisting these students to complete degree requirements at the same rate as their peers without disabilities. However, Vogel and Adelman note that for the nongraduating group of students with learning disabilities, persistently poorer oral language disabilities were present and accounted for one third of the variance in graduation status.

Similarly, Finucci, Gottfredson, and Childs (1985), in their follow-up study of dyslexic boys, reported that those young men who were severely affected and who did not profit from a structured language therapy approach were less likely to earn bachelor's degrees, work in reading-intensive job settings, or have adult literate habits. What is not clear in many of the studies is the nature of the therapeutic experiences of the students, the kinds of educational placements used, and related support services that were provided. In addition, little is known about how therapy was used to address those skills and abilities needed to facilitate academic outcomes.

The experiences of children with language disorders can vary considerably across the school years. The variability occurs as a function of children's inherent abilities and differences, the demands and content of the curriculum, and instructional methods and approaches. From time to time, children with language disabilities will require careful attention. This is especially true during transitions from grade to grade. Throughout the child's school years, the assumption is made that each grade shift assumes that the child can apply, extend, and elaborate previously acquired skills, strategies, and information (Bashir, Kuban, Kleinman, & Scavuzzo, 1984). As a consequence, major grade transitions, such as between kindergarten and first grade or third and fourth grade, will be particularly challenging. As literacy requirements increase and as students are expected to assume responsibility for their own learning, the middle grades as well as transitions to junior and senior high school can be problematic. By this time, administrative decisions can be restrictive, with educational planning limited to a set of reduced educational settings and options.

Persistence and Delay: Synchrony and Demands Capability

There is considerable debate about whether the language productions of children with language disorders reflect simple delays in acquisition or whether the language productions of these children are different and, therefore, suggest abnormalities in underlying language processes and competence. The current evidence suggests that children with language disorders demonstrate a slower rate of acquiring lexical, syntactic, and morphological structures and, in turn, achieve acquisition of language at a later age than their peers (Johnston, 1982). There is also evidence that the persistence of language impairment may extend into adulthood (Gerber & Reiff, 1991; Johnson & Blalock, 1987). Although there are reports of children who produce deviant structures that are not reflected in normal development (Weiner, 1985), the majority of studies demonstrate that problems are associated with late emergence, extended time of acquisition, and reduced frequency of use (Curtiss, Katz, & Tallal, 1992; Johnston, 1982; Lahey, Liebergott, Chesnick, Menyuk, & Adams, 1992; Leonard, 1972). However, recent studies suggest the possible existence of focal areas of linguistic deficiencies (Rice, 1994) and underlying processing-capacity-limitations models to explain specific language learning problems, such as morphology (Leonard, 1992; Watkins, 1994).

In educational planning for children with language disorders, how might issues related to extended time and age of acquisition be understood? How might the presence of focal areas of deficiencies in language help us understand the apparent discrepancies between components of language? How do answers to these questions and others help us plan and treat the student with language problems in a manner that leads to effectiveness in learning and flexibility in adapting to new demands?

Persistence of language problems should not be interpreted as little more than a simple developmental delay. This outlook suggests the possibilities of normalization across time and assumes that only a different rate of growth is the major problem. The persistence of language deficits into the school years does not imply that the children will be all right or that they will get it eventually." For example, the results of the San Diego Longitudinal Study (Rissman et al., 1990) and others (Stark et al., 1984; Strominger, 1983) suggest that children with language disorders do demonstrate growth in learning across the grades, but the learning curves are not equivalent to those of students who are not language disordered. This is especially true in the area of language arts. Furthermore, although there is evidence of change in language behaviors over time, there is also evidence of invariance in the patterns of language impairment observed across time (Aram & Nation, 1975; Bishop & Edmundson, 1987).

For children with language disorders, it is not simply a matter of providing more time or early treatment so that the children will catch up with peers. Ekleman (1994) studied the relationships among speech-language and reading skills in children with a history of speech-language or reading disorders. Surprisingly, nine of her subjects with only articulation problems showed persistence of articulation deficits in the third grade. All but one of the children in her language and speech and language groups continued to show limitations in language.

As part of a study on facilitating reading comprehension in social studies for a group of middle school students with language problems, Conte, Menyuk, and Bashir (1993) assessed the language abilities of seventh-grade students only to find persistence of problems in lexical and syntactic development. For these young students, these types of problems could be noted throughout their early school years.

Using a life-span framework, we can postulate that differences in rates and variations in patterns of language acquisition, in turn, induce qualitative differences and asynchrony in the emergence, consolidation, and structure of behavior (Gould, 1977). These qualitative differences will influence the effectiveness and efficiency with which a behavior can be learned and applied (Bashir et al., 1984). Overall differences in the behavior of a child with a language disorder can be understood as the consequences of interactions among the constraints and differences within the individual and the demands and requirements of different learning tasks and environments (Bashir & Scavuzzo, 1992). The late problems in academic learning experienced by children with language disorders are best understood as a special case of reciprocal causation (Stanovich, 1986).

Using the idea of reciprocal causation, we are in a position to understand the interrelations among such factors as (1) developmental rate, (2) differences in patterns of language behaviors, (3) the time in which basic component processes emerge and the consequences for learning, (4) learning task demands, (5) the overall effects of persistent language disorders on cumulative learning in school (e.g., reading comprehension, writing strategies, and content information), and (6) the effects of achievements in reading and writing as well as content learning on the development of of latter language. Similar arguments have been advanced for students with learning disabilities (Swanson, 1987).

Children develop language competence and performance at varying rates and different levels (Lahey, 1988; Lahey & Bloom, 1994). For children with language disorders, the differential growth in language abilities may or may not be synchronous with the demands of elementary, middle, junior, or senior high school curricula. Clinical experiences suggest that school success for children with language disorders will be predicated on the degree to which the child's cognitive and linguistic abilities are synchronous (consistent) with the assumptions and demands for the learning of a specific task or subject matter (Bashir, 1989).

For many children with language disorders, an asynchrony may exist. For example, one kind of asynchrony occurs because of differences between the child's language abilities and the applications of language required for successful learning (e.g., difficulty with phonological awareness tasks and automatic word recognition abilities). For children with language disorders, specifying the factors that contribute to the asynchrony becomes important in understanding both the maintenance of and onset of other language or learning problems (Bashir et al., 1984). Therefore, defining factors that perpetuate asynchrony between the child's development of language and school-based language requirements—as well as defining the consequences of the asynchrony for the child's development—are basic to understanding the late sequelae of preschool language disorders. This understanding will explain, in part, the continued academic vulnerability of children with language disorders throughout the school years.

How do we understand that for some children learning and academic problems result from the fact that their language knowledge and abilities are not consistent (synchronous) with those required for academic and content learning; that their learning experiences differ from nonaffected peers; that as strategic learners they are less efficient and effective; and that their problems seen initially in language acquisition are later seen as specific problems with literate and social language learning?

Both a developmental and a demands-capabilities perspective help the clinician understand the often persistent nature of language disorders and the late sequelae of academic and social learning. The study of stuttering provides models for demands capabilities (Adams, 1990; Starkweather & Gottwald, 1990); in addition, Lewin's (1935) interaction approach to understanding personality can be applied. Putnam, Deshler, and Schumaker (1993), using Lewin as well as a demands capacity model, the advocate for understanding student outcome behaviors by analyzing the relation between setting (task) demands and the characteristics of the student. This model helps explain why children with developmental language problems might continue to experience problems with academic, content, and social learning. Putnam et al. (1993) suggest that an individual's behavior (successful or not) results from an interaction between the demands of the task or environment (cognitive, motivational, attentional, communicative, linguistic, social) and the capabilities (characteristics) of the person (e.g., cognitive, linguistic).

Using this model to account for the interaction of learning demands and the individual's capabilities, we can begin to understand the influence on academic and social learning of factors such as increased processing time requirements, executive problems, reductions in metalinguistic abilities, reduced lexical development, delayed morphological learning, and difficulty in understanding complex syntactic structures. By understanding context and content demands, for instance, we are provided with the perspectives needed to appreciate the specificity of impairment and the continued vulnerability of children with developmental language disorders. We can then develop appropriate educational and therapeutic solutions and strategies.

Language Disorders and Learning to Read

The problems of developmental synchrony and task demands become clearer when we consider the research on learning to read in children with developmental language disorders. Learning to read and using reading for learning are often particularly difficult for a majority of children with developmental language disorders. Not all preschool children with developmental language disorders have problems learning to read. Important advances are occurring in understanding which children are at risk for reading problems (Bishop & Adams, 1990; Catts, 1991, 1993; Catts, Hu, Larrivee, & Swank, 1994; Liebergott et al., 1989; Menyuk, 1985; Menyuk et al., 1991). When the results of studies of preschool children with language disorders are considered collectively, reading problems (including problems with word recognition and comprehension) occur in 40% to 75% of the children (Aram et al., 1984; Aram & Nation, 1980; Graham, Bashir, Stark, Silbert, & Walzer, 1988; King et al., 1982; Magnusson & Naucler, 1990; Scarborough & Dobrich, 1990; Strominger, 1983; Strominger & Bashir, 1977).

Strominger (1983) studied the relation of language deficits to reading, spelling, and written language production. All 38 children (9 girls, 29 boys) were diagnosed as language impaired before 5 years of age; they ranged in age from 9 to 12 years at follow-up. The majority of the children had problems with linguistically complex tasks of verbal comprehension and, even more so, with expressive language production. None of the 38 children were free of language-related problems, although the range was from mild to moderately severe. The mean achievement on the Gray Oral Reading for boys was a grade equivalent of 3.8 (actual mean grade placement 5.1), and for girls it was 2.7 (actual mean grade placement 4.8). Consistent with previous explanations (Strominger & Bashir, 1977), Strominger argued that when language learning is disturbed in the initial stages of acquisition, there is increased risk for future deficits in the learning of tasks that are language based and require the application of language knowledge.

As is the case in other studies, more boys than girls were reported in Strominger's study. Depending on sampling and definitional criteria, there is now evidence that the percentage of boys to girls with dyslexia may be closer than previously believed (Shaywitz, Shaywitz, Fletcher, & Escobar, 1990). Strominger pointed out that when the girls in her study were affected with language and reading disorders, the girls were more severely involved than the boys. Indeed, this is an intriguing finding and will need further clarification through longitudinal research. In addition, family aggregation effects and differential outcomes in the language abilities of boys and girls need further study (Tallal, Ross, & Curtiss, 1989).

Studies of boys with XXY aneuploidy (Kleinfelter's syndrome) indicate that delays in speech and language development are common and there is an increase in speech and language impairment within the group when compared to nonaffected controls (Neilsen et al., 1981; Puck, Tennes, Frankenburg, Bryant, & Robinson, 1975). Further studies of XXY boys indicate that they develop problems in both language and reading (Graham, Bashir, Walzer, Stark, & Gerald, 1981; Graham et al., 1988; Pennington, Puck, & Robinson, 1980; Robinson, Puck, & Pennington, 1979; Walzer et al., 1978). Graham et al. (1988) studied 14 XXY boys (mean age 9 years and 7 months) who were identified during neonatal cytogenetic screening and a control group of 15 normal boys (mean age 9 years and 3 months); all boys were studied during the third- to fourth-grade transitional period.

The results of the study indicated significant differences between the groups on measures of verbal IQ, expressive language functions, and reading and spelling achievement. Of the 14 boys with XXY, 11 evidenced difficulties with sequencing nonverbal tones at rapid rates of presentation; they also had difficulty preserving the serial order of both speech and nonspeech stimuli. These difficulties correlated with oral language problems (word-finding deficits, problems in syntactic production, narrative production problems), reading deficits, and spelling problems. Performances on the Gilmore Oral Reading Test revealed significant differences, with the XXY boys performing lower on accuracy, speed, and comprehension. On the Gates-McGinitie Silent Reading Test, the mean comprehension of the XXY group was equivalent to grade 2.8 in comparison with a grade 5.7 achievement by the control group.

The association among oral language deficits, reduced language processing, and reading problems is reported in the work of Tallal (1980a, 1980b). What is striking in her work is the finding that children with reading problems and oral language problems have neuropsychological deficits similar to children with language disorders alone (e.g., deficits in temporal processing of information). In fact, studies of Tallal and Stark (1982) indicate that these deficits in temporal processing are absent in a group of reading-impaired children who do not have concomitant oral language deficits or difficulty with phonics. Recent studies by Rissman et al. (1990) indicate that children with receptive language disorders may have more severe reading deficits than other language-impaired children. In his recent work, Catts (1993) indicates the importance of language status on the prediction of reading comprehension. Certainly, further study is needed if we are to understand the differential outcomes for different subtypes of language disorders on learning to read and the contributions of concomitant problems in language processing.

All of the aforementioned studies address reading during the early elementary grades when the child is learning relations between speech and orthographic representation. In Chall's (1983) stages of reading development, these children are within Stages I and II, in which children are developing automatic word recognition abilities as well as practicing reading extensively with different kinds of literature. There is evidence (Catts, 1991, 1993; Graham et al., 1988; Liebergott et al., 1989; Magnusson & Naucler, 1990; Menyuk et al., 1991; Tallal & Stark, 1982) that those children with specific language disorders who evidence concomitant problems in auditory rate processing or metalinguisitc abilities are the same children who will be more likely to have difficulty learning to read during Stages I and II, when word recognition and automaticity of word recognition abilities play a predominant role.

In their study of predictors of reading problems in a group of high-risk premature children and children with specific language impairment, Liebergott et al. (1989) reported that 70% ($n = 23$) of children with language impairment were problem readers; prediction of their reading status was based on the use of a metalinguistic battery that included syllable and phoneme segmentation of words, judgments of grammatical correctness, naming, and story recall. It is interesting to note that 31% of children in the high-risk groups who were not overtly language impaired also had problems with reading and did not succeed on the test battery of metaprocessing tasks. Menyuk and her colleagues (1991), reporting on a group of at-risk children, indicated that language-processing abilities of the children accounted for greater variance in reading tests than did performance on standard language tests. They noted that measures of language awareness were good predictors of later reading performance. However, different measures of awareness predicted differently across groups of children.

Current theory in reading disabilities supports the argument that deficits in phonological processing are basic to understanding the reading problems of children with dyslexia (Catts, 1989a, 1989b, 1989c; Kamhi & Catts, 1986, 1989; Lieberman, 1973; Lieberman & Shankweiler, 1986; Stanovich, 1988, 1993; Wagner & Torgesen, 1987). As the child is required to deal with a phonological analysis task, certain inherent factors may interfere with the child's performance. These include (1) the presence of delays in the emergence of phonological awareness, (2) retrieval latencies, (3) restrictions in verbal processing within short-term memory, and (4) restrictions in the child's ability to produce complex phonological sequences (Catts, 1989b). Given the findings of the aforementioned studies, deficits in phonological awareness and related metalinguistic abilities constitute an important focus in explaining and resolving problems associated with learning to read (Blachman, 1989). Clearly, the phonological processing models, which regard early reading problems as the result of deficits in phonological processing, are useful in explaining why some children with developmental language disorders experience difficulties in the early phases of reading acquisition (Stanovich, 1988, 1993; Tunmer & Hoover, 1993). These phonological process models also can contribute to an appreciation of the deficits in automaticity that are often seen in these children, such as those with word retrieval deficits (Wolf et al., 1986).

However, deficits in phonological processing do not necessarily explain all of the reading problems that children with language disorders encounter, especially by the middle grades. As noted earlier in this chapter, research has shown that children with language disorders do have persistent difficulties in comprehension of syntactic structures, problems in the management of narratives and expository text, deficits in word retrieval abilities, and possible restrictions in range of vocabulary development. The ways in which these deficits in word recognition and language problems contribute to or interact with persistent reading deficits in children with language impairment need systematic clarification and explanation. Menyuk and Flood (1981) have demonstrated the close relationship between oral comprehension of syntactic structures and reading comprehension. Curtis (1980) demonstrated that verbal coding and listening comprehension were both problematic for a group of less skilled readers in the second, third, and fifth grades. As verbal coding speed increased, level of comprehension emerged as a critical predictor of reading abilities.

This is consistent with the simple model of reading, which relates reading comprehension to both word recognition and listening comprehension (Gough &

Tumner, 1986; Tumner & Hoover, 1993). This model is helpful in explaining the differential predictability of language components to later reading. For example, phonological processing abilities may be related more to early reading achievement in language-disordered children and receptive and expressive language abilities to later reading comprehension (Catts et al., 1994). There is a clear need to understand that various components of language may contribute to reading abilities in different ways and degrees and at different stages in learning to read.

Longitudinal research will be needed if we are to understand the relation of language disorders and language processing deficits to reading disorders. We have little information on the emergence and development of reading in children with language disorders. There are those who argue that the later reading problems of school-age children with language disorders reflect a lack of development of higher order language abilities (Wiig & Semel, 1974) and problems with text-level processing (Roth & Spekman, 1989; Westby, 1989). Recent evidence suggests that for both normally developing children and adolescents with language disorders, expository text is more difficult to process than narrative text (Conte, Menyuk, & Bashir, 1992). In the study by Conte et al. (1992), unaffected adolescent boys did significantly better in recall of information from both expository and narrative text than did their language-disordered peers. Familiarity with discourse genre emerges as an important variable in text comprehension for both normal children and adolescents with language disorders.

Finally, we know little about the effects of reduced reading experiences on the later development of language in children with language disorders as well as their development of subject information, although the positive effects of such experiences are well documented for children with appropriate language development (Stanovich, 1986). In discussing the development of differences in readers, Stanovich (1986) notes that "reading itself is an important contributor to the development of many language/cognitive skills" (p. 364). The contribution occurs in vocabulary and syntactic growth as well as general learning, information, and cultural perspectives.

It is reasonable to argue that the continued academic vulnerability in children with language disorders in the middle grades reflects both the persistence of language problems and restrictions on later language development resulting from reduced reading as well as restricted exposure to different texts and text-based information. The long-term effects on general knowledge and information have yet to be determined. However, it is not surprising that teachers often state that these children cannot maintain pace with the rest of the class in content area learning, especially when it is dependent on processing text-based information or applying prior subject knowledge to current learning demands.

The dual consequences and interrelatedness of language disorder and reading disability can best be understood as a special case of reciprocal causation. Stanovich's discussion of Matthew effects must also be considered a way of conceptualizing and understanding the chronic nature of language disorders and the potential problems encountered by these children throughout the school years. Stanovich's arguments are important because they can direct and influence philosophy and approaches used to develop educational practices for children with language disorders.

Summary

Children with developmental language disorders change over time, demonstrating varying degrees of achievement and persistence of problems. These problems are associated with language learning and are expressed in difficulties with the development of reading and writing as well as academic and social development. Consequently, there is variability in outcomes for these children, ranging from normal young lives for some, to academic, social, and personal compromise for others. The life-long vulnerability of individuals with language disorders reflects the continuous need to learn language, to learn with language, and to apply language for academic, vocational, and social development throughout life. Similarly, language is an essential part of personal identity and cultural integration. Clinicians and educators are beginning to understand the specific factors that contribute to this vulnerability, and this is allowing them to provide appropriate education and interventions that facilitate successful learning and adaptation in language-disordered young people.

References

Adams, M. R. (1990). The demands and capacities model I: Theoretical elaborations. *Journal of Fluency Disorders, 15,* 135–141.

Aram, D. M., Ekelman, B. L., & Nation, J. E. (1984). Preschoolers with language disorders: 10 years later. *Journal of Speech and Hearing Research, 27,* 232–244.

Aram, D. M., & Hall, N. E. (1989). Longitudinal follow-up of children with preschool communication disorders: Treatment implications. *School Psychology Review, 18,* 487–501.

Aram, D. M., & Nation, J. E. (1975). Patterns of language behavior in children with developmental language disorders. *Journal of Speech and Hearing Research, 18,* 229–241.

Aram, D. M., & Nation, J. E. (1980). Preschool language disorders and subsequent language and academic difficulties. *Journal of Communication Disorders, 13,* 159–170.

Baker, L., & Cantwell, D. P. (1982). Psychiatric disorder in children with different types of communication disorders. *Journal of Communication Disorders, 15,* 113–126.

Baker, L., & Cantwell, D. P. (1987). A prospective psychiatric follow-up of children with speech/language disorders. *Journal of the American Academy of Child and Adolescent Psychiatry, 26,* 546–553.

Bashir, A. S. (1989). Language intervention and the curriculum. *Seminars in Speech and Language, 10,* 181–191.

Bashir, A. S., Kuban, K. C., Kleinman, S. N., & Scavuzzo, A. (1984). Issues in language disorders: Considerations of cause, maintenance, and change. In J. Miller, D. Yoder, & R. Schiefelbusch (Eds.), *ASHA Reports No. 12* (pp. 92–106). Rockville, MD: American Speech-Language-Hearing Association.

Bashir, A. S., & Scavuzzo, A. (1992). Children with language disorders: Natural history and academic success. *Journal of Learning Disabilities, 25,* 53–65.

Bashir, A. S., Wiig, E. H., & Abrams, J. C. (1987). Language disorders in childhood and adolescence: Implications for learning and socialization. *Pediatric Annals, 16,* 145–156.

Beagley, H. A., & Wrenn, M. (1970). Clinical follow-up of 192 normally hearing children with delayed speech. *Journal of Laryngology and Otology, 84,* 1001–1011.

Berry, M. T. (1969). *Language disorders of children: The bases of diagnosis.* New York: Appleton-Century-Crofts.

Bishop, D. V. M., & Adams, C. (1990). A prospective study of the relationship between specific language impairment, phonological disorders and reading retardation. *Journal of Child Psychology and Psychiatry, 31,* 1027–1050.

Bishop, D. V. M., & Edmundson, A. (1987). Language-impaired 4-year-olds: Distinguishing transient from persistent impairment. *Journal of Speech and Hearing Disorders, 52,* 156–173.

Blachman, B. A. (1989). Phonological awareness and word recognition: Assessment and intervention. In A. G. Kamhi and H. W. Catts (Eds.), *Reading disabilities: A developmental language perspective* (pp. 133–158). Boston: Little Brown.

Blank, M., Rose, S., & Berlin, L. (1978). *The language of learning: The preschool years.* New York: Grune & Stratton.

Catts, H. W. (1989a). Defining dyslexia as a developmental language disorder. *Annals of Dyslexia, 39,* 50–64.

Catts, H. W. (1989b). Phonological processing deficits and reading disabilities. In A. Kamhi & H. Catts (Eds.), *Reading disabilities: A developmental language perspective* (pp. 101–132). San Diego, CA: College-Hill Press.

Catts, H. W. (1989c). Speech production deficits in developmental dyslexia. *Journal of Speech and Hearing Disorders, 54,* 422–428.

Catts, H. W. (1991). Early identification of dyslexia: Evidence from a follow-up study of speech-language impaired children. *Annals of Dyslexia, 41,* 163–177.

Catts, H. W. (1993). The relationship between speech-language impairments and reading disabilities. *Journal of Speech and Hearing Research, 36,* 948–958.

Catts, H. W., Hu, C-F., Larrivee, L., & Swank, L. (1994). Early identification of reading disabilities in children with speech-language impairments. In R. V. Watkins & M. L. Rice (Eds.), *Specific language impairments in children* (pp. 145–160). Baltimore: Paul H. Brookes.

Chall, J. S. (1983). *Stages of reading development.* New York: McGraw-Hill.

Clarke, L. (1973). *Can't read, can't write, can't talk too good either.* New York: Walker and Co.

Conte, B. M. (1993). *The effect of genre, vocabulary, and syntax on the comprehension of expository text in language impaired and non-impaired adolescents.* Unpublished doctoral dissertation, Boston University.

Conte, B. M., Menyuk, P., & Bashir, A. S. (1992, November). *Text comprehension in language impaired and non-impaired adolescents.* Paper presented at the annual meeting of the American Speech-Language-Hearing Association.

Conte, B. M., Menyuk, P., & Bashir, A. S. (1993, November). *Facilitating reading comprehension in middle school students with language disorders.* Paper presented at the annual meeting of the American Speech-Language-Hearing Association.

Curtis, M. E. (1980). Development of components of reading skill. *Journal of Educational Psychology, 72,* 656–669.

Curtiss, S., Katz, W., & Tallal, P. (1992). Delay vs. deviance in the language acquisition of language impaired children. *Journal of Speech and Hearing Research, 35,* 373–383.

de Ajuriaguerra, J., Jaeggi, A., Guignaro, F., Kocher, F., Mauard, M., Roth, S., & Schmidt, E. (1976). The development and prognosis of dysphasia in children. In D. Morehead & A. Morehead (Eds.), *Normal and deficient child language* (pp. 345–385). Baltimore: University Park Press.

Denckla, M. B. (1977). Minimal brain dysfunction and dyslexia: Beyond diagnosis by exclusion. In M. Blaw, I. Rapin, & M. Kinsborne (Eds.), *Topics in child neurology* (pp. 79–86). New York: Spectrum Publications.

Dickinson, D., & McCabe, A. (1991). The acquisition and development of language: A social interactionist account of language and literacy development. In. J. E. Kavanagh (Ed.), *The language continuum: From infancy to literacy* (pp. 1–40). Parkton, MD: York Press.

Ehren, B. J., & Lenz, B. K. (1989). Adolescents with language disorders: Special considerations in providing academically relevant language intervention. *Seminars in Speech and Language, 10,* 192–203.

Eisenson, J. (1972). *Aphasia in children.* New York: Harper & Row.

Ekelman, B. L. (1994). *Examining the relationships among speech-language and reading skills in children with a history of speech-language or reading disorders.* Unpublished doctoral thesis, Case Western Reserve University, Cleveland, OH.

Evans, J. S., & Bangs, T. (1972). Effects of preschool language training on later academic achievement of children with language and learning disabilities: A descriptive analysis. *Journal of Learning Disabilities, 5,* 585–592.

Finucci, J. M., Gottfredson, L. S., & Childs, B. (1985). A follow-up study of dyslexic boys. *Annals of Dyslexia, 35,* 1–20.

Garnett, K. (1986). Telling tales: Narratives and learning disabled children. *Topics in Language Disorders, 6,* 44–56.

Garvey, M., & Gordon, N. (1973). A follow-up study of children with disorders of speech. *British Journal of Disorders of Communication, 8,* 17–28.

Gerber, P. J., & Reiff, H. B. (1991). *Speaking for themselves: Ethnographic interviews with adults with learning disabilities.* Ann Arbor: The University of Michigan Press.

German, D. J. (1979). Word-finding skills in children with learning disabilities. *Journal of Learning Disabilities, 12,* 176–181.

German, D J. (1982). Word-finding substitutions in children with learning disabilities. *Language, Speech, and Hearing Services in Schools, 13,* 223–230.

Gough, P. B., & Tunmer, W. (1986). Decoding, reading and reading disability. *Remedial and Special Education, 7,* 6–10.

Gould, S. J. (1977). *Ontogeny and phylogeny.* Cambridge, MA: Belknap Press.

Graham, J. M., Bashir, A. S., Stark, R. E., Silbert, A., & Walzer, S. (1988). Oral and written language abilities of XXY boys: Implications for anticipatory guidance. *Pediatrics, 81,* 795–806.

Graham, J. M., Bashir, A. S., Walzer, S, Stark, R. E., & Gerald, P. S. (1981). Communication skills among unselected XXY boys. *Pediatric Research, 15,* 562.

Griffiths, C. P. S. (1969). A follow-up study of children with disorders of speech. *British Journal of Disorders of Communication, 4,* 46–57.

Hall, P., & Tomblin, B. (1978). A follow-up study of children with articulation and language disorders. *Journal of Speech and Hearing Disorders, 43,* 227–241.

Howlin, P., & Rutter, M. (1987). The consequences of language delay for other aspects of development. *Clinics in Developmental Medicine, 101/102,* 271–294.

Johnson, D. (1968). The language continuum. *Bulletin of the Orton Society, 18,* 1–11.

Johnson, D. (1991). Written language. In J. F. Kavanagh (Ed.), *The language continuum: From infancy to literacy* (pp. 147–165). Parkton, MD: York Press.

Johnson, D., & Blalock, J. (1987). *Adults with learning disabilities.* New York: Grune and Stratton.

Johnson, D., & Myklebust, H. R. (1967). *Learning disabilities.* New York: Grune and Stratton.

Johnston, J. R. (1982). The language disordered child. In N. A. Lass, L. V. McReynolds, J. L. Northern, & D. E. Yoder (Eds.), *Speech, language and hearing, Vol. II. Pathologies of speech and language* (pp. 780–801). Philadelphia: W. B. Saunders.

Johnston, J. (1988). The nature of change. *Language, Speech, and Hearing Services in Schools, 19,* 314–329.

Johnston, J. R. (1994). Cognitive abilities of children with language impairment. In R. V. Watkins & M. L. Rice (Eds.), *Specific language impairment* (pp. 107–121). Baltimore, MD: Paul H. Brookes.

Johnston J., & Schery, T. (1976). The use of grammatical morphemes by children with communication disorders. In D. Morehead & A. Morehead (Eds.), *Normal and deficient child language* (pp. 239–258). Baltimore: University Park Press.

Kamhi, A. G. (1988). A reconceptualization of generalization and generalization problems. *Language, Speech, and Hearing Services in Schools, 19,* 304–313.

Kamhi, A. G., & Catts, H. W. (1986). Toward an understanding of developmental language and reading disorders. *Journal of Speech and Hearing Disorders, 51,* 337–348.

Kamhi, A. G., & Catts, H. W. (1989). Language and reading: Convergences, divergences, and development. In A. G. Kamhi & H. W. Catts (Eds.), *Reading disabilities: A developmental language perspective* (pp. 1–34). Boston: Little, Brown and Co.

Kastein, S., & Trace, B. (1966). *The birth of language: The case history of a non-verbal child.* Springfield, IL: Charles C. Thomas.

King, R. R., Jones, C., & Lasky, E. (1982). In retrospect: A fifteen-year follow-up report of speech-language disordered children. *Language, Speech and Hearing Services in Schools, 13,* 24–32.

Lahey, M. (1988). *Language disorders and language development.* New York: MacMillian.

Lahey, M., & Bloom, L. (1994). Variability and language learning disabilities. In G. P. Wallach & K. G. Butler, (Eds.) *Language learning disabilities in school-age children and adolescents: Some principles and applications* (pp. 354–372). New York: Merrill.

Lahey, M., Liebergott, J., Chesnick, M., Menyuk, P., & Adams, J. (1992). Variability in children's use of grammatical morphemes. *Applied Psycholinguistics, 13,* 373–398.

Lassman, F. M., Fisch, R. O., Vetter, D. K., & LaBenz, E. S. (1980). *Early correlates of speech, language and hearing: The collaborative perinatal project of the National Institute of Neurological and Communicative Disorders and Stroke.* Littleton, MA: P.S.G. Publishing Co.

Lee, R. F., & Kamhi, A. G. (1990). Metaphoric competence in children with learning disabilities. *Journal of Learning Disabilities, 23,* 476–482.

Leonard, L. (1972). What is deviant language? *Journal of Speech and Hearing Research, 37,* 427–446.

Leonard, L. (1992). The use of morphology by children with specific language impairment: Evidence from three languages. In R. Chapman (Ed.), *Processes in language acquisition and disorders.* St. Louis, MO: Mosby-Yearbook.

Leonard, L. (1994). Some problems facing accounts of morphological deficits in children with specific language impairments. In R. V. Watkins & M. L. Rice (Eds.), *Specific language impairments in children* (pp. 91–105). Baltimore: Paul H. Brookes.

Lewin, K. (1935). *A dynamic theory of personality: Selected papers.* New York: McGraw-Hill.

Lewis, B. A., & Freebairn, L. (1992). Residual effects of preschool phonology disorders in grade school, adolescence, and adulthood. *Journal of Speech and Hearing Research, 35,* 819–831.

Liebergott, J. W., Menyuk, P., Chesnick, M., Korngold, B., D'Agostino, R., & Belanger, A. (1989). *Predicting reading problems in at risk children.* Paper presented at the Speech, Language and Hearing Association, Boston, MA.

Lieberman, I. Y. (1973). Segmentation of the spoken word and reading acquisition. *Bulletin of the Orton Society, 23,* 65–67.

Lieberman, I. Y., & Shankweiler, D. (1986). Phonology and the problems of learning to read and write. *Remedial and Special Education, 6,* 8–17.

Magnusson, E., & Naucler, K. (1990). Reading and spelling in language-disordered children—linguistic and metalinguistic prerequisites: Report on a longitudinal study. *Clinical Linguistics & Phonetics, 4,* 49–61.

Mattis, S., French, J. H., & Rapin, I. (1975). Dyslexia in children and young adults: Three independent neuropsychological syndromes. *Developmental Medicine and Child Neurology, 17,* 150–163.

Maxwell, S. E., & Wallach, G. P. (1984). The language-learning disabilities connection: Symptoms of early language disability change over time. In G. P. Wallach & K. G. Butler (Eds.), *Language learning disabilities in school-age children* (pp. 15–34). Baltimore: Williams & Wilkins.

McGinnis, M. (1963). *Aphasic children.* Washington, DC: Alexander Graham Bell Association for the Deaf.

Meltzer, L. J. (1990). Problem-solving strategies and academic performances in learning disabled students: Do subtypes exist? In L. Feagans, E. Short, & L. Meltzer (Eds.), *Subtypes of learning disabilities* (pp. 163–188). Hillside, NJ: Erlbaum.

Menyuk, P. (1985). Language development and reading. In T. M. Gallagher & C. A. Prutting (Eds.), *Pragmatic assessment and intervention issues in language* (pp. 151–170). San Diego: College-Hill Press.

Menyuk, P., Chesnick, M., Liebergott, J. W., Korngold, B., D'Agnostino, R., & Belanger, A. (1991). Predicting reading problems in at-risk children. *Journal of Speech and Hearing Research, 34,* 893–903.

Menyuk, P., & Flood, J. (1981). Linguistic competence, reading, and writing problems and remediation. *Bulletin of the Orton Society, 31,* 13–28.

Montague, M., Maddus, C. D., & Dereshiwsky, M. I. (1990). Story grammar and comprehension and production of narrative prose by students with learning disabilities. *Journal of Learning Disabilities, 23,* 190–197.

Morley, M. E. (1965). *Development and disorders of speech in childhood,* 2nd ed. Baltimore: Williams & Wilkins.

Myklebust, H. R. (1954). *Auditory disorders in children: A manual for differential diagnosis.* New York: Grune & Stratton.

Myklebust, H. R. (1960). *The psychology of deafness.* New York: Grune & Stratton.

National Advisory Committee on Handicapped Children. (1968). *First annual report, special education for handicapped children.* Washington, DC: U.S. Office of Education, Department of Health, Education, and Welfare.

Neilsen, J., Sorensen, A. M., & Sorensen, K. (1981). Mental development of unselected children with sex chromosome abnormalities. *Human Genetics, 59,* 324–332.

Nelson, N. W. (1984). Beyond information processing: The language of teachers and textbooks. In G. P. Wallach and K. G. Butler (Eds.), *Language learning disabilities in school-age children* (pp. 154–178). Baltimore: Williams & Wilkins.

Nelson, N. W. (1994). Curriculum-based language assessment and intervention across the grades. In G. P. Wallach and K. G. Butler (Eds.), *Language learning disabilities in school-age children and adolescents: Some principles and applications* (pp. 104–131). New York: Merrill.

Nodine, B. F., Barenbaum, E., & Newcomber, P. (1985). Story grammar and comprehension and production of narrative prose by students with learning disabilities. *Journal of Learning Disabilities, 23,* 190–197.

Pennington, B., Puck, M., & Robinson, A. (1980). Language and cognitive development in 47, XXX females followed since birth. *Behavioral Genetics, 10,* 31–41.

Proceedings of the Institute on Childhood Aphasia. (1962). Chicago, IL: National Society for Crippled Children and Adults.

Puck, M., Tennes, K., Frankenburg, W., Bryant, K., & Robinson, A. (1975). Early childhood development of four boys with 47, XXX karyotype. *Clinical Genetics, 7,* 8–20.

Putnam, M. L., Deshler, D. D., & Schumaker, J. B. (1993). The investigation of setting demands: A missing link in learning strategy instruction. In. L. J. Meltzer (Ed.), *Strategy assessment and instruction for students with learning disabilities* (pp. 325–353). Austin, TX: Pro-ed.

Rice, M. L. (1994). Grammatical categories of children with specific language impairments. In R. V. Watkins & M. L. Rice (Eds.), *Specific language impairments in children* (pp. 69–90). Baltimore: Paul H. Brookes.

Rissman, M., Curtiss, S., & Tallal, P. (1990). School placement outcomes of young language impaired children. *Journal of Speech Language Pathology and Audiology, 14,* 49–58.

Robinson, A., Puck, M., & Pennington, B. (1979). Abnormalities of the sex chromosomes: A prospective study on randomly identified newborns. *Birth Defects, 15,* 203–241.

Roth, F., & Spekman, N. (1986). Narrative discourse: Spontaneously generated stories of learning disabled and normally achieving students. *Journal of Speech and Hearing Disorders, 51,* 8–23.

Roth, F. P., & Spekman, N. J. (1989). Higher-order language process and reading disabilities. In A. G. Kamhi & H. W. Catts (Eds.), *Reading disabilities: A developmental language perspective* (pp. 159–190). Boston: Little, Brown and Co.

Rubin, H., Bernstein, S., & Katz, R. B. (1989). Effect of cues on object naming in first-grade good and poor readers. *Annals of Dyslexia, 39,* 116–124.

Rudel, R. G., Holmes, J. M., & Pardes, J. R. (1988). *Assessment of developmental learning disorders: A neuropsychological approach.* New York: Basic Books.

Scarborough, H. S. (1990). Very early language deficits in dyslexic children. *Child Development, 61,* 1728–1743.

Scarborough, H. S. (1991). Early syntactic development of dyslexic children. *Annals of Dyslexia, 41,* 207–220.

Scarborough, H. S., & Dobrich, W. (1990). Development of children with early language delay. *Journal of Speech and Hearing Research, 33,* 70–83.

Scott, C. M. (1989). Problem writers: Nature, assessment, and intervention. In A. G. Kahmi & H. W. Catts (Eds.), *Reading disability: A developmental language perspective* (pp. 303–344). Boston: Little, Brown and Company.

Shaywitz, S. E. (1989). *Developmental changes in learning and behavior: Results of the Connecticut Longitudinal Study.* The Fifth Annual Conference on Learning Disorders: Cognitive, Linguistic, and Developmental Variations. Cambridge, MA: Graduate School of Education, Harvard University.

Shaywitz, S. E., Shaywitz, B. A., Flectcher, J. M., & Escobar, M. D. (1990). Prevalence of reading disability in boys and girls. *Journal of the American Medical Association, 264,* 998–1002.

Sheridan, M. D., & Peckham, C. (1975). Follow-up at 11 years of children who had marked speech defects at 7 years. *Child: Care, Health and Development, 1,* 157–166.

Stanovich, K. E. (1986). Matthew effects in reading: Some consequences of individual differences in the acquisition of literacy. *Reading Research Quarterly, 21,* 360–407.

Stanovich, K. E. (1988). Explaining the differences between the dyslexic and the garden-variety poor reader: The phonological-core variable-difference model. *Journal of Learning Disabilities, 21,* 590–604.

Stanovich, K. E. (1993). Problems in the differential diagnosis of reading disabilities. In R. M. Joshi & C. K. Leong (Eds.), *Reading disabilities: Diagnosis and component processes* (pp. 3–31). Dordrecht, The Netherlands: Kluwer Academic.

Stark, R. E., Bernstein, L. E., Condino, R., Bender, M., Tallal, P., & Catts, H. (1984). Four-year follow-up study of language impaired children. *Annals of Dyslexia, 34,* 49–68.

Starkweather, C. W., & Gottwald, S. R. (1990). The demands and capacities model II: Clinical applications. *Journal of Fluency Disorders, 15,* 143–157.

Strominger, A. Z. (1983). *A follow-up of reading and linguistic abilities in language delayed children.* Unpublished doctoral dissertation, Boston University.

Strominger, A. Z., & Bashir A. S. (1977). *A nine year follow-up of language disordered children.* Paper presented at the American Speech and Hearing Association Meeting, Chicago.

Swanson, H. L. (1987). Information-processing theory and learning disabilities: An overview. *Journal of Learning Disabilities, 20,* 3–7.

Swartz, E. R., & Solot, C. B. (1980). Response patterns characteristic of verbal expressive disorders. *Language, Speech, and Hearing Services in Schools, 21,* 139–144.

Tallal, P. (1980a). Auditory temporal perception, phonics and reading disabilities in children. *Brain and Language, 9,* 182–198.

Tallal, P. (1980b). Language and reading: Some perceptual prerequisites. *Bulletin of the Orton Society, 30,* 170–178.

Tallal, P. (1988). Developmental language disorders. In J. F. Kavanagh & T. J. Truss, Jr. (Eds.), *Learning disabilities: Proceedings of the national conference* (pp. 181–272). Parkton, MD: York Press.

Tallal, P. (1990, March). *A follow-up study of children with language disorders.* Paper presented at The New York Orton Dyslexia Society, New York.

Tallal, P., Ross, R., & Curtiss, S. (1989). Familial aggregation in specific language impairment. *Journal of Speech and Hearing Disorders, 54,* 167–173.

Tallal, P., & Stark, R. E. (1982). Perceptual/motor profiles of reading impaired children with or without concomitant oral language deficits. *Annals of Dyslexia, 32,* 163–176.

Torgeson, J. K., & Licht, B. (1983). The learning disabled child as an inactive learner: Retrospect and prospects. In J. D. McKinney & L. Feagans (Eds.), *Current topics in learning disabilities* (pp. 3–31). Norwood, NJ: Ablex.

Tunmer, W. E., & Hoover, W. A. (1993). Components of variance models of language-related factors in reading disability: A conceptual overview. In R. M. Joshi & C. K. Leong (Eds.), *Reading disabilities: Diagnosis and component processes* (pp. 135–173). Dordrecht, The Netherlands: Kluwer Academic.

Vogel, S. A., & Adelman, P. B. (1990). Extrinsic and intrinsic factors in graduation and academic failure among LD college students. *Annals of Dyslexia, 40,* 119–137.

Wagner, R., & Togesen, J. (1987). The nature of phonological processing and its causal role in the equation of reading skills. *Psychological Bulletin, 101,* 192–212.

Wallach, G. P. (1985). What do we really mean by verbal language proficiency? Higher level language learning and school performance. *Peabody Journal of Education, 62,* 44–69.

Walzer, S., Wolff, P., Bowen, D., Bashir, A. S., Silbert, A., Gerald, P., Richmond, J. (1978). A method for the longitudinal study of behavioral development in infants and children. The early development of XXY children. *Journal of Child Psychology and Psychiatry, 19,* 213–229.

Ward, S., & McCartney, E. (1976). Congenital auditory imperception—A follow up study. *British Journal of Disorders of Communication, 13,* 3–17.

Watkins, R. V. (1994). Grammatical challenges for children with specific language impairments. In R. V. Watkins & M. L. Rice (Eds.), *Specific language impairments in children* (pp. 53–89). Baltimore: Paul H. Brookes.

Weiner, P. S. (1972). The perceptual functioning of dysphasic children: A follow-up study. *Journal of Speech and Hearing Research, 15,* 423–438.

Weiner, P. S. (1974). A language-delayed child at adolescence. *Journal of Speech and Hearing Disorders, 39,* 202–213.

Weiner, P. S. (1985). The value of follow-up studies. *Topics in Language Disorders, 5,* 78–92.

Westby, C. E. (1985). Learning to talk—talking to learn: Oral-literate language differences. In C. S. Simon (Ed.), *Communication skills and classroom success.* San Diego: College-Hill Press.

Westby, C. E. (1989). Assessing and remediating text comprehension problems. In A. G. Kamhi & H. W. Catts (Eds.), *Reading disabilities: A developmental language perspective* (pp. 199–260). Boston: Little, Brown and Company.

Wiig, E. H., & Fleischmann, N. (1980). Knowledge of pronominalization, reflexivization, and relativization by learned disabled college students. *Journal of Learning Disabilities, 12,* 571–578.

Wiig, E. H., & Semel, E. H. (1973). Comprehension of linguistic concepts requiring logical operations by learning disabled children. *Journal of Speech and Hearing Research, 16,* 627–636.

Wiig, E. H., & Semel, E. M. (1974). Development of comprehension of logic-grammatical sentences by grade school children. *Perceptual and Motor Skills, 38,* 171–176.

Wiig, E. H., & Semel, E. M. (1976). *Language disabilities in children and adolescents.* Columbus, OH: Charles E. Merrill.

Wiig, E. H., & Semel, E. M. (1984). *Language assessment and intervention for the learning disabled,* 2nd ed. Columbus, OH: Charles E. Merrill.

Wolf, M. (1982). The word-retrieval process and reading in children and aphasics. In K. Nelson (Ed.), *Children's language, Vol. III.* Hillsdale, NJ: Erlbaum.

Wolf, M., Bally, H., & Morris, R. (1986). Automaticity, retrieval processes, and reading: A longitudinal study in average and impaired readers. *Child Development, 57,* 988–1000.

7

Specific Language Impairment

A Changing Role for Normal Developmental Language Theories During the 1990s

HOLLY K. CRAIG, PH.D.

Introduction

The study of childhood language disorders is an applied discipline. Typically, the theorist examines promising normal language models and theories that are guiding research in related disciplines and that seem to have potential application to the study of children's language problems. The investigator formulates questions and methodologies consistent with these theoretical orientations and then probes how the child with a language problem appears similar or dissimilar to the child with normal language. The motivations for these endeavors derive from the pursuit of two goals: (1) to describe the linguistic and nonlinguistic characteristics of a particular language disorder, and (2) to discover a valid explanation for the nature of the disorder.

This chapter discusses the advantages and limitations of this applied process for the study of one particular type of developmental childhood language disorder: specific language impairment (SLI). Children with this type of problem have been a long-standing research priority in the field of speech-language pathology, and in the past they have been identified as language delayed, language disordered, and language-learning disabled. For the purposes of this chapter, the term *specific language impairment* will reference children defined by the widely used Stark and Tallal (1981) exclusion criteria. Accordingly, children with SLI evidence significant and primary expressive language deficits in the apparent absence of intellectual, sensory, motor, neurological, or emotional problems. The accuracy of the descriptor-specific language impairment is not without controversy (Leonard, 1987) but is retained here as a common reference point because it is so widely used and because no better terminological candidate is available currently.

To focus this discussion, the following questions are posed:

1. What has the application of normal language theory contributed to our understanding of SLI? What are the advantages represented by the continued

application of normal language theories to the study of this particular type of childhood language disorder?

2. Are there ways in which the applied approach restricts theorizing about SLI?
3. Relative to these contributions and restrictions, what are the implications for clinical practice and for future research with this population?

The Contributions of Normal Language Theories

The application of normal developmental theories to the study of children's language problems is historically rooted and is the predominant current approach to inquiry. The contributions of each past major theoretical approach, as well as how each conceptualized the nature of the language problem presented by the child with SLI, are discussed.

Behavioristic Theories

Borrowed from the prominent psychological theories of the 1950s (especially Skinner, 1954, 1968), behaviorism made major contributions to the study of childhood language disorders by focusing on the quantification of differences from a normal language standard. The theoretical assumptions underlying behaviorism emphasized the description of discrete observable behaviors, the conceptualization of complex behaviors as an expansion of simpler behaviors, and the definition of learning as an increase in response strength over time (Holland, 1960; Holland & Skinner, 1961). Applications yielded age-referenced computations of language behaviors, including vocabulary size, sentence length, and phoneme repertoires (McCarthy, 1954; Templin, 1957). Accordingly, children with language problems were considered to be those whose test performances fell short of a norm-referenced, age-based statistical value.

Like most influential theories, behaviorism contributed to its own demise. It supported the generation of enough new knowledge that ultimately its own limitations became clear. In terms of the present discussion, for example, focusing as the theory did on observable behaviors and environmental stimuli, problems in language acquisition were viewed simply as quantitative differences from normal linguistic behavior due presumably to faulty relationships between stimulus and response. In other words, the oral productions of the child with SLI were characterized by limited vocabularies, shorter sentence lengths, and smaller numbers of adult-like phonemes, all due ostensibly to the child's incomplete or inadequate imitations of adult stimulus models available in the environment.

A number of criticisms were eventually directed at the theory, a discussion of which are beyond the scope of this chapter. For the present purposes, however, it became clear that although behaviorism might contribute to an understanding of some aspects of *how* a child acquires language, it offered little to the conceptualization of *what* was or was not being acquired. For the child with SLI, therefore, behaviorism offered little conceptually beyond norm-referenced language tests with which to quantify the amount of impairment, paired with the impressive technology of operant conditioning as a framework for intervention procedures.

(See Craig, 1983, for a more detailed discussion of the contributions of behaviorism to intervention.)

Generative Theories

In a context of mounting dissatisfaction with behaviorism's limitations, during the 1960s prominent generative syntactic theories (Braine, 1963; Chomsky, 1957, 1965; Lenneberg, 1967; McNeill, 1966) were applied to the study of childhood language disorders. Generative syntax emphasized grammatical regularities in language production. Language acquisition was viewed as the development of grammatical systems and the evolution of sets of phrase structure and transformational, morphological, and phonological rules into increasingly adult-like grammars.

From a generative syntactic perspective, the child with SLI was considered to be one whose grammar was unlike that of the child developing language normally. The impact of this theoretical change was profound for speech-language pathology. Assessments dramatically shifted away from the test administrations typical of behaviorism toward the collection and analysis of spontaneous speech and language samples. Based on a host of carefully conducted, labor-intensive investigations (for example, Johnston & Schery, 1976; Lee, 1966; Leonard, 1972; Menyuk, 1964; Menyuk & Looney, 1972; Morehead & Ingram, 1973), the sentence formulation skills of the child with SLI were found to differ from that of the child with normal language skills. Overall, children with SLI demonstrated the production of shorter utterances, simpler syntax, and persistent morphological errors at virtually any age or stage of language acquisition.

During the 1970s, the search for underlying linguistic regularities turned toward the characterization of sentence meanings or functions underlying grammatical expressions. Borrowing from psycholinguistics, generative semantic theories of language acquisition (Bloom, 1970; Bowerman, 1973; Brown, 1973; Chafe, 1970; Schlesinger, 1974; Slobin, 1973) quickly influenced the utterance production goals of intervention program planning so that differences in both utterance content and form were considered important (see especially Bloom & Lahey, 1978). Only a few intermittent studies have been conducted that compare directly the sentence meanings conveyed by word relationships between children with SLI and those with normal language skills. In particular, Leonard and colleagues found that children with SLI differed in their frequency of use of specific semantic categories, such as agent-verb relationships (Leonard, Bolders, & Miller, 1976; Leonard, Steckol, & Schwartz, 1978).

These generative approaches continue to motivate important descriptions of the oral production skills of children with SLI. The works of Fletcher and colleagues (Fletcher, 1991; Fletcher & Garman, 1988; Fletcher & Peters, 1984) are notable examples.

Pragmatic Theories

Other researchers have applied pragmatics (Austin, 1962; Bates, 1976; Searle, 1969) to their search for rule-system differences between SLI and normal language acquisition, principally looking for significant discourse in addition to sentence meaning discrepancies (Brinton & Fujiki, 1982; Craig & Gallagher, 1986; Gallagher & Craig, 1984; Gallagher & Darnton, 1978; Leonard, 1986; Prinz, 1982; Skarakis & Greenfield, 1982; VanKleeck & Frankel, 1981). When analyzing discourse, for example, an utterance may take the form of a statement or code an internal state, but in the context of dialogue it may convey the interactive force of a request. For example, the utterance "I need this open" said by a girl holding a closed box and directed toward her mother could be scored syntactically as a declarative, semantically as coding a state, and functionally as a request for action. Identification of interlocutor regularities and, for SLI, significant differences from normal expectations for the latter types of discourse meanings have been the primary contributions of this line of research.

Pragmatics has been warmly embraced as a theoretical and practical guide for language disorders, so much so that the 1980s have been characterized as the time of a pragmatics "revolution" (Duchan, 1984). As Gallagher (1990) recalls, pragmatic perspectives return us to concerns stated by the earliest scholars: The identification of a language disorder is defined in large part by its significant negative social consequences. Pragmatics offers the theorist a systematic framework within which to investigate the communication failures of children with SLI and to explore their potential grammatical, referential, and/or conversational causes.

Pragmatically, to some extent children with SLI appear similar to the normal language child. Early in development, particularly at the one-word stage, the child with SLI formulates requests and comments and foregrounds and backgrounds information for the listener to the same extent as language-matched controls (Leonard, Camarata, Rowan, & Chapman, 1982; Rowan, Leonard, Chapman, & Weiss, 1983; Skarakis & Greenfield, 1982; Snyder, 1978). In addition, Craig and Evans (1989) observed major similarities among the turn-management characteristics of spontaneous discourse by children with SLI as by age-matched and language-matched control subjects with normally developing language. The subjects' other discourse characteristics—including their narrative production, formulation of conversational repairs, and speech act repertoires at language levels beyond the one-word stage—appear essentially similar to those predicted by a normal comparison group (Blank, Gessner, & Esposito, 1979; Brinton & Fujiki, 1982; Brinton, Fujiki, Winkler, & Loeb, 1986; Gallagher & Craig, 1984; Gallagher & Darnton, 1978; Liles, 1985, 1987; Prinz, 1982; VanKleeck & Frankel, 1981). Further, Leonard (1986) found that children with SLI at the one-word stage were even more responsive and used a greater variety of responses than normal language-matched controls.

The above-mentioned research in a number of ways represents another generative approach. These pragmatic studies reflect many of the same assumptions as generative theory (syntax and semantics) in that they posit a small but comprehensive set of discourse regularities or rules and envision the ultimate formulation of a discourse schema evolving across development into increasingly mature, adult-like grammatical systems. Most generative pragmatic research focuses on the search for a conversational analogue to phonology, morphology, syntax, and semantics. Viewed from this perspective, the literature indicates that children with SLI present the same profile of discourse functions as those developing language normally but do exhibit ongoing difficulties in using linguistic forms for their expression. It is possible to conclude, therefore, that children with SLI are as pragmatically intact as one would predict they could be based on their limited linguistic resources (Johnston, 1988).

The conversational analogue approach is only one perspective on pragmatics, however, and a more functionalist approach (Bates, 1976; Bates & MacWhinney, 1987, 1989; Bates, Thal, & MacWhinney, 1991; MacWhinney, 1987, 1991) focuses on interactions between systems, especially the connections among functions and forms. Functionalism may isolate as yet undetected but basic conversational-linguistic deficits for SLI. Research of this type with this population will require specific research design controls not apparent in most prior investigations of pragmatics. Most critically, these will include task controls for ensuring that subjects with SLI evidence the necessary linguistic forms and discourse functions in their oral productions prior to experimentally probing to see how they try to link the two (Craig, 1995).

Pursuing pragmatics from a functionalist perspective seems warranted because the pragmatic profile for SLI emerging within conversational analogue approaches is not a consistent one. In particular, some children with SLI do seem to experience more interactional difficulties than predicted by their linguistic form deficits. They evidence more differences from the patterns presented by normal language children than even other children with SLI of comparable ages and expressive skill levels (Craig & Evans, 1989; Craig & Evans, in press; Craig & Washington, 1993). Further, a number of studies reveal considerable performance heterogeneity within small subject samples (see, for example, Craig & Evans, 1989; Fujiki, Brinton, & Sonnenberg, 1990; VanKleeck & Frankel, 1981). The source of this variability remains unknown at this time, but as I have suggested elsewhere, different processing skills may be responsible in part for the finding that some children with SLI function pragmatically like their normal language peers whereas others present quantitative and probably qualitative differences (Craig & Evans, 1993; Craig & Washington, 1993). There may be an identifiable subgroup of children with SLI who, in functionalist terms, present basic pragmatic deficits by failing to integrate forms and functions.

Considerable additional research is needed, however, to distinguish whether these conversational differences reflect a paucity of forms for demonstrating a conversational function, something more generalized like slow and sluggish encoding and decoding, or a failure to acquire rules for selecting among lexical, syntactic, and semantic alternatives when forming specific conversational-linguistic matches. Outcomes like each of these would imply explanations for discourse differences in terms of a research design problem, a pragmatic performance problem, or a pragmatic competence problem, respectively (Craig, 1995). Overall, from a pragmatic perspective, the child with SLI is considered to be one who is an ineffective communicator, although the linguistic, conversational, or conversational-linguistic basis for that ineffectiveness remains under debate.

Advantages of Applying Normal Language Models

As Kuhn (1970) has discussed, the process of scientific inquiry is fundamentally inductive in nature. It involves the systematic acquisition of theory-driven "facts" and then the affirmation, modification, or rejection of these facts with each new theory, thereby resulting over time in the accumulation of a generally well-accepted knowledge base. The application of normal language theories to the study of SLI has mirrored this process and contributed a well-established set of facts about the functioning of this population. Accordingly, the cumulative facts garnered from behavioristic, generative syntactic, semantic, and pragmatic perspectives have contributed the following to our current characterization of children with SLI:

- They typically perform lower on standardized tests than age-referenced standards predict for normally developing children.
- They acquire language at a slower rate, and the period for acquisition is more protracted.
- Grammatical rules are immature for their age, and complex syntax and morphology may remain problematic across development.
- Their phoneme, vocabulary, and morpheme repertoires are typically smaller than their chronological age peers and more like those of younger children with normal language skills.
- Their utterances reflect the same relational semantic categories as those of their normal language peers, although frequencies of occurrence vary.
- Many children with SLI evidence the same discourse meanings as normal language peers and essentially similar turn-management skills, and they are responsive.
- Aspects of discourse that differ from normal expectations reflect problems with grammatical errors, semantic relatedness, and informational completeness.

Exclusion criteria define language as the problem domain for SLI (Stark & Tallal, 1981) and, as the preceding list of descriptors indicates, the language characteristics themselves reveal at least quantitative differences from patterns of normal acquisition. The application of normal language theories, therefore, has offered valuable assistance to the central SLI research goals: to describe the specific linguistic and nonlinguistic characteristics of this particular childhood language disorder.

Future Contributions of Normal Language Theories

In their seminal work on language disorders, Bloom and Lahey (1978, p. 35) emphasized a distinction made earlier by Kenneth Pike (1967) between etic and emic approaches to describing language behaviors. The language characteristics listed in the previous section resulted from etic analyses. Etic approaches use units available in advance, allow the formulation of predictions when applied to another type of language data, and offer a way to gain initial access to regularities in a particular language system. In contrast, emic approaches use units discovered during the analysis of the language system and probe their interactions.

Bloom and Lahey noted that beginning studies of normal language acquisition were etic in approach in that their starting point was a set of language behaviors derived from adult usage. Etic approaches, however, gave way to emic ones that used relevant child-based variables and looked for their interrelationships in child language data. Bloom and Lahey observed that a strictly etic approach is inherently limited and a strictly emic approach may be unsystematic. Instead, they recommended a more dynamic etic-emic-etic process for the study of language acquisition. As they discussed, this allows initial access to language systems to be guided by a priori hypotheses and results in all the systematicity that such an approach would represent but also permits the in-process discovery of unique variables relevant to eventually understanding a particular language system. Accordingly, these emic language variables would be used to make predictions about larger samples of the population or novel patterns of behaviors, which then could be tested and replicated.

Bloom and Lahey raised these issues at the time when (etic) adult models were defining the study of language usage by children. The same concerns pertain, however, to contemporary study of children's language disorders. The application of normal language theories to the study of language disorders constitutes an essentially etic approach. Categories of behavior now discovered from the study of children's normal language acquisition serve as a priori hypotheses about disordered language processes. As Miller (1991) observes, the primary research question for SLI has been, "Do children with language disorder do 'X' or have/perform 'X'?" (p. 4). The X variable in this question derives in advance from normal theories. Using this paradigm, Miller concludes that the answer to this question is usually yes, although with specific quantitative differences. As he summarizes, children with SLI evidence a later onset of language skills, progress more slowly in developing language, and may never achieve adult linguistic competence.

The application of etic/normal language models to the study of disorders has been advantageous in providing initial access to the domain of language disorder. It has provided a nonlinguistic and linguistic characterization of SLI that reveals a number of developmental trouble spots. The etic/normal application approach to language disorders should continue to prove valuable as a first-step research strategy when encountering characteristics of SLI not studied previously. A new promising application at this time, for example, involves studying the social skills of this population (Craig, 1993; Craig & Washington, 1993; Gallagher, 1991; Hadley & Rice, 1991; Rice, Sell, & Hadley, 1991; Roth & Clark, 1987).

Social skills are developmentally important in their own right. Depending as they do on intact language formulation and processing skills, these skills are at risk in children with language disorders. This new line of inquiry derives practical impetus from the day-to-day interactive difficulties observed for many children with SLI, and it also derives theoretical motivation from a logical extension of SLI pragmatic research (Prutting, 1982). As a first step, social skills of known developmental value have been identified from the normal language literature. These include peer relationships and, more specifically, interpersonal responsiveness or interactive behaviors when entering play groups. These social skills have been applied to the study of SLI, and discrepancies have been observed. This process is again etic in nature and reveals quantitative differences from normal developmental expectations. The strength of the etic approach is to isolate and describe characteristics differing from a predetermined standard and to identify variables for future exploration. The social skills studies, although currently few in number, have been successful in revealing that peer interactions by children with SLI are problematic and, therefore, warrant future in-depth investigation. Obviously, they are important developmental tools for a variety of other achievements.

Summary

Normal language theories, in their role as etic applications, have made important contributions to our understanding when applied to the study of SLI. They have provided a foundation to describe SLI quantitatively based on normal language expectations. As a way to gain initial access into the functioning of a particular language system, etic applications will continue to be useful as new language variables become the focus of investigation.

The Limitations of Normal Language Applications

Applications of normal language theories have yielded a well-accepted body of facts about SLI, but the etic approach is not well suited to the accomplishment of two other vital tasks. The etic approach seems unlikely to uncover unique features of disordered language or to explain the problem of specific language impairment. With normal developmental models serving as the sole prototype, the observation of any unique characteristics associated with SLI is precluded. Our current etic views of SLI are in essence a series of subtractions from normal development, a definition by default. They tell us what children with SLI are not doing rather than what they are doing; what language disorder is not rather than what it is.

Applications of normal language models also deemphasize those systems functioning within normal limits and reflect a general inattention to interactive effects between systems. An emic approach permits the exploration of performance outcomes and, thus, interrelationships between systems. Indeed, a more emic approach to inquiry is necessary to foster the discovery of new variables within the process of analysis and then the discovery of interrelationships among them. The language characteristics of SLI have been described quantitatively particularly as late onset, slow progress, and perhaps a ceiling on achievement. Outcomes other than these quantitative differences from normal are unlikely from an etic analysis of language disorder. As in any research endeavor, the choice of methods directly affects the kinds of results obtained. The application of etic approaches by its nature, therefore, is likely to constrain our ability to characterize any differences from normal that are more than quantitative. Other approaches may be more beneficial.

Johnston's (1988) comprehensive review of SLI presents a research agenda that is consistent with a more etic-to-emic approach, like that originally recommended by Bloom and Lahey. Noting that most research with the SLI population has examined one linguistic domain at a time, Johnston offered two critical examples of developmental asynchronies between language systems. First, she observed that a developmental gap exists between morphology and syntax when morphological errors apparent for children with SLI are compared to normally developing children whose mean lengths of utterance (MLUs) are comparable. Second, she proposed that older children with SLI (who by definition have normal IQs) should use vocabulary items that are more mature than their syntax, and yet this is not the case. Their vocabulary and syntax are comparable at various language levels, indicating another developmental gap.

As part of a search for interrelationships, Johnston and Kamhi (1984) profiled syntactic, morphological, semantic, and pragmatic behaviors of 5-year-old children with SLI and made comparisons to normal language controls. The children with SLI formulated sentences containing ellipsis, pronominalization, and imperatives like their MLU-matched subjects but made more morphological errors and produced fewer sentences with embedded propositions. Johnston's (1988) review allows us to ask why children with SLI acquire different aspects of language at different rates. This is a daunting question and one not readily approachable within a strictly etic approach.

How might one move beyond current tactics and take a more emic approach to inquiry for SLI? In Chapter 2 of this book, Bjorklund and Schwartz argue for the integrity of developmental periods, a proposal with clear potential for grounding emic approaches. Rather than viewing development as a progression from immature/inefficient to mature/efficient states, they propose that serious consideration be given to the view that young normal language children's immature cognition is well suited to the learning tasks they face.

Is There Integrity in the Developmental States of Children with SLI?

The relationship between cognition and language is an interesting place to begin to address this question and one for which considerable empirical data are available for understanding both systems. By definition, children with SLI evidence nonverbal IQ scores within normal ranges, but current theorizing does little with this information beyond citing its role as an exclusion criterion for diagnostic purposes. Although a number of researchers have questioned whether subtle cognitive deficits not tapped by traditional IQ tests are present for SLI and, thus, play a causal role (see recent observations made by Johnston, 1991; Kamhi, this volume), the general intellectual function of these children appears to be within normal limits. If SLI performance reflects developmental integrity, then how does normal cognition act to affect language development in this population? Are there co-occurring influences which may account in part for the profile of language characteristics currently ascribed to SLI?

Consider again the report of persistent difficulties with morphology in this population even when syntax develops. Leonard (1989) has proposed that learnability theory (Pinker, 1984) accounts for the SLI morphological problems. Accordingly, some morphemes have low phonetic substance and, therefore, are predictably more difficult to acquire by individuals with SLI who evidence perceptual limitations (Stark & Tallal, 1981; Tallal, Stark, Kallman, & Mellits, 1981). However, for reasons discussed by Kamhi in this volume as an application of normal language theory to disorder (and by MacWhinney, 1991, more generally), learnability theory falls short in explanatory power. Indeed, the fact that it is another etic application suggests that this approach can only offer our understanding of SLI more of the same. Similarly, learnability theory as applied to the study of SLI is a conceptually weak approach because it has little to contribute to the current research edge of the field. The performance of children with SLI may represent some interesting tests of assumptions specific to learnability theory without informing our understanding of SLI. Future research needs to isolate unique characteristics of the disorder, including unusual interrelationships between linguistic systems and ultimately the reasons underlying anomalous patterns not predicted by current theory.

Alternatively, the developmental gaps between syntax and morphology have been described for other populations as well. Newport (1990) observed discrepancies between word-order acquisition and other grammatical structures for individuals learning a primary language (specifically, American Sign Language) and second-language learners of English. She found that although constraints on word order were readily mastered, morphology was affected by the age of learning. In an important examination of the long-standing critical periods hypothesis, she proposed that the ability to learn language declines with maturation for the same reason that cognitive abilities advance. She noted that young children focus more on parts than wholes. The cognitive saliency of components of all types in the young child is an advantage when learning involves componential analyses (e.g., for language, those components involved in the learning of morphology). Accordingly, cognition in young children seems specially suited to the learning of morphological rules. Cognitively, the older child finds wholes rather than parts more salient, so broad conceptualizations and the integration of ideas are facilitated. For language, the cognitive saliency afforded wholes is advantageous for older learners, including efforts to fit language into larger interactive schemes, to advance world knowledge, and to expand vocabulary and alternative discourse genres. The older learner may be disadvantaged, however, when the analysis of componential parts is involved, again as in the case of morphology. By implication, older and basically cognitively intact children with SLI may never master morphology as a consequence of being a more mature learner. The cognition of the 2- to 3-year-old is well suited to learning morphology, but the cognition of the 12-year-old is not. Perhaps the grammatical look, therefore, to the nature of SLI is defined less by morphological properties than by age of the population at testing.

Again, for the purposes of this chapter, etic approaches are not conducive to this kind of questioning, whereas emic approaches that probe interrelationships are. As the Bjorklund and Schwartz proposals underscore, instead of focusing on those behaviors not yet present in SLI, we ought to assume that the functional status of children with SLI reflects a developmental integrity and then determine the co-occurring influences operating among these systems.

The Bjorklund and Schwartz viewpoints require that future theorizing address the ways in which different systems interact in SLI. For example, in what ways do more intact motor and cognitive systems influence language outcomes? If articulation and cognition are more preserved in SLI, how do these enhance and degrade the acquisition of linguistic systems? Continued broad-based application of normal developmental theories may not allow researchers to ask the most sensitive questions. At this time, a shift to emic-oriented approaches would foster consideration of the functioning of children with SLI in their own right rather than as a subtraction from normal language patterns.

Implications for Future Research

An emic orientation to inquiry for SLI will require fundamental changes in our research protocols. It is unclear at the outset what changes this may entail, but two possibilities are suggested in this section. First, the selection of control groups in research designs warrants reconsideration. Typical research protocols involve two control groups: one matched for chronological age (and presumably mental age and social maturity) and one for language status (usually defined by MLU). An increasing number of researchers have suggested that a standard control group protocol applied uniformly across studies may have little utility for understanding SLI (Conti-Ramsden, 1985; Craig, 1995; Johnston, 1988; Miller, 1991), but instead controls should be selected for their potential contrastive value specific to particular questions or hypotheses. For example, the MLU match continues to have merit when research questions require a contrast reasonably indexed by changes in average utterance length. It fails to be informative when social skills, receptive skills, or other nongrammatical behaviors are the investigative focus. Johnston (1988) has asked specifically that we reexamine reliance on MLU-defined control subjects in instances when linguistic forms are not the focus. However, Newport's (1990) proposals considered in concert with those of Bjorklund and Schwartz (in this volume) further imply that no valid control group can be found for any language system when studying SLI because these systems are codetermined by others. Considerable future deliberations will be required to ensure that research designs employ maximally informative experimental contrasts.

Second, we may need to attend more to error patterns in performance profiles. Fletcher (1991) asks, "Are there features of the language-impaired data that are being missed, when our perspective is limited to what is sufficient for an account of normal development?" (p. 173). He goes on to suggest that mazes (self-corrections), formulation problems, and grammatical errors may be particularly rich sources of information for understanding the syntax profiles of children with SLI. Newport (1990) found that younger learners and older learners make different types of errors in the early stages of language learning. The errors of late learners reflected unanalyzed wholes and evidenced difficulties in breaking complex structures into component parts, whereas young learners made componential errors in which only parts of structures were produced and whole morphemes were omitted. Error analyses represent an emic approach to inquiry and, therefore, should be pursued as an alternative approach to prior etic normal theory applications. Overall, Miller (1991) proposes that error analyses may be necessary to document different types of language disorders.

Implications for Clinical Management

Etic approaches to understanding SLI provide the clinician with a template for identifying language disorder. The syntactic, semantic, and pragmatic taxonomies available in the literature detail the behaviors presented by the child with SLI that will most likely differ from normal language expectations. This information is invaluable when asking the basic assessment question: Does this child have a language problem?

Current etic characterizations unfortunately, however, provide little clinical insight into the developmental integrity of the communication skills presented by the child with SLI. The clinician has little guidance from the extant literature as to which principles are governing the kinds of linguistic choices that the child with SLI makes when speaking or when processing another's speech. The clinical consequences of this paucity of more etic-emic information about SLI are profound. Viewing the child with SLI from an etic perspective implies that we have excellent tools available to detect differences from normal language expectations and can diagnose SLI with reasonable confidence. Viewing the child with SLI from an etic-emic perspective, we have much less confidence about the nature of the developmental problem requiring clinical management.

If the functioning of children with SLI reflects as much (albeit different) developmental integrity as any other maturing organism, then some alternative clinical strategies are implied. First, once assessments have established that the child is performing differently than predicted by normal language expectations and in what language domains, additional normative comparisons are unwarranted. Instead, it should be more fruitful for the clinician to try to determine how and why the child's performances are different. The co-occurring effects of intact motor skills and age-appropriate cognition seem especially relevant for children with SLI. Accordingly, assessments need to include testing of these nonlinguistic domains to develop a comprehensive profile of the child with SLI. Intervention goals then can be set with all of these systems considered together.

In our Outpatient Clinic at the University of Michigan, for example, we recently assessed a 16-year-old male incarcerated in a juvenile detention center who was referred for extremely limited language expression. For the purposes of this discussion, I will name this client Max. Our assessment of Max's communication skills revealed key problems with expression, such that his utterances were typically two- and three-word combinations without any evidence of mastery of complex syntax. His comprehension skills were also below age level, and his speech was extremely unintelligible. Pragmatically, however, he assumed both initiator and respondent roles, and his nonverbal performance IQ indicated average functioning. Viewing Max's functioning from a perspective of developmental integrity simply emphasizes the need to consider all systems at the same clinical decision point. There is nothing radically different in this assessment and intervention goal-setting approach. When considered together, this profile led to the formulation of intervention goals designed to increase the length, complexity, and clarity of Max's utterance formulation.

Second, maturing cognition may impose a pedagogic ceiling on some types of language learning. Consider again the clinical example of Max. One strategy for improving his utterance formulations would be to focus on morphology, syntax, and phonology in parallel. Accordingly, intervention might be directed toward eliminating specific phonological processes and toward including omitted morphosyntactic forms so that grammatical relationships are expressed more completely and correctly. This strategy is incompatible, however, with a perspective that emphasizes the developmental integrity of Max's functioning. Targeting phonological processes and grammatical constituents ignores his chronological age and the relatively adult-like cognition that his 16 years represent. Without the developmental integrity perspective, it would be possible to consider intelligence and receptive language performances as exclusionary criteria for diagnosing the language disorder and poor intelligibility as a complicating parallel factor. A second strategy that seems more consistent with the developmental integrity approach was adopted after the first strategy produced only limited results. This second strategy acknowledged that Max's cognitive maturity would have diminished the saliency of parts of larger components (e.g., of morphemes and phonemes as parts of utterances). Alternatively then, we focused on utterances as whole interactive units in contexts designed to exploit Max's ability to be a respondent. Intervention used interactive response routines developed to be relevant for vocational and classroom communications. Utterance repertoires were established, and Max was encouraged to approximate the prosodic, phonological, and grammatical shape of the clinician's model when formulating them as responses. Max was responsive to patterning whole utterances, and his ability to communicate effectively in his educational and living environments improved dramatically. Overall, the developmental integrity approach suggests some exciting new directions for conceptualizing clinical management with older children and adolescents.

Third, error analyses can be informative for clinical purposes as well as for research. VanKleeck and Richardson (1986) discuss how clinicians' responses to children's errors are a critical part of intervention but not yet an integral component of the lesson plan. Practically, errors may offer clues about the nature of the difficulty the child is having during intervention and conceptually provide insights about the special constraints that govern language use in SLI.

Conclusion

This chapter highlights the contributions of normal language theories to our understanding of SLI and speculates about the contributions and limitations of this primary approach to inquiry. It is suggested that applications of normal language theories offer an informative initial strategy when approaching new language systems but are limited beyond that type of contribution. An understanding of SLI will remain critically incomplete until any unique characteristics associated with the disorder are discovered and until a credible explanation for the nature of the impairment is offered that accounts for both quantitative differences from normal and more unique features. Approaches which anchor themselves in the behavior of the child with SLI and only secondarily look to normal language patterns for interpretive assistance should prove more valuable in addressing these key unknowns. Current characterizations of SLI indicate that the applications of normal language theories have been successful in providing linguistic and nonlinguistic outlines, but more in-process analyses are necessary to complete the SLI profile and to explain its existence.

References

Austin, J. (1962). *How to do things with words.* Oxford, UK: Oxford University Press.
Bates, E. (1976). *Language and context.* New York: Academic Press.

Bates, E., & MacWhinney, B. (1987). Competition, variation and language learning. In B. MacWhinney (Ed.), *Mechanisms of language acquisition* (pp. 157–194). Hillsdale, NJ: Erlbaum.

Bates, E., & MacWhinney, B. (1989). Functionalism and the competition model. In B. MacWhinney & E. Bates (Eds.), *The crosslinguistic study of sentence processing* (pp. 3–73). New York: Cambridge University Press.

Bates, E., Thal, D., & MacWhinney, B. (1991). A functionalist approach to language and its implications for assessment and intervention. In T. M. Gallagher (Ed.), *Pragmatics of language: Clinical practice issues* (pp. 133–161). San Diego: Singular Publishing Group, Inc.

Blank, M., Gessner, M., & Esposito, A. (1979). Language without communication: A case study. *Journal of Child Language, 6,* 329–352.

Bloom, L. (1970). *Language development: Form and function in emerging grammars.* Cambridge, MA: MIT Press.

Bloom, L., & Lahey, M. (1978). *Language development and language disorders.* New York: Wiley.

Bowerman, M. (1973). Structural relationships in children's utterances: Syntactic or semantic? In T. Moore (Ed.), *Cognitive development and the acquisition of language* (pp. 197–213). New York: Academic Press.

Braine, M. D. S. (1963). The ontogeny of English phrase structure: The first phase. *Language, 39,* 1–13.

Brinton, B., & Fujiki, M. (1982). A comparison of request-response sequences in the discourse of normal and language-disordered children. *Journal of Speech and Hearing Disorders, 47,* 57–62.

Brinton, B., Fujiki, M., Winkler, E., & Loeb, D. (1986). Responses to requests for clarification in linguistically normal and language-impaired children. *Journal of Speech and Hearing Disorders, 51,* 370–378.

Brown, R. (1973). *A first language.* Cambridge, MA: Harvard University Press.

Chafe, W. (1970). *Meaning and the structure of language.* Chicago: University of Chicago Press.

Chomsky, N. (1957). *Syntactic structures.* The Hague: Mouton.

Chomsky, N. (1965). *Aspects of the theory of syntax.* Cambridge, MA: MIT Press.

Conti-Ramsden, G. (1985). Mothers in dialogue with language-impaired children. *Topics in Language Disorders, 5,* 58–68.

Craig, H. K. (1983). Applications of pragmatic language models for intervention. In T. Gallagher & C. Prutting (Eds.), *Pragmatic assessment and intervention issues in language* (pp. 101–127). San Diego, CA: College-Hill Press.

Craig, H. K., & Gallagher, T. M. (1986). Interactive play: The frequency of related verbal responses. *Journal of Speech and Hearing Research, 29,* 375–383.

Craig, H., & Evans, J. (1989). Turn exchange characteristics of SLI children's simultaneous and nonsimultaneous speech. *Journal of Speech and Hearing Disorders, 54,* 334–347.

Craig, H. K., & Washington, J. A. (1993). Access behaviors of children with Specific Language Impairment. *Journal of Speech and Hearing Research, 36,* 322–337.

Craig, H. K. (1993). Social skills of children with specific language impairment: Peer relationships. *Language, Speech, and Hearing Services in Schools, 24,* 206–215.

Craig, H. K. (1995). Pragmatic impairments. In P. Fletcher & B. MacWhinney (Eds.), *Handbook of child language* (pp. 633–640). Oxford, UK: Blackwell Publishers.

Craig, H., & Evans, J. (1993). Pragmatics and SLI: Within group variations in discourse profiles. *Journal of Speech and Hearing Research, 36,* 777–789.

Duchan, J. (1984). Language assessment: The pragmatics revolution. In R. Naremore (Ed.), *Language science* (pp. 147–180). San Diego, CA: College-Hill Press.

Fletcher, P., & Peters, J. (1984). Characterizing language impairment in children: An exploratory study. *Language Testing, 1,* 33–49.

Fletcher, P., & Garman, M. (1988). Normal language development and language impairment: Syntax and beyond. *Clinical Linguistics and Phonetics, 2,* 97–113.

Fletcher, P. (1991). Evidence from syntax for language impairment. In J. Miller (Ed.), *Research on child language disorders.* Austin, TX: Pro-ed.

Fujiki, M., Brinton, B., & Sonnenberg, E. (1990). Repair of overlapping speech in the conversations of specifically language-impaired and normally developing children. *Applied Psycholinguistics, 11,* 201–215.

Gallagher, T. M., & Darnton, B. (1978). Conversational aspects of the speech of language-disordered children: Revision behaviors. *Journal of Speech and Hearing Research, 21,* 118–135.

Gallagher, T. M., & Craig, H. K. (1984). Pragmatic assessment: Analysis of a highly frequent repeated utterance. *Journal of Speech and Hearing Disorders, 49,* 368–377.

Gallagher, T. M. (1990). Clinical pragmatics: Expectations and realizations. *Journal of Speech-Language Pathology and Audiology, 14,* 3–6.

Gallagher, T. M. (1991). Language and social skills: Implications for clinical assessment and intervention with school-age children. In T. M. Gallagher (Ed.), *Pragmatics of language: Clinical practice issues* (pp. 11–41). San Diego: Singular Publishing Group, Inc.

Hadley, P. A., & Rice, M. L. (1991). Conversational responsiveness of speech- and language-impaired preschoolers. *Journal of Speech and Hearing Research, 34,* 1308–1317.

Holland, J. G. (1960). Teaching machines: An application of principles from the laboratory. In A. A. Lumsdaine & R. Glaser (Eds.), *Teaching machines and programmed learning* (pp. 215–228). Washington, DC: National Educational Association.

Holland, J. G., & Skinner, B. F. (1961). *The analysis of behavior.* New York: McGraw-Hill.

Johnston, J., & Schery, T. (1976). The use of grammatical morphemes by children with communication disorders. In D. Morehead & A. Morehead (Eds.), *Normal and deficient child language.* Baltimore: University Park Press.

Johnston, J. L. (1991). Questions about cognition in children with specific language impairment. In. J. Miller (Ed.), *Research on child language disorders* (pp. 299–307). Austin, TX: Pro-ed.

Johnston, J. R., & Kamhi, A. G. (1984). Syntactic and semantic aspects of the utterances of language-impaired children: The same can be less. *Merill-Palmer Quarterly, 30,* 65–85.

Johnston, J. R. (1988). Specific language disorders in the child. In N. Lass, L. McReynolds, J. Northern, & D. Yoder (Eds.), *Handbook of speech-language pathology and audiology* (pp. 685–715). Philadelphia: W. B. Saunders.

Kuhn, T. (1970). *The structure of scientific revolutions,* 2nd ed. Chicago: The University of Chicago Press.

Lee, L. (1966). Developmental sentence types: A method for comparing normal and deviant syntactic development. *Journal of Speech and Hearing Disorders, 31,* 311–330.

Lenneberg, E. (1967). *Biological foundations of language.* New York: Wiley.

Leonard, L. (1972). What is deviant language? *Journal of Speech and Hearing Disorders, 37,* 427–446.

Leonard, L., Bolders, J., & Miller, J. (1976). An examination of the semantic relations reflected in the language usage of normal and language disordered children. *Journal of Speech and Hearing Research, 19,* 371–392.

Leonard, L., Steckol, K., & Schwartz, R. (1978). Semantic relations and utterance lengths in child language. In F. Peng & W. von Raffler Engel (Eds.), *Language acquisition and developmental kinesics* (pp. 93–105). Tokyo: University of Tokyo.

Leonard, L., Camarata, S., Rowan, L., & Chapman, K. (1982). The communicative functions of lexical usage by language-impaired children. *Applied Psycholinguistics, 3,* 109–125.

Leonard, L. (1986). Conversational replies of children with specific language impairment. *Journal of Speech and Hearing Research, 29,* 114–119.

Leonard, L. (1987). Is specific language impairment a useful construct? In S. Rosenberg (Ed.), *Advances in applied psycholinguistics: Vol. I. Disorders of first language development* (pp. 1–39). New York: Cambridge University Press.

Leonard, L. (1989). Language learnability and specific language impairment in children. *Applied Psycholinguistics, 10,* 179–202.

Liles, B. (1985). Cohesion in the narratives of normal and language disordered children. *Journal of Speech and Hearing Research, 28,* 123–133.

Liles, B. (1987). Episode organization and cohesive conjunctives in narratives of children with and without language disorder. *Journal of Speech and Hearing Research, 30,* 185–196.

MacWhinney, B. (1987). The competition model. In B. MacWhinney (Ed.), *Mechanisms of language acquisition* (pp. 249–308). Hillsdale, NJ: Erlbaum.

MacWhinney, B. (1991). Connectionism as a framework for language acquisition theory. In J. Miller (Ed.), *Research on child language disorders: A decade of progress* (pp. 73–103). Austin, TX: Pro-ed.

McCarthy, D. (1954). Language development in children. In P. Mussen (Ed.), *Carmichael's manual of child psychology.* New York: Wiley.

McNeill, D. (1966). Developmental psycholinguistics. In F. Smith & G. Miller (Eds.), *The genesis of language: A psycholinguistic approach* (pp. 89–91). Cambridge, MA: MIT Press.

Menyuk, P. (1964). Comparison of grammar of children with functionally deviant and normal speech. *Journal of Speech and Hearing Research, 7,* 109–121.

Menyuk, P., & Looney, P. (1972). A problem of language disorder: length vs. structure. *Journal of Speech and Hearing Research, 15,* 264–279.

Miller, J. F. (1991). Research on language disorders in children: A progress report. In. J. Miller (Ed.), *Research on child language disorders* (pp. 3–22). Austin, TX: Pro-ed.

Morehead, D., & Ingram, D. (1973). The development of base syntax in normal and linguistically deviant children. *Journal of Speech and Hearing Research, 16,* 330–352.

Newport, E. L. (1990). Maturational constraints on language learning. *Cognitive Science, 14,* 11–28.

Pike, K. (1967). *Language in relation to a unified theory of the structure of human behavior.* The Hague: Mouton & Co.

Pinker, S. (1984). *Language learnability and language development.* Cambridge, MA: Harvard University Press.

Prinz, P. (1982). An investigation of the comprehension and production of requests in normal and language-disordered children. *Journal of Communication Disorders, 15,* 75–93.

Prutting, C. (1982). Pragmatics as social competence. *Journal of Speech and Hearing Disorders, 47,* 123–134.

Rice, M. L., Sell, M. A., & Hadley, P. A. (1991). Social interactions of speech- and language-impaired children. *Journal of Speech and Hearing Research, 34,* 1299–1307.

Roth, F. P., & Clark, D. M. (1987). Symbolic play and social participation abilities of language-impaired and normally developing children. *Journal of Speech and Hearing Disorders, 52,* 17–29.

Rowan, L., Leonard, L., Chapman, K., & Weiss, A. (1983). Performative and presuppositional skills in language-disordered and normal children. *Journal of Speech and Hearing Research, 26,* 97–106.

Schlesinger, I. (1974). Relational concepts underlying language. In R. L. Schiefelbusch & L. L. Lloyd (Eds.), *Language perspectives—Acquisition, retardation, and intervention* (pp. 129–151). Baltimore: University Park Press.

Searle, J. (1969). *Speech acts.* Cambridge, UK: Cambridge University Press.

Skarakis, E., & Greenfield, P. (1982). The role of new and old information in the verbal expression of language-disordered children. *Journal of Speech and Hearing Research, 25,* 462–467.

Skinner, B. F. (1954). The science of learning and the art of teaching. *Harvard Educational Review, 24,* 86–97.

Skinner, B. F. (1968). *The technology of teaching.* New York: Appleton-Century-Crofts.

Slobin, D. (1973). Cognitive pre-requisites for the acquisition of grammar. In C. A. Ferguson & D. I. Slobin (Eds.), *Studies of child language development* (pp. 175–208). New York: Holt, Rinehart and Winston.

Snyder, L. (1978). Communicative and cognitive abilities and disabilities in the sensorimotor period. *Merrill-Palmer Quarterly, 24,* 161–180.

Stark, R., & Tallal, P. (1981). Selection of children with specific language deficits. *Journal of Speech and Hearing Disorders, 46,* 114–122.

Tallal, P., Stark, R., Kallman, C., & Mellits, D. (1981). A re-examination of some nonverbal perceptual abilities of language-impaired and normal children as a function of age and sensory modality. *Journal of Speech and Hearing Research, 24,* 351–357.

Templin, M. (1957). Certain language skills in children. *Institute of Child Welfare Monograph Series,* No. 26. Minneapolis: University of Minnesota Press.

VanKleeck, A., & Frankel, T. (1981). Discourse devices used by language disordered children: A preliminary investigation. *Journal of Speech and Hearing Disorders, 46,* 250–257.

VanKleeck, A., & Richardson, A. (1986). What's in an error? Using children's wrong responses as language teaching opportunities. *NSSLHA Journal, 14,* 25–50.

8

Atypical Cognitive, Linguistic, and Social Development in Children with Pervasive Developmental Disorders of Childhood

DIANE M. KIRCHNER, PH.D.

Introduction

The complexity of presentation in many children diagnosed with a form of language or communication disorder seems to be increasing rapidly. At the same time, our understanding of the origins of atypical development and the principles governing the capacity for change with intervention proceeds more slowly. Children with atypical profiles seem unusual and uneven in their development. These are children who appear to fit no particular diagnostic category yet are clearly distinguishable from the norm on the basis of their clinical presentation. They are also children who fit no particular educational setting and are nonresponsive to usual practices and approaches to intervention. Many children who present with substantially more than minor or transient departures from the usual developmental course or pattern of behavior with respect to language and social interaction are eventually diagnosed with a Pervasive Developmental Disorder (PDD).

Children with PDD fail to develop despite exposure to the typical patterns of social-communicative interaction that parents provide naturally and usually outside the context of any medically or technologically identifiable neurobiologic explanation. For all the progress and clarification our current models of development represent, in many ways these same models contribute little to capturing the nature of atypical processes. Minimally, further refinements in our models of atypical development are needed. More radically, there is cause for great concern regarding the viability of models of normal growth and advancement as a way of understanding or clarifying the origins and course of atypical development. What is needed is a distinctive kind of understanding which goes beyond the external descriptors leading to the taxonomic grouping of children with complex developmental disorders. Etiologic statements of PDD on the basis of a genetic marker, metabolic disorder, or specific neurological process are far from complete. Explanatory research is important and necessary; as well, there is a rather urgent need to capture the essential features of the disorder in a way that allows practitioners to move forward with interventions, develop and implement appropriate educational programs, and initiate appropriate medical management and follow-up. This chapter defines those essential features, provides a theoretical framework embedded within the broader scope of human development, and makes recommendations for assessment and intervention plans for the child with atypical language and a pervasive developmental disorder of development.

Diagnosis and Classification

The category of PDD was originally established to cover autism and similar disorders which were previously considered to be a type of schizophrenia, a variant of infantile psychosis, or a form of developmental psychopathology. In recognition of the fact that "autism is a disorder of development and not a psychosis . . . it seemed inappropriate to treat autistic children as if they had an emotional disorder or were mentally ill" (Rutter & Schopler, 1992, p. 469). In practice, there appears to be an increasing number of children with atypical profiles who fit the taxonomic classification of PDD. However, there is no cohesive model for conceptualizing the clinicopathologic processes which form the basis for atypical patterns of development. Even more important, we have failed to identify a set of principled approaches underlying interventions for children who fit these categories at least descriptively. One reason that these fundamental tasks have proven difficult is a lack of consensus on criteria for classification based on the vast range of clinical features possible in children given a diagnosis of PDD (Szatmari, 1992b).

The goal of the most recent revision of the *Diagnostic and Statistical Manual of Mental Disorders* (DSM-IV; American Psychiatric Association [APA], 1994) was to focus on the "clinical, research, and educational purposes . . . supported by an extensive empirical foundation . . . [and to] provide a helpful guide to clinical practice" (p. iv). Toward that end, there has been a substantial revision and elaboration of diagnostic classification within the broad set of features which define the Pervasive Developmental Disorders of Childhood, and the most recent version includes the following diagnostic groups:

1. Autistic Disorder (299.0)
2. Rett's Disorder (299.80)
3. Childhood Disintegrative Disorder (299.10)
4. Asperger's Disorder (299.80)
5. Pervasive Developmental Disorder–Not Otherwise Specified (NOS), including Atypical Autism (299.80).

The core feature of Autistic Disorder, or variations which fall into the category of PDD-NOS, is one of impaired social interaction in at least three specific areas. The broad domains of atypicality which characterize the generic PDD group include the following: (1) qualitative impairment in reciprocal social interaction;

(2) qualitative impairment or deviance in social and reciprocal communication; and (3) stereotypic or repetitive patterns of behavior in the presence of a restricted range of interests and lack of imaginative activity (Rutter & Schopler, 1992; Szatmari, 1992b). The clinical manifestations of this triad (Wing, 1981a, 1981b, 1988; Wing & Gould, 1979) of symptoms are highly variant in form, severity, and course. However, and regardless of the diversity or variation of the behavioral expression depending on developmental stage, there is agreement that these three core features are pathognomic to a diagnosis of autism and are always present. The qualitative impairments that define these conditions must, however, be distinctly deviant relative to the individual's developmental level or mental age. These disorders are usually evident in the first years of life and may or may not be associated with global cognitive impairment; a PDD may or may not be associated with a range of other medical conditions, such as chromosomal abnormalities, congenital infections, and structural abnormalities of the central nervous system (APA, 1994). Table 8–1 shows the essential features of the disorders within the category of PDD on the basis of DSM-VI classification.

A diagnosis of Rett's Disorder centers on the development of multiple and specific deficits following a period of normal functioning after birth. Between the ages of 5 and 48 months, there is a deceleration of growth in head circumference. Between 5 and 30 months of age, there is a loss of previously acquired purposeful hand skills, subsequent development of characteristic stereotyped hand movements which resemble hand wringing or hand washing, a diminished interest in the social environment in the first few years following onset of the disorder, and an emergence of poor coordination of gait or trunk movements. In association with the previous set of symptoms, there is also a severe impairment in expressive and receptive language development with severe psychomotor retardation. In Rett's Disorder, although there is a diminishing of social interest after the onset of the disorder, in some cases social interaction develops later in the course. Rett's Disorder is typically associated with severe or profound mental retardation, abnormal electroencephalogram (EEG), and/or nonspecific abnormalities after brain imaging. What appears to differentiate Rett's from other forms of PDD is a distinctive pattern of developmental regression prior to age 4 and usually in the first 1 or 2 years of life. Rett's is progressive and persistent over the lifespan, although modest developmental gains are sometimes observed in later childhood and adolescence (APA, 1994).

Childhood Disintegrative Disorder as a subclassification of PDD is also characterized by regression across areas of functioning following at least 2 years of apparently normal development. These children seem to develop age-appropriate verbal and nonverbal communication, social relationships, and play and adaptive behavior in the first 2 years of life. There is then a significant loss of function in at least two of the following areas: expressive/receptive language, social skills or adaptive behavior, bowel or bladder control, play, or motor skills. The social and communicative deficits of children in this diagnostic classification resemble those of children with a diagnosable Autistic Disorder, and the Childhood Disintegrative Disorders are also termed Heller's syndrome, dementia infantilis, or disintegrative psychosis. A diagnosis of Childhood Disintegrative Disorder is usually associated with mental retardation (APA, 1994); in addition, there is an increased frequency of EEG abnormality which is suggestive of central nervous system (CNS) disorder. No precise etiologic mechanism has been identified, and unfortunately onset (between 3 and 4 years old) can be insidious or abrupt. In some cases, there is an increase in activity level, irritability, and/or anxiety coinciding with the loss of speech and other skills. The disorder is, however, progressive and lifelong (APA, 1994).

Asperger's Disorder (299.80) is characterized by a severe and sustained impairment in social interaction and the development of restricted, repetitive patterns of behavior, interests, and activities. With the exception of social interaction, adaptive behavior and curiosity are well developed. Asperger's Disorder is usually recognized later than Autistic Disorder and may be associated with motor delays or clumsiness in the preschool period. Although Asperger's Disorder is often conceptualized as a variant of Autistic Disorder and there is considerable evidence for a relationship between the syndromes, one of the primary differences between these two groups is language acquisition. In the DSM-IV classification, Asperger's Disorder is diagnosed in the absence of clinically significant delays in language acquisition. Within DSM-IV, the statement that that there is no "clinically significant general delay in language" refers to the fact that children with Asperger's Disorder are not delayed in the onset of language marked by milestones such as the emergence of single words and the emergence of phrases and simple sentences, which are general criteria. Once expressive language emerges, there is often a rather "rapid transition to adult-like, formalistic expression" (Frith, 1992, p. 46) which often masks the essential features of the primary deficit. The literature is replete with clinical and empirical accounts of significantly impaired communication and language when more complex levels of analysis are undertaken. In fact, the majority of children with Asperger's Disorder do have atypical language with respect to verbal and nonverbal communicative criteria.

Atypical language development has been identified in children with Asperger's Disorder in the syntactic, semantic, and pragmatic aspects of language. Frith (1992), however, has reported that syntactic errors are relatively rare in Asperger's Disorder and always occurred in association with semantic errors which distort meaning in context (e.g., neologisms, lexical selection). The pragmatic aspects of language are often measured on the dimension of "appropriateness" (Prutting & Kirchner, 1983, 1987) with respect to the communicative context. Happe (1992) suggests that despite adequate, and perhaps even exceptional, ability to process linguistic surface structure, children diagnosed with Asperger's Disorder may be unable to process or absorb information and important aspects of context. In this case, the child's unusual talents for rote memorization and storage of information may produce a reliance on such abilities in a way which is compensatory but neglects the processing of meaning and context. In a population of subjects with Asperger's Disorder studied by Frith (1992), two thirds of the Asperger's group had pragmatic deficits which were characterized by having poor perspective—violations of social convention, idiosyncratic speech, violations of boundaries of familiarity or intrusiveness, inappropriate or poor use of speech acts, and deficits in nonverbal communication (e.g., speech prosody, facial expression, gaze, gesture). Clinically, children with Asperger's Disorder have profound deficits at the

Table 8–1. Pervasive Developmental Disorders of Childhood

Autistic Disorder (Infantile Autism; Kanner's Syndrome)	*Rett's Disorder*	*Childhood Disintegrative Disorder (Heller's Syndrome)*	*Pervasive Developmental Disorder-NOS (Including Atypical Autism)*	*Asperger's Disorder*
Onset: In infancy or early development but always before age 3. A minority of cases report normal development in the first 1–2 years. Ratio 4–5:1 males over females. Prevalence is 2–5 in 10,000.	**Onset:** Essential feature is the development of multiple specific deficits following a period of normal functioning after birth. Onset is prior to 5 years and usually in first or second year of life. Females only to date; about 1500 cases worldwide.	**Onset:** Primary difference from Autistic Disorder is "late onset." Mean age is 3.36 years (range: 1.2–9.0 years); always before 10. Insidious or abrupt. Epidemiological studies are limited but reported more commonly in males.	**Onset:** Infancy and before age 3; typically around age 2. "Subthreshold" classification for children with features of autistic disorder but failing to meet the full criteria for AD. "Atypical Autism" includes presentations that do not meet the criteria for Autistic Disorder in DSM-IV.	**Onset:** Later than Autistic Disorder at least or recognized later.
Features and Course: Qualitative impairment in social interaction such as use of multiple nonverbal behaviors to regulate social interaction, failure to develop peer relationships at developmental level, lack of spontaneous seeking to share enjoyment, interest, and lack of social/emotional reciprocity. Impaired communication includes delay in or failure to develop spoken language without attempts to compensate through alternative modes such as gesture or mime, when speech is present impairment in initiation or sustaining conversation, stereotyped and repetitive use of	**Features and Course:** Apparently normal prenatal and perinatal periods; deceleration of head growth between 5 months and 4 years; loss of acquired purposeful hand skills between 6 and 30 months replaced by stereotypic use of hands; rubbing or mouthing automatisms; severe psychomotor retardation including gait apraxia and truncal apraxia/ataxia between 1–4 years; social withdrawal; some with accompanying clinical seizures or abnormal EEG tracings. "Autistic" features of shorter duration than with the Disintegrative Disorders of Childhood. Dx may be tentative until 4–5 years of age. Dx requires	**Features and Course:** Marked regression in communication skills, social interaction deficits, stereotypic movements, resistance to change, compulsive behaviors, overactivity, disturbances in affective modulation such as excessive fearfulness or anxiety, and deterioration in adaptive skills. Seizure disorder can be a major complication. Differs from Autistic Disorder on basis of developmental regression and associated "organicity"; differs from Rett's in that motor function is rarely impaired; regression is between 3–4 years vs. 6–12 months in Rett's. Deterioration is to a much lower level of functioning followed by a plateau of	**Features and Course**: Sometimes referred to as "atypical autism" or "subthreshold" classification with features similar to but failing to meet full criteria for AD. Range of deficits is similar though children diagnosed with PDD-NOS typically exhibit more differentiated social relatedness, cognitive development, and communicative skills than most autistic children. May or may not have restricted range of interests and levels of attachment; eye contact and patterns of affective engagement are usually higher than children with Autistic Disorder.	**Features and Course:** Motor delays or clumsiness in the preschool period, difficulties in social interaction at school, and idiosyncratic interests. No clinically significant delays reported in acquisition of early language milestones, cognition, or adaptive behavior. Dx requires at least 2 criteria in qualitative impairment of social interaction—impairment in use of multiple nonverbal behaviors, failure to develop peer relationships at developmental level, lack of spontaneous seeking to share enjoyment, interest, and lack of social or emotional reciprocity. At least one criterion must be identified in the category of restricted repetitive and stereotyped patterns of

Table 8–1. *(continued)*

Autistic Disorder (Infantile Autism; Kanner's Syndrome)	*Rett's Disorder*	*Childhood Disintegrative Disorder (Heller's Syndrome)*	*Pervasive Developmental Disorder-NOS (Including Atypical Autism)*	*Asperger's Disorder*
language or idiosyncratic language, lack of spontaneous make-believe play or social imitative play at developmental level. Interests are restricted and may include preoccupation with one or more stereotyped or restricted interests, adherence to specific, nonfunctional routines or rituals, stereotyped and repetitive motor mannerisms, and/or persistent preoccupation with parts of objects. Diagnosis (Dx) requires at least 6/12 features with at least two in the area of qualitative impairment of social interaction and one in each of the following: qualitative impairment in communication and restricted, repetitive, and stereotyped patterns of behavior, interest, and activity.	that all criteria are met.	development and limited degrees of recovery.		behavior, interests, and activities.
Linguistic-Cognitive Profile: May have no mode of communication—verbal or nonverbal; higher functioning autistics may have sophisticated expressive language with deficits in form or content of speech, marked	**Linguistic-Cognitive Profile:** Severely impaired expressive and receptive language. Rudimentary language prior to regression; words, but few develop word combinations; poor eye contact; little awareness of others;	**Linguistic Profile:** Many reported to have spoken clearly and in sentences prior to onset of regression; more likely than "late onset" autistics to be mute following a prior progression to point of using sentences. Higher	**Linguistic-Cognitive Profile:** Features overlap with those diagnosed with Autistic Disorder. Early preverbal/gestural systems of communication fail to develop at 12–15 months; oversensitivities to sensory stimuli. Continuum of	**Linguistic-Cognitive Profile:** Clinically significant language and cognitive delays are not present in the first 1–3 years. Language and communication deficits are thought to be primarily social rather than linguistic in origin. Syntactic

deficits in ability to initiate or sustain a conversation, echolalia. Abnormal non-verbal communicative behavior; poor eye contact; poor use of gesture; abnormal prosody; abnormal facial expression. In older children, long-term memory can be excellent; information is repeated again and again regardless of appropriateness. Behavioral disorders range from mild to severe; may have self-injurious behavior. Can be diagnosed with normal nonverbal IQ or with global cognitive delays.	restricted range of nonverbal expressions of communicative intent. Little or no imitation due to dyspraxia; output constraints may mask higher comprehension.	IQ late onset autistics never progress past single words or use of phrases. When present, language is characterized by lack of ability to initiate or sustain conversation, stereotyped repetitive use of language, and disorders of syntax, semantics, and pragmatics.	relationship and affect expression abnormalities. Rigid and idiosyncratic characteristics. Delays in both receptive and expressive language; some have deficits in visual/spatial processing as well. May have well-developed rote capacities—reciting numbers, alphabet, colors, recitation of songs and dialogue from books or television programs. Some appear to be hyperlexic.	and semantic deficits are not diagnosed in all Asperger's individuals and when present may be an expression of a distinct language disorder. Pragmatic deficits are severe and are observed at the level of appropriateness, nonverbal communication, use of speech acts, and discourse. Communication and social skills co-vary; evaluate both linguistically and in the social context.
Outcome: Variable severity; long-term prognosis related to language level and overall cognitive level. Behavior may improve or deteriorate during adolescence; 25% may develop a seizure disorder in adolescence.	**Outcome:** Severe global developmental delay with little or no change in cognitive, motor, or linguistic domains with age.	**Outcome:** Long-term differences in IQ with CDD children exhibiting lower IQ than "late onset" autistics; limited recovery; progressive in 25% of cases; static in 75% of cases. Loss of skills seems to reach a plateau unless associated with a progressive neurological condition.	**Outcome:** Variable severity; long-term prognosis related to IQ and development of language and social skills.	**Outcome:** The duration of the disorder is lifelong and continuous. As adults, problems with empathy and social interaction persist. May pursue interests privately rather than in social contexts, and social deficits persist. At risk for depression, antisocial behavior, and suicide in severe cases. Social adjustment and eventual outcome depends on levels of support and intervention. Outcome tends to be good.

Adapted and integrated from *DSM-IV*, 1994; Rutter & Schopler, 1992; Mayes, Volkmar, Hooks, & Cicchatti, 1993; Volkmar, 1992; VanAcker, 1991; Tsai, 1992; Woodyatt & Ozanne, 1992; Firth, 1992; Szatmari et al., 1990; Burd, Fisher, & Kerbeshian, 1989; Szatmari, Bremmer, & Nagy, 1989; Szatmari, Bartolucci et al., 1989.

level of discourse—"naturally occurring connected spoken or written discourse" (Stubbs, 1983, p. 67)—wherein there is a requirement for the organization of language at the textual level rather than at the level of the sentence or clause.

Finally, the last classification within the broad category of Pervasive Developmental Disorder is PDD-NOS (299.80). Children diagnosed as PDD-NOS may demonstrate language, communication, and social interaction deficits but not meet the criteria for diagnosis of Autistic Disorder on certain dimensions such as restricted range of interests; others may simply fail to meet the number and distribution of positive symptoms needed for a diagnosis of Autistic Disorder under the current guidelines set forth within DSM-IV.

The DSM-VI is a categorical approach to classification which divides mental disorders into types based on sets of defining features, but "there is no assumption that each category is completely discrete . . . with absolute boundaries dividing it from other mental disorders" (APA, 1994, p. xxii). As such, there is a need for a diagnostic category which includes atypical autism and other forms of PDD which do not meet the criteria for diagnosis in any of the other categories. DSM-IV guidelines for categorical grouping do not eliminate the need for a rich description of clinical features and informed clinical judgment when making recommendations for a course of treatment or educational plan. These classifications are based on presentation of symptoms (not etiology) and reflect the consensus of a range of health professionals who contributed to the most recent revision.

A review of the literature suggests that there are particular and often clear clinical differences between children with PDD-NOS, Asperger's Disorder, Autistic Disorder, and those disorders with overlapping features but which coexist with positive neurological findings. Children with PDD-NOS "tend to have fewer autistic symptoms, greater fluency in language, and later age of onset" (Szatmari, 1992, p. 507), and children with Asperger's Disorder present a clinically distinct profile which has been documented extensively (Bishop, 1989; Frith, 1992; Ghaziuddin, Tsai, & Ghaziuddin, 1992; Szatmari, Bartolucci, Bremner, Bond, & Rich, 1989; Szatmari, Bremner, & Nagy, 1989; Szatmari, Tuff, & Finlayson, 1990). Over the past several years, however, the category of PDD-NOS has been used interchangeably with the classification sometimes referred to as Autistic Spectrum Disorder (ASD; Szatmari, 1992a,b), and this practice has been challenged on the basis of the potential loss of information both clinically and in research (Rutter & Schopler, 1992) when such broad descriptions are used. Consequently and coinciding with the revision of DSM-IV, there have been a series of debates among researchers and clinicians alike to stipulate which symptoms and symptom clusters should and should not be included in this category. The revisions in DSM-IV are published as the current *International Classification of Diseases*, ninth edition (ICD-9-CM) is under revision toward the publication of ICD-10 (World Health Organization, 1990). A close coordination of effort among the two groups has led to a compatibility of codes and terms between the two diagnostic classification systems. It is thought that ICD-10 will eventually appear in both a clinical and research version in an effort to distinguish further among categories within the broad category of Pervasive Developmental Disorder. A number of conditions wherein the constellation of symptoms on presentation or during the course overlap with core features of the PDD (e.g., Rett's Syndrome, the Childhood Disintegrative Disorders) but which have clear neurological or genetic etiologies are now distinguished within both classification systems.

The peculiarity of the language and patterns of communicative competence in social contexts is central to a diagnosis of PDD. In addition, language is a measurable aspect of performance which provides a way of making inferences about underlying psychological processes or cognitive abilities, which are not always available for inspection directly, and for that reason often becomes the focus of an assessment and intervention plan (Frith, 1989, 1992). On this basis, evaluating to define and remediate the child's communicative competence—nonverbally (e.g., gesturally, prosodic characteristics) or verbally—is a complex and important aspect of the more comprehensive effort to provide an appropriate management for the child with PDD.

Prevalence and Epidemiology

Gillberg and Coleman (1992) make the distinction between "nuclear" (resembling Kanner's original syndrome) and "non-nuclear" autism (closely resembling Kanner's syndrome but with a few atypical traits) on the basis of the original work of Lotter (1966). Lotter's finding of four to five cases of autism per 10,000 children was eventually confirmed in two epidemiological studies worldwide (Brask, 1970; Wing & Gould, 1979). Wing and Gould (1979) produced data which showed that classic autism in its most severe form and most closely resembling Kanner's original description is present in 2:10,000 children. In the same study, however, these authors identified social impairment in an additional 62 of the children they studied under the age of 15 years who could not be diagnosed with a typical autism. Therefore, nuclear and non-nuclear children with severe disorders of social impairment were identified in 21 per 10,000 children, and this study is thought to be one of the best epidemiological studies in autism to date (Gillberg & Coleman, 1992). It seems, however, that the frequency of severely mentally retarded and normally intelligent children has increased, and this is attributed to better detection rather than to an increase in frequency (Gillberg & Coleman, 1992). Recent studies suggest that the frequency may be as high as 10 to 13 per 10,000 children when Asperger's Disorder and cases of atypical autism are included.

The prevalence of Autistic Disorder in DSM-IV is given as two to five cases per 10,000 individuals. Other forms of PDD are less frequent. Rett's Syndrome has been identified on a case-by-case basis and is reported only in females. Likewise, Childhood Disintegrative Disorder is rare and is now thought to be more common in males, although initial studies found an equal sex ratio. Asperger's Disorder without mental retardation has been reported in 10 to 26 per 10,000 children, with lower rates of .4 and 1.7 per 10,000 in children with associated mild mental retardation (see Gillberg & Gillberg, 1989, for a review). Information on the prevalence of Asperger's Disorder is limited, but it appears to be more common in males.

The language impairment in children with Autistic Disorder includes but is not confined to the pragmatic aspects of language use for social interaction. In fact, the deficits are severe in the syntactic and semantic domains as well. Least clearly defined as a distinct entity for either clinical or research purposes is the broad and large group of children diagnosed as PDD. Although children with PDD may be clinically distinct from both of the other two categories, the presentation and constellation of symptoms manifested by children within this group could hardly be more diverse. The aggressive effort directed toward modifying current classification systems is a product of an increasing awareness of the wide range of variation in etiology and outcome, which comprises the clinical population falling under the broad category of Pervasive Developmental Disorder.

Etiology

The majority of clinical scientists conducting investigations into the origin of PDD would agree that a neurobiologic explanation for the manifestations of the disorder is increasingly likely. In addition, there would most likely be agreement that within the broad category of PDD, the differences among those individuals who are relatively high functioning compared to those whose symptoms are more severe is one of variation in expression of the same underlying deficit (Frith, 1992; Gillberg, 1989). However, precise neurobiologic explanations of atypical development are not possible with present knowledge and technology; in practice, we continue to rely on behavioral manifestations and external indicators of development which are suggestive of underlying organic dysfunction in atypical children. In part, the failure to identify a particular neurobiologic etiology is related to the enormous range of potential causes and a correspondingly wide variation in outcome from any single cause.

Even "careful neurobiological analyses" (Gillberg, 1992, p. 122) are inconclusive, but when 23 children with a diagnosis of Autistic Disorder or Asperger's Disorder were studied (Gillberg, 1989), 61% of children with a diagnosable Autistic Disorder and 78% of children with Asperger's Disorder revealed indications of brain damage or dysfunction. There is some neuroradiographic evidence of cerebellar hypoplasia in autistic youngsters with and without mental retardation (Murakami, Courchesne, & Press, 1989), and evidence of brainstem dysfunction has recently been identified in groups of autistic children using magnetic resonance imaging (MRI) and Brainstem Auditory Evoked Potentials (BAEPs) (Hashimoto et al., 1992; McClelland, Eyre, Watson, Calvert, & Sherrard, 1992). The presence of ventricular enlargement in a subgroup of patients with autism has been reported using computed tomography (CT) methods (Campbell et al., 1982; Caparulo et al., 1981; Damasio, Maurer, Damasio, & Chui, 1980). At the same time, other studies provide detailed measures which confirm the presence of ventricular enlargement in a small proportion of children with autism but do not show any consistent difference in comparison to controls (Rosenbloom et al., 1984). Single photon emission computer tomography (SPECT) imaging reveals decreased cerebral blood flow in autistic subjects, particularly in the "right lateral temporal and right, left, and midfrontal lobes" compared with age-matched controls (George, Costa, Kouris, Ring, & Ell, 1992, p. 413). Increasingly, then, the behavioral expression of PDD seems to suggest a neurobiologic origin, but for as many affected children with positive neuroradiographic evidence there is an equal number with symptoms but no evidence of conclusive CNS pathology.

"The main problem with anatomical investigations is that they have not so far produced evidence that would exclude general pathology or show an effect of specific pathology, possibly over and above the general impairment" (Frith, 1989, p. 72).

Obstetric complications are cited more frequently in autistic children than in their nonautistic siblings, twins, or normal controls (Deykin & MacMahon, 1980; Finegan & Quadrington, 1979; Folstein & Rutter, 1977; Gillberg & Gillberg, 1982; Torrey, Hersch, & McCabe, 1975). However, when larger populations are considered, there is no consistent of pattern of obstetric complication accompanying the diagnosis of PDD. Prenatal complication may have direct etiologic significance or exacerbate the expression of symptoms over the course of development. However, the specific deficits attributable to prenatal variables would depend on the nature of the complication and the timing of the exposure or event. In addition, prenatal exposure and insult during pregnancy are associated with a range of CNS anomalies (c.f. Hakosalo & Saxen, 1971) neither limited to nor specific to the manifestation of symptoms classifiable as PDD.

Genetic studies of Autistic Disorder and its related disorders have produced a body of scientific data which suggest, but do not confirm, a genetic inheritance (see Smalley, 1991, or Hagerman, 1990, for a review). In part, speculations about genetic inheritance in autistic disorders have grown out of studies which examine overlapping symptom expression in children with known genetic diagnoses, such as fragile-X or tuberous sclerosis, and twin studies. Twin studies are strongly suggestive of a genetic component in some cases of autism (Bolton & Rutter, 1990; Folstein & Rutter, 1977; Ritvo et al., 1985; Steffenburg et al., 1989), but there is no definitive evidence that a broad autism phenotype is inheritable (Gillberg, 1992). The most comprehensive review of the biologic bases of the autistic syndromes is from Gillberg and Coleman (1992), and the reader is referred to this work for a more in-depth treatment of this research.

Studies of Neuropsychological Function and Cognitive Process

Neuropsychological studies have been conducted on groups of children who are higher functioning as a way of obtaining data suggestive of underlying brain dysfunction. Several studies have identified patterns of performance which are consistent with frontal lobe dysfunction in higher functioning youngsters diagnosed with Asperger's Disorder (Oznoff, Pennington, & Rogers, 1991; Rumsey, 1985; Rumsey & Hamburger, 1988). Frontal lobe disorders are thought to produce a cluster of symptoms which have become known as "executive function deficits" (Oznoff et al., 1991, p. 1081). The cluster includes symptoms such as rigidity and inflexibility, perseverative or narrow range of interests, stereotypic behavior, poor ability to apprehend future or long-term effects of actions, poor metacognitive abilities (e.g., self-reflecting, self-monitoring), and poor response inhibition (Oznoff et al., 1991). Within the context of the neuropsychological battery, these children perform in perseverative ways on measures such as the Wisconsin Card Sorting Test (Rumsey, 1985; Rumsey & Hamburger, 1988) and reveal selective deficits on tasks which tap executive function, theory of mind, emotional perception, and verbal memory (Oznoff et al., 1991). Oznoff et al. (1991)

suggest that the constellation of deficits identified in children with Asperger's Disorder implicate the prefrontal cortex, which regulates both executive functions and emotional behavior. The Wisconsin Sorting Test seems to be a good measure of processing carried out by the frontal lobe. The specific task is one of sorting a set of cards on three dimensions accompanied by a series of changes which require that the Subjects shift the dimensions of the sort and make use of examiner feedback in making the appropriate shift. One can differentiate between deficits in acquiring the initial set of associations with specific feedback from the examiner and deficits which are more specific to an interruption of those associations to shift when the dimensions of anticipation and expectation are interrupted.

A recent study (Berger et al., 1993) addressed the issue of cognitive shifting as an indicator of prognosis in groups of high-functioning autism with normal or near-normal IQ on standard measures. Berger et al. (1993) used a series of card-sorting tasks to compile measures of cognitive shifting (problem solving, concept formation, and set shifting in the absence of external guidance) and relate scores on these measures to progress on measures of social understanding. Even with near-normal IQ, social progress is poor in the majority of autistic individuals, and the correlation between IQ and social understanding on standard measures was negligible. There were, however, significant differences among subjects who made social progress and those who did not on the basis of the cognitive shifting measures. Berger et al. (1994) interpret these findings to suggest that one's ability to develop self-initiated strategies to adapt to changing environmental contingencies may be related to poor social comprehension.

Recent research into the cognitive bases for children with PDD has produced a body of intriguing and important data in two areas: (1) theory of mind (Astington, Harris, & Olson, 1988; Leslie, 1987) and (2) relevance theory (Sperber & Wilson, 1988). The theory-of-mind work centers on the development of pretense and one's ability to infer the mental states of others (e.g., their intentions, beliefs, desires). It appears that the capacity for a theory of mind may be fundamental to the development of social interaction. In fact, Bruner (1990) suggests that "even before language takes over as the instrument of interaction, one cannot interact humanly with others without some protolinguistic 'theory of mind.'" (p. 75). What is needed is a larger body of developmental and normative research, a clearer determination of whether and in what ways such a theory can be assessed in young children, and the formulation of a developmental sequence of how one's ability to infer the mental states of others changes with age and experience. It seems that explanatory theories of PDD on the basis of a theory of mind must take developmental information into account to determine the ways in which the manifestation of such deficits in high-functioning children with PDD varies from the norm. Theory-of-mind tasks which rely on verbal explanations about the beliefs of others cannot be conducted before the age of 4 (Wimmer & Perner, 1983), but there is recent evidence that such beliefs can be situationally assessed as early as 2 and 3 years of age and one may be able to use this information diagnostically (Chandler, Fritz, & Hala, 1989). By the age of 8, and perhaps before, a variety of measures can be developed to assess a theory of mind (Baron-Cohen, 1989a,b; Baron-Cohen, Leslie, & Frith, 1986; Flavell, Flavell, & Green, 1983; Johnson & Wellman, 1982;

Perner, Frith, Leslie, & Leekam, 1989; Perner & Wimmer, 1985; Wellman & Estes, 1986).

Compatible with the theory-of-mind accounts, relevance theory (Sperber & Wilson, 1988) is a cognitive theory designed to assess the expression and perception of intentions in human communication. Relevance theory includes a description of the role of cognitive economy in allocating resources for information processing, as well as a series of hypotheses about the ways in which the recognition and expression of communicative intent are related to the grammatical coding of intentions in syntactic or grammatical form. Failure to process at the contextual level leads to inappropriate and unsuccessful communication along with substantial cost to cognitive economy in the form of processing of unrelated and irrelevant information rather than that which is central to the purpose of communication. The result is an on-line failure to recognize and disambiguate meaning in expression because the child is unable to determine what is relevant to communicate and, thus, how to organize his or her ideas in expression.

In a recent study, Happe (1994) presented autistic subjects with a set of vignettes or stories about everyday situations in which people say things they do not mean literally. The stories were not imaginative or highly fictional. Rather they were simple accounts of events dealing with a range of different motivations behind everyday utterances that are not true in the literal sense but that are distinguished by context, emotional expression, and the relationship between the speaker and hearer. Happe (1994) used stories which were unambiguous to avoid multiple interpretations; some of the stories were physical stories which involved unforeseen outcomes with a mechanical-physical cause, and some of the stories were strange stories which involved judgment of mental states. The performance of the autistic subjects on the story measure and a battery of theory-of-mind tasks was then compared to younger normal children, normal adults, and subjects with mental handicaps. The results of the study showed that the physical stories were easy for the subjects in all groups, and the groups did not differ in their ability to answer whether a statement was true or not (linguistic comprehension) which pertained to content in the story. The autistic subjects, however, differed significantly from the other groups when their justifications were scored in response to why questions concerning mental or physical states. Somewhat surprisingly, however, even the autistic subjects used mental state language in their justifications, which suggests that even autistic individuals recognized that the stories required answers in the realm of mental state language. The difference between the autistic subjects and either of the other two groups was on the basis of appropriateness or accuracy of the mental states attributed. The strange stories were successful in differentiating between the control subjects and those autistic subjects who failed all of the theory-of-mind tasks. The data revealed that the strange-stories battery taps the same underlying ability as the theory-of-mind tasks, despite the difference in format and materials. Even those subjects who passed all of the theory-of-mind tests provided characteristic inappropriate mental state answers. Happe (1994) proposed that a deficit in "central coherence" (deficits in extracting global information versus a preference for processing local information) similar to that seen in failure of right-hemisphere-damaged patients (Brownell, Michel, Powelson, & Gardner, 1983; Bryan, 1988;

Kaplan, Brownell, Jacobs, & Gardner, 1990) on tasks of story comprehension may be the more universal or persistent deficit in autism than the inability to attribute mental states alone. Happe (1994) suggests that the single property of relevance makes information processing work for humans engaged in interaction or learning. Toward that end, there are mechanisms which allow one to manage complex, diverse, and changing conditions. Ideally, one would automatically apply or divert attention to that which is most relevant. Failure to engage in such selective processing is at considerable cost from an information processing point of view. In my view, deficits may lie at several levels of accurately determining that which is relevant and then deploying attention to that which is relevant while suppressing attention to that which is not. There is a potential for a deficit both in recognition and selection as well as execution and allocation of resources. Each would seem to be a different type of deficit and lead to a distinctly different intervention.

Explanatory research may be far from complete, but studies of neuropsychological mechanisms, cognitive process, and a theory of mind have provided important data and raised a number of areas that deserve exploration from both neurobiologic and cognitive-psychological perspectives. There are important ways in which these findings may lead to a broader understanding of the core of dysfunction in PDD and eventually to innovative and more effective treatments in the long term. Relying on what we do know, the failure to develop and describe innovative and successful approaches to clinical assessment and intervention is often less complicated by the limits or difficulties of taxonomic classification than by a lack of appreciation for the processes at work in the creation of atypical profiles and the effects of intervening to facilitate growth or change in that context.

As with most clinical evaluations of this nature, the neuropsychological assessment of young children is complicated by the need to relate performance to developmental and neurological processes as well as the effects of environment on performance and outcome. Therefore, the process of delineating which symptoms are constitutional and which are reflective of development and interaction with the environment is complex and often difficult. In addition, the question of causality and primacy of deficits remains open. In my view, however, neuropsychological assessment is an essential component of evaluation which contributes significantly to the practical matters of clinical intervention, instruction, and educational planning.

The Misapplication and Intended Purposes of Clinical Diagnosis

There are good reasons for forming distinct categories in clinical practice, education, and research. On the other hand, there is a tragic side to the application of a categorical model and the subsequent empowerment through diagnosis. Diagnostic classification was never meant to suggest a "therapeutic package" (Rutter & Schopler, 1992, p. 463), nor is there agreement that diagnosis on the basis of behavior without regard for etiology or course (c.f. Waterhouse, Wing, Spritzer, & Siegel, 1992) is within the bounds of acceptable standards of practice. It seems that there is a great potential for clinical error in making diagnoses solely on the basis of the presence or absence of symptoms, without acknowledging that the constellation of behaviors needed for a diagnosis of Autistic Disorder may be present as a manifestation of other neurodevelopmental process. With respect to education and intervention, it also seems inappropriate to view the profiles of very young children with a diagnosis of PDD-NOS as a definitive expression of their potential in the long term. Placing a limit on the eventual level of achievement of 2- to 5-year-old children on the basis of a single observation or evaluation and prescribing a uniform approach to intervention on the basis of an assigned diagnostic label exceeds the practical limits of our knowledge. Clinically, there may be a great risk in making such predictions in the absence of understanding the neurobiologic processes of atypical development and the potential for change as a function of an appropriate type and intensity of intervention. A prescription for intervention biased on the basis of a diagnosis or predictions of outcome, particularly for children under the age of 5, may deprive those same children of the opportunity for full expression of potential in the long term.

There are, however, certain ways in which a diagnosis may be important. Appropriate taxonomic classification is critical to research as a way of specifying groups of children under study so that findings can be replicated and generalized. In addition, a diagnosis is often critical to securing appropriate medical care, obtaining appropriate educational placements, providing children with access to appropriate interventions, and distinguishing among clinical subpopulations in a way which unifies our understanding of the ways in which these children are both similar and different from children in other diagnostic categories (Rutter & Schopler, 1992). There are ways, however, in which assigning a diagnosis—particularly to very young children—is not helpful in securing appropriate interventions, educational placements, or long-term medical and developmental management.

In one of his most compelling works, "The Mismeasure of Man," Gould (1981) presents a written account of the origins and subsequent misuse of psychometric practices to label and consequently limit (rather than expand) opportunities for children diagnosed as functioning outside the normal range of variation. Gould offers a critique of formal theories of strict hereditarian approaches to defining and determining intellectual capacity, and therein lies a theoretical position which I believe is fundamental to the way in which we generally view clinical populations. Gould (1981) states that

> hereditarians view their measures of intelligence as markers of permanent, inborn limits. Children, so labeled, should be sorted, trained according to their inheritance and channeled into professions appropriate for their biology. Mental testing becomes a theory of limits. Antiheriditarians, like Binet [himself], test in order to identify and help. Without denying the evident fact that not all children, whatever their training, will enter the company of Newton and Einstein, they emphasize the power of creative education to increase the achievements of all children, often in extensive and unanticipated ways. Mental testing becomes a theory for enhancing potential through proper education. . . . How can we help a child if we label him as unable to achieve by biological proclamation? . . . Binet believed . . . that special education must be tailored to the individual needs of disadvantaged children: it must be based on "their character and their aptitudes, and on the necessity for adapting ourselves to their needs and their capacities" ([1909, pg. 15]. (pp. 152–153))

In 1909 and with great clarity, Binet prearticulated the spirit and original purpose of the current legislation under Public Law (P.L.) 94-142 and P.L. 99-457 and what that means in terms of a child's entitlement to an appropriate intervention.

Just as the purpose of measurement should be to "identify in order to help and improve, not to label in order to limit" (Gould, 1981, p. 152), so might the same danger be present in our reliance on prognostication or predetermined recommendations for level, type, and intensity of an intervention on the basis of diagnosis alone. Rutter and Schopler (1992) state that the variability which resides within the diagnostic category of PDD itself makes it "manifestly absurd to suppose that their educational requirements will be the same" (p. 463).

The next section of this chapter will outline a set of principled guidelines which can be incorporated into the practice of assessment and intervention with children who have been diagnosed with PDD-NOS and are under the age of 5. I will not address older children or children with more severe, clinically diagnosable forms of Autistic Disorder or Asperger's Syndrome. I will not address those groups of children with an overlapping expression of symptoms in the context of a medical diagnosis of Rett's Syndrome or Childhood Disintegrative Disorder. Each of these diagnostic groups is distinct in a way which deserves study on its own merit relative to the social, cognitive, and linguistic characteristics of the disorder, their etiologic origin, and developmental course. With respect to Asperger's Syndrome, there is a way in which this group of children must be differentiated from those with a diagnosable Nonverbal Learning Disability (Pennington, 1991; Rourke, 1989) when overlapping characteristics are present. In addition, the nature and scope of atypical language in Asperger's Disorder is complex and requires a different level of analysis in assessment and approach to treatment (Frith, 1992).

Theoretical Foundations of a Process-Oriented Approach to Assessment and Intervention: A Broad Framework

Focusing on children with PDD-NOS, three broad areas of research and principles derived from an interdisciplinary perspective of the processes related to growth, change, and outcome in development are valuable in thinking about assessment and intervention questions with this population of children. Unquestionably, there is a need to define populations on the basis of a common set of criteria both in clinical research and clinical practice. An applied interest which concentrates on classification to the exclusion of understanding the processes which interfere with natural development as well as contribute to advancement both naturally and in the context of an intervention is inadequate. In a collaborative relationship between medicine, developmental psychology, neuropsychology, and clinical linguistics, it is possible to enter more deeply into an understanding of what underlies both. The risks of not doing so are even greater than the commitment to an interdisciplinary study, lest we end up severely narrowed in our thinking and failing to meet the needs of the children we diagnose. Medawar (1991) reminds us that it is "individual people, not populations that are . . . in need of treatment" (p. 270) and that must be our focus.

What may be fruitful is a reintegration of what we do know about some broad principles of human development and neuromaturation into our current thinking about children with PDD NOS. Toward that end, I would suggest that there are at least three areas of study which deserve a scholarly and clinical investment if we are to appreciate the concept of what it means to be atypical and all that the notion entails. First and fundamental to an understanding of atypical patterns of development in children with PDD-NOS is that one consider the broad neurobiologic context in which these children experience the world and respond to intervention. These are children who do not exhibit simply an immature system or one resembling the child who has simply lived for a shorter period of time and, thus, has experienced less. Rather, these are children with qualitatively different patterns of development and whose constellation of symptoms cannot be equated with younger children (Parker, 1982).

Second, although children with PDD-NOS display a wide variety of symptoms, the same forces that are at work in all of development are also operative here as well, even though the course of development may be characterized by an unevenness of ability, differences in rate of acquisition, and substantial variation in timing and sequence of developmental achievements. Third, with respect to assessment and intervention, the normal developmental model and our traditional ways of measuring progress as the result of a clinical intervention are inherently inadequate as a framework for appropriately addressing the therapeutic needs of children diagnosed with an unspecified form of PDD-NOS. Until we begin to focus our diagnostic and research efforts on the unique properties of the disorder and the neurodevelopmental context in which the disorder resides, our efforts to provide appropriate interventions will be incomplete. We are presented with a group of children with profiles clearly distinguishable from the standard population and few clinical approaches which can be mobilized to modify and enhance the functioning of children with pervasive disorders of development.

Neurobiologic Context of Atypical Development

The traditional arguments for the relationships between innate, constitutional predispositions and the effects of the environment on development embody two fundamental positions with respect to the role of the neurobiologic context in development. Although proponents of maturational (Gesell, Thompson, & Amatruda, 1934; Knobloch & Passmanick, 1975) and epigenetic theories (Piaget, 1969) recognize the ways in which neurobiologic and environmental factors affect development in certain fundamental ways, their emphasis is different. Maturational perspectives assign the more primary role to biologic unfolding and regulation, whereas epigenetic accounts stress that interaction with the environment and practice is not only critical but necessary for progress toward maturation. Mehler (1982) offers a more dynamic interpretation and suggests that developmental achievements in any domain are influenced by the joint functioning of innate and learned capacities; that is, environment provides the occasion or context for an innate capacity to be developed or manifest itself.

Murphy (1985) suggests that neither maturational nor epigenetic theories alone may be sufficient to explain individual variation and behavioral outcomes in children with atypical developmental patterns. Based on the cross-species accounts of Waddington's theory of development (Waddington, 1962) and Wolff's later work (1981), Murphy (1985) attempted to map the role of the neurobiologic and environmental contexts on atypical development. In doing so, he drew not only on Waddington (1962) but also on more recent theories of development, which attempt to define the ways in which physiological or biologic maturation and experience interact to affect the course of human growth (Bradley & Caldwell, 1982; Sameroff & Chandler, 1975). In Waddington's (1962) original proposal, development is biologically channeled along certain pathways and, over time, certain abilities (which could include linguistic and cognitive skills) become more clearly defined or "canalized." Murphy also proposed that as certain abilities or skills become canalized, they are more fixed and there is a biologically driven tendency for the organism to resist stimuli capable of disturbing or altering those capacities, skills, or forms of adaptation. Basically, this is a theory of developmental plasticity and flexibility which has been elaborated in recent comprehensive accounts of the relationship between biology and behavior (Gazzaniga, 1992). It seems fair to stipulate that integrity in at least three broad areas—neurological structure, neurological function, and neurodevelopmental maturation—will affect the course of both normal and atypical development. Bradley and Caldwell (1982) propose that over the long term, the potential effects of the environment remain fairly constant, but what changes is the child's responsivity to the external forces of change. For example, early in development, there may be an insufficient maturity of fundamental neuronal systems to be responsive to environmental stimulation of skills higher on the ontogenetic ladder, such as language and cognition. As the child becomes more capable and there is progress toward the development of a more mature neurobiologic system, there is a corresponding increase in ability to make use of input and experience.

With respect to the particular case of language acquisition, innate theories (Chomsky, 1956, 1965) are based on the assumption that language needs no motive other than itself, no specialized support from the environment, nothing except some sort of self-initiating "bioprogram" to unfold (Bickerton, 1990). Bruner (1990) himself argues persuasively that a child acquiring language naturally and along a typical course is predisposed and driven to construct meaning. But, Bruner also states that "the child's acquisition of language requires far more assistance from and interaction with caregivers than Chomsky . . . had suspected. Language is acquired not in the role of the spectator but through use. Being 'exposed' to the flow of language is not nearly so important as using it in the midst of doing" (p. 70). So Bruner (1990) does make clear the necessity of biologic priming. However, he also emphasizes that whatever predisposition is present, language can only be mastered initially "from participation in language as an instrument of communication" (p. 73) and that such mastery is accomplished in a social context. Children with atypical profiles of development present with a range of deficits which are fundamentally social and interactive in nature. These children do not commonly participate in and make use of the experience to which they are exposed as a way of acquiring early and foundational skills across cognitive, linguistic, and social domains. Given this framework, there are particular ways in which this view of the interaction between the neurobiologic context and the environment would affect our decisions relative to the timing, intensity, and type of intervention offered to children with atypical profiles.

Abundant support has been accumulated for early, intensive intervention before atypical features become deeply canalized and subsequently require more extreme interventions to alter the pattern and symptoms of the disorder. Failure to intervene early in development may result in a system which is unalterable in presentation regardless of the intensity or nature of the intervention. Recognizing that the general notion of a critical period or "critically timed phases" (Locke, 1994, p. 297) is not new, for children with atypical development it takes on special meaning relative to new views of intervention-aided processes of development.

Locke (1994) has provided an integrated theory of the relationship between neuromaturation and language acquisition. Locke proposes that there is a "critical period for activation of species-typical linguistic mechanisms" (p. 612) and that the presence of delay in the acquisition of an initial lexicon results in "too little stored utterance material to activate the analytic mechanism at the optimum biological moment, and when sufficient words have been learned, the viability of this specialized capability has already begun to decline" (p. 613). Therefore, on the basis of "reduced access to relevant data" at a point in maturation wherein the capacity for change is greatest, linguistic capacity will develop but "will have to be assembled from mechanisms less specialized for, and under most circumstances less adept at, the grammars of language" (p. 613). Locke's proposal is entirely consistent with Bradley and Caldwell's (1982) account of the effects of the maturity of basic neuronal systems relative to the child's responsivity to certain types of input and learning. Locke is extending this broad principal to the specific instance of the development of a linguistic grammar. He proposes that the acquisition of such grammar is ultimately dependent on the acquisition of enough stored utterance material to activate a species-specific analytic mechanism and at a time in development wherein the child is most responsive. Beyond this, however, Locke also proposes that neurodevelopmental delay itself may alter brain structure permanently and in a way that normal or typical linguistic development is never possible. Quantitative and qualitative differences in outcome are ultimately attributable to the effects of delayed onset, slow rate, and improper timing in development as well as the system's effort to compensate for asynchronous development when it occurs (Kirchner & Skarakis-Doyle, 1983; Locke, 1994).

The important practical implication of a neurobiologic framework is that a goal of assessment should be to identify periods when rate of change or capacity for growth is greatest. Intervention during periods when successful mobilization of the forces of change is possible will have the greatest impact on advancement. Successful intervention is, therefore, a combination of a skillful appraisal of the child's neurobiologic potential and the immediate need to determine which processes or structures can be replaced, which must be eliminated, and which can be elaborated or enhanced by applying intervention procedures. In the next section, mechanisms of change which have meaning for normal maturation and the way in which we should be thinking about intervention for children with a pervasive developmental disorder are presented.

Processes of Change

Throughout development, the forces of change are generated internally through the normal process of neurobiologic maturation. New forces are introduced and, as a result, new competencies emerge. To the extent that we have discussed in the previous section, there are also environmental and social inducers (Kagan, 1981) which facilitate patterns of development across domains. Kagan (1981) proposes four classes of change which can be evaluated empirically: enhancement, derivation, replacement, and disappearance. These broad classes can be used as a framework for thinking about the mechanisms responsible for change as a result of an intervention. Enhancement and derivation imply continuity in progress toward more mature and fully elaborated forms of behavior. Replacement and disappearance imply discontinuity.

The enhancement of particular processes or structures (e.g., neurological, linguistic, cognitive, motor, emotional, and social) occurs when such processes or structures undergo qualitative changes in the form of elaboration, efficiency of execution, or the way in which a particular skill is articulated. But what we are assuming here is that the fundamental nature of the process or structure retains the key features by which it is defined. Derivation, on the other hand, implies that at points in development new processes or structures emerge from an earlier ones in a way that the original or derivative process/structure is transformed in qualitative ways. Derivation as a mechanism of change is fundamental to ontogenetic theories of development. The third class of change is replacement. Kagan (1981) suggests that when one structure or process is replaced by another, the ontogenetic parent vanishes. Importantly, the new entity is not contingent on the earlier structure or process; the new form of structure or process is not determined by the parent form. Finally, the fourth class of change is disappearance, wherein a structure, stage, or process vanishes, not to be replaced by other processes or structures.

The promise that these principles hold for understanding atypical development is dependent on reexamining old notions of development as limited to forward movement along the curve. Taking phonological acquisition as an example, it has been suggested (Eimas, Sigveland, Jusczyk, & Vigorito, 1971) that advancement in phonology can be considered a successive disappearance of potential capabilities present at birth, with the net result being a successive narrowing of the repertoire in a way that is particular to the language spoken by the child. Additionally, there are countless examples in which undifferentiated behavior ceases to be active and eventually disappears or reemerges in a more autonomous or differentiated fashion (e.g., gesture); capacities transform themselves from global to specific, from concrete to abstract, and so forth (Mehler, 1982). This suggests that an understanding of developmental progress must include an appreciation of the mechanisms leading to regression as well as progression in neural function and structure—both are essential to normal and atypical ontogenetic development (Prechtl, 1982).

Developmental theories of the natural processes of change are potentially valuable as a framework which can be used to guide clinical practice for children who are diagnosed with a developmental disorder of unspecified origin. In practice, good assessments allow the practitioner to identify processes that interfere with development and consequently fail to allow the child to make advancements in cognitive, social, and/or linguistic domains. The same assessment should also lead to an appropriate intervention wherein the practitioner's focus is to recruit or mobilize (Kagan, 1981) the constructive processes at work within the child's profile and in the interaction as the basis for the corrective or supportive process. I propose that each of the four developmental processes operative in the broader context about which Kagan speaks are also related to change in the context of remediation and that any intervention should incorporate strategies which lead to the following:

1. Enhancement and elaboration of those aspects of the child's profile which are present in more primitive forms and which can be recruited or mobilized in service of developmental advancement
2. Derivation of new capabilities from existing, foundational processes or capabilities which are present within the child's profile
3. Replacement of atypical, nonadaptive behaviors with more adaptive skills and processes
4. Elimination of those atypical or interfering behaviors which serve no foundational function in the long or short term and which may be unproductive or even impede the process of change.

I am not talking here about particular methodologies (e.g., incidental teaching, social interaction therapy, behavioral instruction). The emphasis is on the broader scope of the goals of an intervention and the principles of change. The way in which these changes will be achieved must be individualized depending on the unique characteristics of the child's profile. In doing so, we must acknowledge and appreciate forward movement and the advancement of development as well as what appear to be periods of developmental stasis. Statis may in fact be reflective of failure to progress or a slowing of development at a particular point in time. Furthermore, static periods may serve a particular functioning by allowing for a consolidation and integration of ability, which leads to a qualitative change level of functioning at some time in the future. Process (typical and atypical) is complex, cumulative, and driven by a complex relationship between the child's innate capacities, prior experience, and the demands and context of learning.

Is the Normal Developmental Model Sufficient?

In view of the vast accumulation of the normative facts of development, the arguments for using the normal developmental model as a metric against which to judge children with atypical profiles have been persuasive. However widespread the application of a normal developmental model to atypical populations has been, it is perhaps time to save face and address what it means to be atypical. Atypical children with PDD-NOS represent something more than a departure from the norm or a simple form of human variation which explains the ways in which we differ from one another. These are children who present with the most challenging of social, cognitive, and linguistic profiles and who are likely to "perplex, confuse, frustrate, and undermine purposeful, interactive communication of even very competent parents. . . . Parents are not prepared for a toddler who looks away or withdraws" (Greenspan, 1992, p. 4). These are children who, before our eyes, disengage with the world and seem to "withdraw more idiosyncratically into their own" (Greenspan, 1992, p. 4).

Children with pervasive disorders of development present with profiles which are highly variable. They are often reciting the alphabet, naming colors, repeating dialogue from videotapes or conversations previously heard, and even spelling words in the context of very poor performance or absence of skills thought to be acquired ontogenetically earlier (e.g., visually regarding others, making social eye contact, using gestural communication, participating in reciprocal interaction even with familiar adults, imitating, and/or indexical referencing). The marked unevenness in development is clear, and in remediation there is simply no theoretical justification for the generally unchallenged application of literature on normal acquisition to the child with atypical development. The child with PDD-NOS may not respond to the strategies which have been demonstrated as effective for normally developing children or strategies developed for children who are judged as being delayed but who display a typical and ontogenetically predictable course. Children with PDD-NOS may require different or, at various stages, highly specific and intrusive interventions which are quite different in type and intensity than that which is observed in the normal patterns of exposure or interaction at any stage in interactions with children developing in typical ways. Perhaps most important, there is no evidentiary base to support any claim that simply exposing the atypical child to more of what the child developing normally or even the child with delayed but not atypical language receives is sufficient to promote advancement or qualitative changes in the way in which the child processes, stores, or makes use of what is taught. Locke (1994) points out that "the behavior of clinicians is a powerful sociobiological force . . . [and] it is reasonable to suppose that remediation—undertaken early and pursued rigorously—reorganizes the brain" (p. 614). However, he also suggests that the hope of creating a more favorable long-term outcome depends on the application of appropriate, early intensive interventions before the optimal period of biologic viability begins to decline.

The remaining sections of this chapter are devoted to the parameters of assessment, intervention, and measurement of change in very young children with PDD-NOS. There will be some suggestions relative to the broad parameters of assessment as well as some specific principles which can be applied to the clinical context.

Parameters of Assessment: General

In making appropriate assessment, one must take the context of those assessments into account. Neither assessment contexts which are exclusively spontaneous and naturalistic nor those contexts which are exclusively structured will be sufficient to develop an intervention plan or to gain an accurate appraisal of the child's profile. The limitations of each lie in the potential for either an underestimation or overestimation of the child's capabilities without extensive experience in examining both typical and atypical developmental patterns.

Naturalistic studies minimize the constraints placed on the child and allow one to make determinations about the child's spontaneous preferences or interests, which reveal the ways in which these children interact with other persons and their environment (Hand, 1981). Tunnell (1977) has outlined three criteria for naturalness as follows. The behavior is natural if it is part of the person's existing repertoire; the setting is natural if it is one in which the person normally spends time, and the treatment is natural if it is an event that would have occurred independent of the study in progress. Certainly there is a truth to the argument that constrained and structured assessments will not capture certain aspects of the way in which children are typically responsive or unresponsive to their natural circumstances. Structured observations and assessments provide another, though qualitatively different perspective, on the child's developmental level—that is, the ways in which he or she reacts to the evaluator's attempts to control or limit contextual factors which are left free to vary in the natural context. Hand (1981) suggests that there is a danger in failing to detect the child's competence or infer whether a child possesses a particular skill from naturalistic observations of spontaneous behavior. This argument centers primarily on the ways in which the open-endedness of the context or setting itself allows too much variation when one is attempting to draw conclusions about one's highest potential rather than base an assessment on an observation of ability which may or may not remain the same if the context were different. Hand (1981) also argues that there is the possibility of overestimating competence in naturalistic contexts. In a naturalistic setting, a child can demonstrate a capability but be unable to generate that same behavior with similar competence in more structured circumstances or on demand. For example, when linguistic, cognitive, or behavioral shifting is required, to initiate an action or change in behavior, one must first inhibit action or behavior which is ongoing (Kosslyn & Koenig, 1992). Therefore, the presence of a particular behavior or skill which is in evidence spontaneously demonstrates capability, but the extent to which the child can make conscious, intentional use of that same capacity as a strategy on demand or for interacting or learning is not clear on the basis of spontaneous use alone.

On the other hand, structured assessments may result in a disregard for variations in performance or development in favor of an excessively rigid and narrow view of developmental stage or skill, which surfaces only with considerable prodding or support (Damon, 1977). Hand (1981) suggests that failure to generate performances under conditions of greater situational constraint may be evidence that the skill is neither flexible nor well controlled. Naturalistic, context-sensitive, and ecologically valid modes of assessment provide the opportunity examine "naturally occurring cognition" (Gardner, 1993), which is observable only in situ—in the ordinary environment. Without question, however, an assessment can be structured to a particular purpose or outcome without being standardized. Gardner (1993) proposes that "it is essential that there be a departure from standardized testing" as the foundation for educational and intervention decisions. He suggests that assessment environments should "invite individuals to deploy their various competencies" in meaningful contexts and "make use of intrinsically interesting and motivating materials" which, although sensitive to individual differences, "engage the specific competences" which are under study.

This discussion of both perspectives leads to the stipulation that an appropriate and representative assessment cannot be accomplished without making both naturalistic and structured observations. In this way, it is possible to contrast the child's capabilities to reveal what he or she can do with and without support or under conditions which resemble the instructional context to which the child will be exposed and the natural environments in which the child will be expected to use acquired skills. This constitutes assessment in the zone of proximal development (Bjorkland & Schwartz, Bruner, 1984; Olswang, Bain, & Johnson, 1992; Vygotsky, 1962, 1978, 1986; Wertsch, 1985a, 1985b). Chapter 2 of this volume; Assessments will be collected, and some will be standardized. There is little harm to come from standard assessments used judiciously, for certain purposes, and with a carefully constructed naturalistic, contextualized assessment. What matters is the use to which the data are put and the interpretation of the data which are collected.

Assessment Procedures: Specific

Children with PDD-NOS are often initially referred for assessment and diagnosed between the ages of 2 and 3. This is often related to the fact that these children appear to be developing relatively normally until close to the age of 2, when parents begin to notice differences in the quality of the child's linguistic and communication development, patterns of social interaction with parents and peers, and/or differences in the child's object use or play. At this young age, the process of assessment should be completed across contexts and should be structured and research based, although the assessment does not need to be standardized to develop an intervention plan. In my view, an appropriate assessment for a child with a pervasive developmental disorder of any age would have to be interdisciplinary. These are children with multisystem developmental dysfunction (Greenspan, 1992) who require cross-disciplinary assessment for accurate diagnosis and intervention planning, both initially and as the course of development unfolds. A comprehensive assessment may include all or several of the following: pediatric neurodevelopmental assessment, a developmental psychological assessment, a neuropsychological assessment, psychiatric assessment, language assessment, and sensorimotor assessment.

Assessment should emphasize early identification, and there is some evidence that accurate diagnosis of autism and related syndromes can be accomplished as early as 18 months (Baron-Cohen, Allen, & Gillberg, 1992). These authors developed the CHAT (Checklist for Autism in Toddlers) which is a questionnaire containing 14 questions—nine of which are answered by parents and five of which are answered by physicians. The 87 children passing four or more key developmental areas at 18 months developed normally, and four who failed on two or more key areas at 18 months were diagnosable as autistic by 30 months. In addition to the benefits of early identification, the opportunity for prospective monitoring, and early intervention, the CHAT scale was also found to differentiate between those toddlers who were later diagnosed as autistic from those who were later diagnosed as having more generalized cognitive and developmental delays. This suggests that certain early behaviors may be more specifically predictive of autism than other forms of developmental delay.

With regard to the assessment of language, communication, and the related social/cognitive deficits which are fundamental to a diagnosis of PDD-NOS for children under 5, there are a number of formalized assessment procedures which may be appropriate but which should be selected on the basis of their applicability to each child (see Table 8–2). Children with PDD-NOS often seem not to comprehend much, may produce little language, resist the process of evaluation, resist engagement, and frequently lack the prerequisite skills to participate in standardized assessments in any way which could yield useful information. These are the complications of a difficult assessment which must be taken into account in both choice of evaluation procedures and interpretation of results. What is needed is a resourceful approach to clinical assessment which requires drawing on the published literature, interview formats, language and communication samples, and scales which are reliable and valid but which rely on parent report or careful observation in sed interactive contexts. Because of the difficulty in administering many standard instruments to children diagnosed with PDD-NOS, there is a requirement an assessment wherein goodness of fit is relative to the suitability of the assessment to provide accurate, comprehensive, and useful diagnostic information for the child in question. On this basis, successful assessment often requires an extrapolation of tasks from the literature which have provided empirical guidelines for assessing in a range of domains. For example, Stiles-Davis (Stiles-Davis, Janowsky, Engel, & Nass, 1988) and Stiles and Nass (1991) have developed a set of tasks and criteria for evaluating the development of spatial cognition and drawing ability in very young children with and without focal brain injury. The procedures from this research allow the clinician to assemble a range of tasks which tap spatial integrative functions in constructional and drawing tasks; even 3-year-old children demonstrate their sensitivity to the elements of spatial form and overall configuration (c.f. Fenson, 1985). Given the potential relationship between skills typically associated with right-hemisphere functioning in children with various forms of PDD, early evidence of deficits in parsing elements of the forms drawn or an early inability to organize those elements into integrated spatial configurations carries important diagnostic weight.

Within the language domain, a communication sample of 75 to 100 verbal and nonverbal communicative acts (not restricted to spoken utterances) provides a rich context for the description of communicative behavior as well as the range of socially meaningful behaviors demonstrated by the child, purposeful versus nonpurposeful interactions, initiative, responsiveness, behavioral organization, comprehension, and regulatory patterns. However, the way in which the sample is collected and the way in which the results are interpreted is more critical than the fact that the sample has been collected. The same is true of assessment in other areas of development which overlap with the assessment of language and cognition. In the communicative domain, there is research which addresses the relationship between the development of gesture and language in typical and atypical development (Thal & Bates, 1988; Thal & Tobias, 1992; Thal, Tobias, & Morrison, 1991). A systematic application of the procedures developed for this research allows the clinician to examine the use of gestures by type (e.g., associated with common objects; enactive naming through gestures, deictic gestures, gestural routines) and then relative to the broader relationships between gestural acquisition and imitativeness, communicative status, social responsiveness, conceptual progress, and motor planning.

Finally, because the developmental patterns and presentation of children with PDD-NOS are atypical and not easily characterized in a developmental context,

Table 8–2. Resources for the Assessment of Young Children with PDD-NOS

Resource	*Description*
Fenson, L., Dale, P., Reznick, S., Thal, D., Bates, E., Hartung, J., Pethick, S., and Reilly, J. (1993). *The MacArthur Communicative Development Inventory.* San Diego: Singular Publishing.	The MacArthur Communicative Development Inventory is comprised of two scales which assess gesture, imitation, lexical acquisition, and the transition to early syntax in young children. The scales are normed for children between 9 and 30 months of age. Parent report.
Schaefer, C.E., Gitlin, K., and Sandgrund, A. (1991). *Play Diagnosis and Assessment.* New York: Wiley.	A cross-disciplinary, applied compilation of developmental play scales, diagnostic play scales, parent-child interaction scales, peer interaction scales, projective play assessments, and play therapy scales.
Weatherby, A., and Prizant, B. (1992). *Communication and Symbolic Behavior Scales (CSBS).* Chicago: The Riverside Publishing Company.	Standardized assessment of communicative and symbolic behaviors of children at a communication age between 8 and 24 months of age but whose chronological age may be 72 months or more. Sampling of the child's communication during natural adult-child interactions and in structured and unstructured contexts.
Greenspan, S.I. (1992). *Infancy and Early Childhood: The Practice of Clinical Assessment and Intervention with Emotional and Developmental Challenges.* Madison, CT: International Universities Press, Inc.	Assessment by history and direct observation of regulatory, relational, organizational, representational, symbolic, communicative, sensory, behavioral, and emotional development in children under 5 years of age.

there are a range of parameters sometimes referred to as temperment, which are also important to a clear and accurate description of functioning in the very young child with PDD-NOS. In a way, these are stylistic characteristics which will have a dramatic effect on prescriptive programs and their implementation even when other aspects of objective skill or objective cognitive performance are held constant. Nine general categories were originally part of the New York Longitudinal study to identify and categorize individual differences and their significance in the developmental process (Chess & Thomas, 1992; Thomas & Chess, 1977, 1980). These nine categories are as follows: (1) activity level—high or low; (2) rhythmicity—regularity, predictability or unpredictability in function; (3) approach or withdrawal—nature of the initial response to new stimuli; (4) adaptability—responses to new or altered situations and less concern with the initial response but with the ease with which the response is modifiable in the desired direction; (5) threshold of responsiveness—intensity of stimulation needed to evoke a response regardless of the form of the response; (6) intensity of reaction—energy level of response irrespective of quality or direction; (7) quality of mood—pleasant, friendly behavior contrasted with unpleasant, unfriendly behavior; (8) distractibility—level of interference of extraneous environmental stimuli on direction of ongoing behavior; and (9) attention span and persistence—length of attention span and continuation of activity in the face of obstacles. A clear understanding and description of the child's level of functioning on these dimensions will have an enormous effect on the way in which one plans and implements an intervention—regardless of the domain of focus, whether it be language, social, or cognitive. When the goals and objectives of an intervention are identified, these aspects of individual variation will distinguish the child who needs an intervention which is provided during short periods of graduated exposure to new activities or information from the child who will benefit from a more focused or intensive program.

When we know a priori that the child is atypical in development, the purpose of the assessment is less to confirm that atypicality is present than to map the child's competencies and limitations in a way that leads to an in intervention or educational program. What is important, however, is that any assessment should result in both a description of the child's abilities and disabilities and a clear understanding of how the child learns. An assessment which only provides a description of the child's disabilities, developmental differences, or deficits is incomplete and fails at the level of purpose and scope: to have an appreciable effect on the formulation of a plan for an intervention or on the implementation of that plan.

Intervention: Contexts and Principles

When one intervenes to promote change in the child with PDD-NOS, a complex array of domain-specific and domain-related skills will be addressed, including comprehension, cognition, information processing, strategies for acquiring new skills outside the context of intervention, expressive language, social interaction, and (with the latter the patterns of engagement) regulation of affect and the non-verbal aspects of communication. To what extent the qualitative aspects of functioning in each of these domains which lie outside the range of normal variation can be remediated in the long term is an open question in the absence of well-designed studies of treatment effects. Thus, the clinician must engage in a process of discovery which will lead to a description of what this unique child will learn and how he or she will learn it (Kirchner, 1991). In my view, the distinction between centering on the form of what is taught outside the context of an understanding of the processes or principles of change (c.f. Kagan, 1981) is not trivial. What we are dealing with is a long-standing conceptual incongruity between clinical practice and the neurobiologic context of the child we are treating. The result is a lack of fit—and perhaps even more seriously—a lack of understanding of a number of broad concepts fundamental to designing an appropriate and effective intervention for children who display atypical patterns of learning and engagement or pervasive developmental disorders. When one provides an assessment or attempts to design an intervention for children with atypical profiles, it is necessary to understand both the ways in which their development resembles and deviates from the ordinary or typical course. This appreciation for both similarities and individual variation is the focus of an assessment and leads to an effective intervention.

There is one impressive and consistent finding which speaks directly to the intervention needs of children with a diagnosable PDD. Whether this is a diagnosis of PDD-NOS or a clinically diagnosable Autistic Disorder, early, intensive, one-on-one intervention (preferably before the age of 3 and always before age 5) is essential. There have been compelling reports of remarkable gains in language, cognition, and social interaction using both social interactive therapies (Greenspan, 1992) and behavioral intervention (Lovaas, 1987; Lovaas & Smith, 1988; McEachin, Smith, & Lovaas, 1993).

Greenspan (1992, 1993) proposes that children diagnosed with PDD-NOS fall into two broad categories of disorder: (1) regulatory disorders, and (2) multisystem developmental delay. Children with regulatory disorders show fundamental deficits in processing input of varying types and may demonstrate sensory reactivity, deficits in sensory processing, and/or deficits in motor tone and processing. Despite such variations, these children are often able to relate to others and communicate with relatively good skill. Children with multisystem developmental delay demonstrate more severe regulatory dysfunctions in addition to poor social interaction and communication. Greenspan (1992) suggests that these terms are not only more descriptive of the child's presenting features but "do not carry with them the negative connotations of autism or PDD [and with that the] . . . assumption that these types of children are not capable of love, warmth, and comfort with dependency" (p. 4).

In support of interaction-based, "relational" interventions, Greenspan (1992) offers the following:

> The traditional pessimistic prognosis for PDD has been based on experience with children who tend to begin treatment at slightly older ages [later than between 18 and 30 months], and who received more mechanical, structured treatment approaches rather than relationship, affect cuing based approaches. The possibility must be considered that approaches which do not pull the child into "spontaneous" joyful, relationship patterns may intensify, rather than remediate the child's difficulty. (p. 3)

In fact, Greenspan (1992) suggests that overly rigid and structured behavioral approaches which provide tangible rewards for performance, such as candy or other treats, may "support rather than remediate mechanical behavior" (p. 5), causing the child to develop or sustain more stereotypic or perseverative behavior in the long term. At the same time, Greenspan (1992) makes it clear that a relationship-oriented therapy which "ignores the child's core needs and developmental level" (p. 7) would not succeed. Effective interactive intervention is more than "positioning oneself near a child and commenting on what the child is doing" (p. 8). The child may not be engaged or may not comprehend what is being said. Greenspan (1992) states that "a therapist and child may go on in this fashion for weeks, months, and possibly even years, with very little movement or gain" (p. 5). Equally ineffective are fragmented treatment approaches, which teach isolated, overlearned, rote splinter skills even though the child may have an identified propensity for skills such as memorization, the repeated answering of questions, letter recognition, and other such skills. Effective interactive interventions are those which incorporate an appreciation for the child's developmental level, emphasize reciprocal interaction, and provide structured yet experientially based contexts for skill acquisition, generalization, and abstraction.

According to Greenspan (1993), the goal of intervention for children with PDD-NOS is to mobilize the core developmental capacities of (1) shared attention and engagement, (2) two-way intentional gesturing, and (3) representational elaboration and differentiation in play, cognition, and the interpersonal use of language. Greenspan (1993) proposes that the more challenging the child becomes and the greater the disengagement, the more likely the parent is to stop offering supportive, structured developmental contexts for learning. The unfortunate consequence of the parent's withdrawal from the child is fewer, not more frequent, opportunities to develop core developmental capacities.

A successful intervention depends both on a proper implementation and intensity, which would include interactive play therapy three to five times per week, language intervention three to five times per week, and sometimes sensorimotor therapy two to five times per week—all in addition to placement in an integrated preschool. Greenspan (1992) reports a dramatic response to a well-designed, intensive, interactively oriented program for some children diagnosed with PDD-NOS who receive intervention between the ages of 18 and 30 months: "At 5 to 7 years of age, these same children are fully communicative [using complex sentences adaptively], warm, loving, and joyful. They attend regular schools and are mastering the early academic tasks, are enjoying friendships, and are especially adept at imaginative play" (p. 3).

Many children with PDD-NOS who have acquired a basic level of competence in the foundational skills of engagement, reciprocical interaction, and representation continue to demonstrate profound linguistic deficits which require a more direct and specific remediation. The ways in which supported, predictable, interactive contexts can be structured to develop particular skills such as language and communication have also been identified. Kirchner (1991) described a discourse-based intervention strategy for children with PDD-NOS, wherein the clinician constructs highly situated but meaningful dialogues as a context for language intervention. This intervention strategy represents an application of Vygotsky's (1962, 1978, 1986) view of learning as an outgrowth of the skillful collaboration between the child and partner who is more skilled. It is the context of this partnership that allows the child to practice, understand, organize, and internalize aspects of a skill until eventually the skill or knowledge becomes the child's own.

The fundamental premise of the approach is that what makes language learnable to the child with PDD-NOS in this context is that the material is "embedded in a contextually rich and interest holding activity, is structured, is predictable, and is contextually relevant" (Kirchner, 1991, p. 91). This is an approach which incorporates a compensatory approach to learning from the outset and uses the child's identified strength in verbal imitation to promote "verbal scaffolding" (Snow, Perlman, & Nathan, 1987) and "discourse borrowing" (Clark, 1974, 1977, 1978, 1980) as a way of participating in the interaction and using language in a meaningful context. In doing so, however, the child is also learning to attend to the prior utterance produced by the communicative partner, respond meaningfully to the prior utterance, and make use of cues in the dialogue itself rather than some external source, such as an instruction to verbalize from a teacher or the stimulus properties of the materials themselves.

For children with profound expressive and linguistic formulation deficits, the language needed to be responsive is present and immediately recoverable from the prior utterance and the predictable, textual content of the discourse. Using repetition in a compensatory way from the outset circumvents formulation deficits, creates a continuity of meaning, allows even the most language-impaired child to participate in interactive activities, and makes use of a developmentally early learned skill which permits children with very little in the way of expressive language to learn it. The specific linguistic structures which are taught are selected for both the communicative slot that they fill in the dialogue as well as their linguistic structure. Particular to this approach, and somewhat unique to other developmental approaches, is that it is not necessary for a child to comprehend all linguistic targets selected for production at the outset. In addition, the intervention makes use of capacities which may be incorrectly viewed as isolated, rote, and having little immediate value. Kirchner (1991) suggests that use, repeated association with a meaningful context, and the action sequence which accompanies the dialogue facilitate understanding in the long term, even when such understanding is not present at the outset. In this way, it is the actual pronouncement of language in context which permits the learner to participate in the structured dialogue or discourse activity, learn new material, or practice material which is newly acquired or in need of consolidation. This approach makes explicit the important relationship between the activity, the child's participation in that activity, and the nature of the instructional discourse provided by the adult partner as he or she guides the activity. This is methodology which draws on the general cognitive principle of discovery through active manipulation—in this case, the manipulation of linguistic structure in a meaningful context.

Although this is an intervention which is derived from social-interactive theory, it is both structured and intensive. For children with PDD-NOS, exposure and opportunity alone are insufficient to facilitate significant growth in language acquisition, and there is a point at which suggestions such as following the child's lead have virtually no impact on the direct remediation of specific linguistic, cognitive, or information processing deficits which sustain the child's disorder. Additionally, there is a point at which goals must address linguistic advancement with respect to structure and meaning as well as communicative competence. When this is the case, procedures similar to those described by Kirchner (1991) constitute the intervention of choice. This is an example of a way in which the larger goals of linguistic elaboration and conversational participation can be achieved by constructing small, structured segments of discourse in a way which resembles the intractive exchanges used in ordinary interaction. Teaching compensation for acquisition and use exploits the adaptive skill of young children with atypical development, allowing the child to master linguistic and discourse goals which may have been unachievable using traditional approaches (Bjorkland and Schwartz, this volume).

Using an approach which is in dramatic contrast to Greenspan's (1992, 1993) interactive therapy, researchers employing intensive, behavioral interventions for very young children with an Autistic Disorder are also producing well-documented and extraordinary results (Lovaas, 1987; Lovaas & Smith, 1988; McEachin et al., 1993). These are typically not children with PDD-NOS and who have less severe manifestations of the social, language, and behavioral deficits which accompany a diagnosis of Autistic Disorder. Proponents of behavioral interventions have affirmatively discounted relational-interactive therapies for children with autism in the absence of well-controlled studies which provide evidence of a successful and durable outcome.[1] At the Early Childhood Autism Clinic at UCLA, under the direction of Dr. Ivar Lovaas, children diagnosed with Autistic Disorder participate in a 40-hour-per-week, behaviorally based intervention program. Lovaas (1987, 1988) treated and evaluated treatment outcome in three groups of autistic children under 46 months of age who differed on the variable of intensity of treatment. Outcome studies were completed at 7 (Lovaas & Smith, 1988) and 13 years of age (McEachin et al., 1993). All children in the intensive intervention program received 40 hours per week of one-on-one behavioral treatment for 2 or more years. At 7, all had gained an average of 20 IQ points and demonstrated significant gains in educational achievement; at 13 years of age, all subjects who received the intensive treatment program maintained their increased level of intellectual functioning and all had significantly higher levels of functioning on measures of adaptive behavior and personality. Nine of the 19 children who received the intensive intervention and were identified as "best outcome" in the first study (Lovaas, 1987) were assessed as being average in intelligence and adaptive functioning. Of these best-outcome subjects, eight of nine attend regular education classrooms and are described as "indistinguishable from average classmates on tests of intelligence and adaptive behavior" (McEachin et al., 1993, p. 359). Without question, these findings are astonishing and have generated a good deal of controversy among experts (c.f. Baer, 1993; Foxx, 1993; Kazdin, 1993; Mesibov, 1993; Munday, 1993; Schopler, Short, & Mesibov, 1989). There continues to be a need for substantial research, particularly with respect to replication of outcome, detailed subject descriptions, and detailed descriptions of the procedures used. Nevertheless, it would be impossible to ignore these extraordinary findings and the promise this research holds for treatment of one of the most severe and profoundly disabling conditions of early childhood.

We have two different treatment approaches and a description of a specific methodology used to facilitate language acquisition which combines the essential principles of social interaction with the need for predictability, structure, salience, and frequent opportunities for practice in meaningful contexts. Each provides either clinical or experimental evidence of an impressive outcome for individual children or groups of children who present unquestionable clinical challenge for even the most skilled clinicians. Having acknowledged the vast differences between pure forms of interactive and behavioral approaches, the commonality of the two broad methodologies lies in three important areas, which may ultimately prove to be more related to successful outcome than to the methodology itself: (1) establishing a level of engagement and participation on the part of the child which allows an intervention to proceed, (2) age at the time

[1]Behavioral research has historically ignored the case study as a source of evidence for scientifically validated treatment effects. However, rich descriptions in the form of case studies may offer important direction for future experimental research. In addition, the individual case study is the appropriate forum for conveying the insight and methodologies based on the extensive clinical experience of master clinicians.

of intervention, and (3) intensity of program. In both cases, the child is an active participant in the learning process, interventions are implemented at the earliest appropriate age, and the programs are intensive. Regardless of approach, there is no basis for delaying treatment in a "wait-and-see" approach (Greenspan, 1992). Infrequent or intermittent exposure to any intervention will have little, if any, effect on the developmental course of children with PDD. Conversely, all indications are that the only hope of inducing neurological or behavioral compensation or reorganization is early in development. This is a view which is entirely compatible with the fundamental concepts relating to the effect of neurobiologic maturation on development and critical periods, in which responsiveness to treatment may be greatest. The important clinical decision, however, concerns which intervention should be applied to which children. There is a need for research which specifies a set of criteria for making such judgments. We are in great need of objective, well-controlled experimental research which documents the efficacy of particular intervention approaches. However, we are also in need of a rich descriptive database which provides an opportunity for a more thorough and in-depth study of individual children and the processes associated with measurable change rather than point differences on standardized measures. Such differences may support some type of incremental improvement but say nothing about the ways in which a child changes or which specific aspects of development have undergone the greatest transformation as a result of an intervention.

In the next section, some criteria for what might constitute a clinically relevant and useful approach to documenting change in atypical children is presented. We are not concerned with drawing inferences or making statements which are applicable to large groups of children with common diagnoses. Rather, we are concerned with the need for systematic collection of data in the clinical environment which supports benefit from any intervention, regardless of theoretical orientation.

Measurement and Individual Growth Curves

In many ways, the evaluation of change in children with atypical development requires a unique approach which differs in significant ways from incremental measurements, such as pre- and posttest comparisons on standardized test scores. Fletcher et al. (1991) provide an excellent summary of the complexities associated with documenting the course of development or change. It is well known that change can be quantitative or qualitative. Quantitative differences are indexed by rate and trajectory effects—how rapidly a particular concept or construct is acquired when measured at different intervals (e.g., mean length of utterance, language quotients, IQ scores). Qualitative changes are those differences in development which represent movement from one stage or developmental period to another.

When quantitative measures such as numerical values are used, one must determine if a 3-, 5-, or even 10-point difference in a test score is significant, and making such appraisals "presumes knowledge of the magnitude of clinically significant change, [and] poorly handles problems of measurement error" (Fletcher et. al, 1991, p. 1269). It is not known, when two children both show different scores of equivalent values, if similar variables or processes are responsible for the measurable growth.

The course of development and the child's response to intervention are varied and diverse. There is no evidence that the the normal developmental model is sufficient to predict or explain change in this group of children or that change is always linear. When this is the case, intra-individual differences and the meaning of those differences for that child will contribute more toward what defines progression, stasis, or regression in development. This is the clinical equivalent of a within-subject research design, and what one is able to define is the unique response of a particular child to a particular intervention and a more precise description of individual growth rather than a comparison to norms from groups of children which are unlike the child with PDD. Fletcher et al. (1991) provide the example of "standard score indications of declines in intelligence when an inspection of raw scores shows that the child is actually improving on each assessment. Generally, the child is growing at a slower than normal rate, so that the standardized IQ scores decline even though the child is actually continuing to develop" (p. 1275).

If one views change, whether as a result of an intervention or natural, as a continuous process, then one is more interested in the trajectory of growth (which reflects process) rather than the simple difference in amount of change between two arbitrary points in time (Francis, Fletcher, Stuebing, Davidson, & Thompson, 1992). Using carefully selected measures and repeated observations over time, patterns in the treatment data can be discerned and changes can be documented with little concern for the influence of maturation. As Kazdin (1992) points out, "maturational changes are not likely to be abrupt and large" (p. 485) and, having established stability of the deficits in the past, can remove the suspicion that the target behaviors were episodic in nature to begin with and may have changed on their own. Whatever argument can be made for the inadequacy of individual growth curves as a methodology used to make inferences about larger populations of children is not an issue here. When the aim is to demonstrate the effectiveness of a particular approach with a particular child, the broader question of applicability to diagnostic populations in general is neither the focus nor purpose of measurement.

Conclusion

The atypical profile of the child with PDD will not resolve spontaneously with the passage of time, and there is no justification for delaying intervention after identifying the constellation of symptoms and behaviors. An intervention should be immediate and intensive; which aspects of the disorder will be treated and which approach will have an effect depend on both the presenting profile and the neurodevelopmental maturity of the child. In many ways, it is impossible to define an intervention plan which takes the unique traits of the atypical child into account without entering more deeply into an understanding of what underlies the dysfunction to begin with. This is a difficult task even for the most experienced clinician.

As practioners, however, we must be neither syntactic nor pragmatic, structured nor unstructured. Interventions should not categorically or exclusively be delivered as consultation or in the classroom as opposed to one-on-one instruction. Altering aberrant and unproductive patterns of interaction, attempting to teach children to want to engage with others, and creating effective solutions to the barriers of learning which are present in children with PDD is a difficult clinical challenge. But even more problematic on a day-to-day basis are two other important variables: (1) a lack of fiscal support for implementing programs even with research which supports their necessity; and (2) the misguided but widespread eagerness of clinicians and administrators within the educational or medical milieu to recommend and fund consultative models or brief interventions rather than intensive, direct service.

In many ways, the two are related. Despite overwhelming evidence that children with PDD require intensive, one-on-one intervention, and despite laws which stipulate the right to appropriate treatment, the financial resources to implement such programs have not been made available. The administrative response at local, state, and federal levels has been to deliver services only as resources permit or to attempt to get more out of existing resources, which are already inadequate to meet the demands of treating or educating those children with complex disorders. Within the educational milieu, those who stress consultation rather than direct service have also embraced the notion that the place where instruction is provided (e.g., within the classroom) is important rather than the content and scope of the intervention which is provided. As Craig (1983) states, "It seems simplistic to assume that there is anything inherently good or bad about conducting intervention in a clinic . . . [and] specialized learning situations allow intensive individualized interventions and should not be abandoned prematurely" (p. 114). Terms such as *consultation, collaborative-classroom based,* and *full inclusion* refer to service delivery models, not intervention plans or treatment strategies, and a service delivery model cannot be uniformly adopted to meet the needs of all children with the range of diagnoses I have outlined in this chapter. Acceptable standards of clinical practice are defined and developed to ensure that appropriate interventions are developed and implemented and to avoid the implementation of broad interventions to large populations of children. PDD children are an enormously heterogeneous population, and it is unlikely that there is a single intervention appropriate to these children as a group on the basis of a common diagnosis. It is equally unlikely that enrollment or placement in an educational setting which is broadly configured or employs general or nonspecific early childhood or special education curriculum can provide the individualized and unique intervention that children with PDD require. Such an approach fails to incorporate new data and persuasive evidence that unless programs are intensive and uniquely suited to meeting the needs of the child with atypical development, little progress can be expected. One must approach intervention as an entirely individual endeavor. Similarily, the way in which treatment outcome is documented and intervention is justified requires a precise description of individual change relative to the child's own profile of assets and liabilities.

Within the health care system, many of the questions about when, how, and how long to serve children are addressed quickly. Children with developmental disabilities are uniformly denied access to treatment benefits to remediate their deficits directly. Because the expense associated with the scope and intensity of service often lies at the core of debate, it seems reasonable to ask whether there is any fiscal advantage to denying access to early, effective interventions. This seems particularly relevant in that there is every reason to believe that early, intensive interventions will ultimately reduce the need for more restrictive placements and even more costly treatments in the long term.

With or without the practical barriers of implementation, more children than ever are being diagnosed with some form of pervasive developmental disorder. Each presents a complex and often perplexing profile; each requires intensive intervention with substantial personal contact and financial commitment within the first 5 years (Greenspan, 1992). A majority of these children have been poorly evaluated and may be receiving treatments which are inadequate at best; some treatments may place the child at risk for intensifying or sustaining rather than remediating the child's expression of deficits, resulting in a failure to progress to potential. In many ways, we have been poor at assimilating or translating research into clinical practice in a way which benefits those children with atypical development. This chapter has presented a framework for moving away from discovering generalities and commonalities among children. It is unlikely that a greater appreciation for the needs of children with pervasive developmental disorders of childhood will be achieved by drawing conclusions and/or making a series of simple deductions from our observations of normal or typical acquisition. More likely, it will be the discovery of the unique, often remarkable, and atypical capacities of these young children which will serve as the foundation for understanding what to teach and how to teach it.

References and Suggested Readings

American Psychiatric Association. (1994). *Diagnostic and statistical manual of mental disorders* (4th ed., rev.). Washington, DC: Author.

Astington, J. W., Harris, P. L., & Olson, D. R. (1988). *Developing theories of mind.* New York: Cambridge University Press.

Baer, D. (1993). Commentaries on McEachin, Smith and Lovaas: Quasi-random assignment can be as convincing as random assignment. *American Journal of Mental Retardation, 97*(4), 385–391.

Baron-Cohen, S. (1988). Social and pragmatic deficits in autism: cognitive or affective? *Journal of Autism and Developmental Disorders, 18,* 379–402.

Baron-Cohen, S. (1989a). Are autistic children behaviorists? An examination of their mental-physical and appearance-reality distinctions. *Journal of Autism and Developmental Disorders, 19,* 579–600.

Baron-Cohen, S. (1989b). The autistic child's theory of mind: A case of specific developmental delay. *Journal of Child Psychology and Psychiatry, 30,* 285–297.

Baren-Cohen, S. (1989c). Perceptual role-taking and proto-declarative pointing in autism. *British Journal of Developmental Psychology, 7,* 113–127.

Baron-Cohen, S. (1991). The development of a theory of mind in autism: Deviance and delay? *Psychiatric Clinics of North America: Pervasive Developmental Disorders, 14*(1), 33–51.

Baron-Cohen, S., Allen, J., & Gillberg, C. (1992). Can autism be detected at 18 months? The needle, the haystack, and the CHAT. *British Journal of Psychiatry, 161,* 839–843.

Baron-Cohen, S., Leslie, A. M., & Frith, U. (1985). Does the autistic child have a "theory of mind"? *Cognition, 21,* 37–46.

Baron-Cohen, S., Leslie, A. M., & Frith, U. (1986). Mechanical, behavioral, and intentional understanding of picture stories in autistic children. *British Journal of Developmental Psychology, 4,* 113–125.

Bates, E., Thal, D., Whitesell, K., Fenson, L., & Oakes, R. (1989). Integrating language and gesture in infancy. *Developmental Psychology, 25,* 1004–1019.

Berger, H., Spaendonck, K., Horstink, M., Buytenjuijs, E., Lammers, P., & Cools, A. (1993). Cognitive shifting as predictor of progress in social understanding in high functioning adolescents with autism: A prospective study. *Journal of Autism and Developmental Disorders, 23*(2), 341–359.

Bertenthal, B. I. (1981). The significance of developmental sequences for investigating the what and how of development. *New Directions for Child Development, 12,* 43–53.

Bickerton, D. (1981). *Roots of language.* Ann Arbor, MI: Karoma.

Bickerton, D. (1990). *Language and species.* Chicago: University of Chicago Press.

Bishop, D. V. M. (1989). Autism, Asperger's syndrome and semantic-pragmatic disorder: Where are the boundaries? *British Journal of Disorders of Communication, 24,* 107–121.

Bolton, P., & Rutter, M. (1990). Genetic influences in autism. *International Review of Psychiatry, 2,* 67–80.

Bradley, R. H., & Caldwell, B. M. (1982). The consistency of the home environment and its relation to child development. *International Journal of Behavioral Development, 5,* 433–444.

Brask, B. H. (1970). *A prevalence investigation of childhood psychosis.* Paper presented at the Scandanavian Congress of Psychiatry, Oslo, Norway.

Brownell, H. H., Michel, D., Powelson, J., & Gardner, H. (1983). Surprise but not coherence; sensitivity to verbal humour in right hemisphere patients. *Brain and Language, 18,* 20–27.

Bruner, J. (1984). Vgotsky's sone of proximal development: The hidden agenda. In B. Rogoff & J. V. Wertsch (Eds.), *Children's learning in the zone of proximal development* (pp. 93–97). San Francosco: Jossey-Bass.

Bruner, J. (1990). *Acts of meaning.* Cambridge, MA: Harvard University Press.

Bryan, K. L. (1988). Assessment of language disorders after right hemisphere damage. *British Journal of Disorders of Communication, 23,* 111–125.

Burd, L., Fisher, W., & Kerbeshian, J. (1989). Pervasive disintegrative disorder: Are Rett syndrome and Heller dementia infantilis subtypes? *Developmental Medical Child Neurology, 31,* 609–616.

Campbell, M., Rosenbloom, S., Perry, R., George, A. E., Kricheff, I. I., Anderson, L., Small, A. M., & Jennings, S. J. (1982). Computerized axial tomography in young autistic children. *American Journal of Psychiatry, 139,* 510–512.

Caparulo, B. K., Cohen, D. J., Rothman, S. L., Young, J. G., Katz, J. D., Shaywitz, S. E., & Shaywitz, B. A. (1981). Computed tomographic brain scanning in children with developmental neuropsychiatric disorders. *Journal of the American Academy of Child Psychiatry, 20,* 338–357.

Chandler, M., Fritz, A. S., & Hala, S. (1989) Small-scale deceit: Deception as a marker of two-, three-, and four-year-olds' theories of mind. *Child Development, 60,* 1263–1272.

Chess, S., & Thomas, A. (1992). Dynamics of individual behavioral development. In M. Levine, W. Carey, & A. Crocker (Eds.), *Developmental-behavioral pediatrics* (2nd ed., pp. 84–94).

Chomsky, N. (1956). *Syntactic structures.* The Hague: Mouton.

Chomsky, N. (1965). *Aspects of a theory of syntax.* Cambridge, MA: MIT Press.

Clark, R. (1974). Performing without competence. *Journal of Child Language, 11,* 1–10.

Clark, R. (1977). What's the use of imitation? *Journal of Child Language, 1,* 341–358.

Clark, R. (1978). Some even simpler ways to learn to talk. In N. Waterson & C. Snow (Eds.), *The development of communication* (pp. 121–148). New York: Wiley.

Clark, R. (1980). Errors in talint to learn. *First Language, 1,* 7–32.

Craig, H. (1983). Applications of pragmatic language models for intervention. In T. A. Gallagher & C. A. Prutting (Eds.), *Pragmatic assessment and intervention issues in language* (pp. 101–127). San Diego: College-Hill Press.

Damasio, H., Maurer, R. G., Damasio, A. R., & Chui, H. C. (1980). Computerized tomographic scan findings in patients with autistic behavior. *Archives of Neurology, 37,* 504–510.

Damon, W. (1977). *The social world of the child.* San Francisco: Jossey-Bass.

Deykin, E. Y., & MacMahon, B. (1980). Pregnancy, delivery, and neonatal complications among autistic children. *American Journal of Diseases in Children, 134,* 860–864.

Eimas, P., Sigveland, E. P., Jusczyk, P., & Vigorito, J. (1971). Speech perception in infants. *Science, 171,* 303–306.

Fenson, L. (1985). The transition from construction to sketching in children's drawing. In N. H. Freeman & M. V. Cox (Eds.), *Visual order: The nature and development of pictorial representation* (pp. 374–384). New York: Cambridge University Press.

Fenson, L., Dale, P., Reznick, S., Thal, D., Bates, E., Hartung, J., Pethick, S., & Reilly, J. (1993). *MacArthur communicative development inventories.* San Diego: Singular.

Finegan, J., & Quadrington, B. (1979). Pre-, peri-, and neonatal factors and infantile autism. *Journal of Child Psychology and Psychiatry, 20,* 119–128.

Fischer, K. W. (1980). A theory of cognitive development: The control and construction of hierarchies of skills. *Psychological Review, 87,* 477–531.

Fischer, K. W. (1983). Developmental levels as periods of discontinuity. *New Directions for Child Development: Levels and Transitions in Children's Development, 21,* 5–19.

Flavell, J. H., Flavell, E., & Green, F. L. (1983). Development of the appearance-reality distinction. *Cognitive Psychology, 15,* 95–120.

Fletcher, J. M, Francis, D. J., Pequegnat, W., Raudenbush, S. W., Bornstein, M. H., Schmitt, F.,

Brouwers, P., & Stover, E. (1991). Neurobehavioral outcomes in diseases of childhood: Individual change models for pediatric human immunodeficiency viruses. *American Psychologist, 46*(12), 1267–1277.

Folstein, S., & Rutter, M. (1977). Genetic influences and infantile autism: A genetic study of 21 twin pairs. *Journal of Child Psychology and Psychiatry, 18*, 297–321.

Foxx, R. M. (1993). Sapid effects awaiting independent replication. *American Journal on Mental Retardation, 97*(4), 375–376.

Francis, D. J., Fletcher, J. M., Stuebing, K. K., Davidson, K. C., & Thompson, N. M. (1992). Analysis of change: Modeling individual growth. In A. E. Kazdin (Ed.), *Methodological issues and strategies in clinical research* (pp. 607–630). Hyattsville, MD: American Psychological Association.

Frith, U. (1989). *Autism: Explaining the enigma.* Oxford, UK: Blackwell.

Frith, U. (1992). *Autism and Asperger's syndrome.* New York: Cambridge University Press.

Gardner, H. (1993). *Multiple intelligences: The theory in practice.* New York: Basic Books-HarperCollins.

Gazzaniga, M. S. (1992). *Natures mind: The biological roots of thinking, emotions, sexuality, language, and intelligence.* New York: Basic Books.

George, M., Costa, D., Kouris, K., Ring, H., & Ell, P. (1992). Cerebral blood flow abnormalities in adults with Infantile autism, *Journal of Nervous and Mental Disorders, 180*, 413–417.

Gesell, A., Thompson, H., & Amatruda, C. S. (1934). *Infant behavior: Its genesis and growth.* New York: McGraw-Hill.

Ghaziuddin, M., Tsai, L, & Ghaziuddin, N. (1992a). Brief report: A comparison of the diagnostic criteria for Asperger Syndrome. *Journal of Autism and Developmental Disorders, 22*(4), 643–649.

Ghaziuddin, M., Tsai, L., & Ghaziuddin, N. (1992b). Brief report: A reappraisal of clumsiness as a diagnostic feature of Asperger Syndrome. *Journal of Autism and Developmental Disorders, 22*(4), 651–656.

Gillberg, C. (1989). *Diagnosis and treatment of autism.* New York: Plenum.

Gillberg, C. (1992). Clinical and neurobiological aspects of Asperger syndrome in six family studies. In U. Frith (Ed.), *Autism and Asperger syndrome* (pp. 122–145). New York: Cambridge University Press.

Gillberg, C., & Coleman, M. (1992). *The biology of the autistic syndromes* (2nd ed.). London: Mac Keith Press.

Gillberg, C., & Gillberg, I. C. (1982). Infantile autism: A total population study of reduced optimality in pre-, peri-, neonatal period. *Journal of Autism and Developmental Disorders, 13*(2), 153–166.

Gillberg, C., & Gillberg, I. C. (1989). Asperger's syndrome—some epidemiological considerations: A research note. *Journal of Child Psychology and Psychiatry, 30*, 631–638.

Gould, S. J. (1981). *The mismeasure of man.* New York: W. W. Norton.

Greenspan, S. (1992). Reconsidering the diagnosis and treatment of very young children with autistic spectrum or pervasive developmental disorder. *Zero-Three: National Center for Clinical Infant Programs, 13*(2), 7–9.

Greenspan, S. I. (1993). *Infancy and early childhood: The practice of clinical assessment and intervention with emotional and developmental challenges.* Madison, CT: International Universities Press, Inc.

Hagerman, R. J. (1990). Chromosomes, genes and autism. In C. Gillberg (Ed.), *Autism: diagnosis and treatment: The state of the art* (pp. 105–131). New York: Plenum.

Hakosalo, J. K., & Saxen, L. (1971). Influenza epidemic and congenital defects. *Lancet, 2*, 1346–1347.

Hand, H. (1981). The relation between developmental level and spontaneous behavior: The importance of sampling contexts. *New Directions for Child Development, 12*, 55–67.

Happe, F. G. E. (1992). The autobiographical writings of three Asperger syndrome adults: Problems of interpretation and implications for theory. In U. Frith (Ed.), *Autism and Asperger syndrome* (pp. 207–242). New York: Cambridge University Press.

Happe, F. G. E. (1994). An advanced test of theory of mind: Understanding of story characters thoughts and feelings by able autistic, mentally handicapped, and normal children and adults. *Journal of Autism and Developmental Disorders, 24*(2), 129–154.

Hashimoto, T., Tayama, T., Miyazaki, M., Sakurama, N., Yoshimoto, T., Murakawa, K., & Kuroda, Y. (1992). Reduced brainstem size in children with autism. *Brain and Development, 14*(2), 94–97.

Johnson, C. M., & Wellman, H. M. (1982). Children's developing conceptions of the mind. *Child Development, 53*, 222–234.

Kagan, J. (1981). Perspectives on continuity. In R. M. Lerner & N. A. Busch-Rossnagel (Eds.), *Individuals as producers of their development: A life-span perspective* (pp. 26–74). New York: Academic Press.

Kanner, L. (1943). Autustic disturbances of affective contact. *The Nervous Child, 2*, 217–250.

Kaplan, J., Brownell, H. H., Jacobs, J. R., & Gardner, H. (1990). The effects of right hemisphere damage on the pragmatic interpretation of conversational remarks. *Brain and Language, 38*, 315–333.

Kazdin, A. E. (1992). Drawing valid inferences from case studies. In A. E. Kazdin (Ed.), *Methodological issues and strategies in clinical research* (pp. 475–490). Hyattsville, MD: American Psychological Association.

Kazdin, A. E. (1993). Replication and extension of behavioral treatment of autistic disorder. *American Journal on Mental Retardation, 97*(4), 377–379.

Kirchner, D. M., & Skarakis-Doyle, E. A. (1983). Developmental language disorders: A theoretical perspective. In T. M. Gallagher & C. A. Prutting (Eds.), *Pragmatic assessment and intervention issues in language* (pp. 215–246). San Diego: College-Hill Press.

Kirchner, D. M. (1991). Using verbal scaffolding to facilitate conversational participation and language acquisition in children with pervasive developmental disorders. *Journal of Childhood Communication Disorders, 14*(1), 81–98.

Knoblock, H., & Passmanick, B. (1975). Some etiological and prognostic factors in early infantile autism and psychosis. *Pediatrics, 55,* 182–191.

Kosslyn, S. M., & Koenig, O. (1992). *Wet mind: The new cognitive neuroscience.* New York: The Free Press.

Leslie, A. M. (1987). Pretense and representation: The origins of "theory of mind." *Psychological Review, 94,* 412–426.

Locke, J. L. (1994). Gradual emergence of developmental language disorders. *Journal of Speech and Hearing Research, 37,* 608–616.

Lotter, V. (1966). Epidemiology of autistic conditions in children. I. Prevalence. *Social Psychiatry, 1,* 124–137.

Lovaas, I. (1987). Behavioral treatment and normal educational and intellectual functioning in young autistic children. *Journal of Consulting and Clinical Psychology, 55,* 3–9.

Lovaas, I., & Smith, T. (1988). Intensive behavioral treatment with young autistic children. In B. B. Lahey & A. E. Kazdin (Eds.), *Advances in Clinical Child Psychology* (Vol. 11, pp. 285–324). New York: Plenum.

Mayes, L., Volkmar, F., Hooks, M., & Cicchetti, D. (1993). Differentiating pervasive developmental disorder not otherwise specified from autism and language disorders. *Journal of Autism and Developmental Disorders, 23*(1), 74–90.

McClelland, D. G., Eyre, D., Watson, D., Calvert, G. J., & Sherrard, E. (1992). Central conduction time in childhood autism. *British Journal of Psychiatry, 160,* 659–663.

McEachin, J. J., Smith, T., & Lovaas, I. (1993). Long-term outcome for children with autism who received early intensive behavioral treatment. *American Journal on Mental Retardation, 97*(4), 359–372.

McTear, M., & Conti-Ramsden, G. (1992). *Pragmatic disability in children.* San Diego: Singular.

Medawar, P. (1991). *The threat and the glory: Reflections on science and scientists.* Oxford, UK: Oxford University Press.

Mehler, J. (1982). Unlearning; Dips and drops—a theory of cognitive development. In J. Mehler (Ed.), *Regressions in mental development: Basic phenomena and theories* (pp. 133–152). Hillsdale, NJ: Erlbaum.

Mesibov, G. B. (1993). Treatment outcome is encouraging. *American Journal on Mental Retardation, 97*(4), 379–380.

Miller, A. (1991). Cognitive-developmental systems theory in pervasive developmental disorders. *Psychiatric Clinics of North America: Pervasive Developmental Disorders, 14*(1), 141–163.

Murkami, J. W., Courchesne, E., & Press, G. A. (1989). Reduced cerebellar hemisphere size and its relationship to vermal hypoplasia in autism. *Archives of Neurology, 46,* 689–694.

Munday, P. (1993). Normal versus high functioning status in children with autism. *American Journal on Mental Retardation, 97*(4), 381–384.

Murphy, T. F. (1985). Atypical infant development: Interacting neurological and environmental factors. In L. Siegel, & J. M. Frederick (Eds.), *Cognitive development in atypical children: Progress in cognitive developmental research* (pp. 143–172). New York: Springer-Verlag.

Oznoff, S., Pennington, B., & Rogers, S. (1991). Executive function deficits in high functioning autistic individuals: Relationship to theory of mind. *Journal of Child Psychology and Psychiatry, 32,* 1081–1105.

Parker, D. (1982). Determinate and plastic principles in neuropsychological development. In J. Dickerson & H. McGurk (Eds.), *Brain and behavioral development: Interdisciplinary perspectives on structure and function* (pp. 203–232). Surrey, UK: Surrey University Press.

Pennington, B. (1991). *Diagnosing learning disorders: A neuropsychological framework.* New York: Guilford.

Perner, J., Frith, U., Leslie, A. M., & Leekam, S. R. (1989). Exploration of the autistic child's theory of mind: Knowledge, belief, and communication. *Child Development, 60,* 689–700.

Perner, J., & Wimmer, H. (1985). "John thinks that Mary thinks that . . .", Attribution of second order beliefs by 5–10 year old children. *Journal of Experimental Child Psychology, 39,* 437–.

Piaget, J. (1969). Operational structures of the intelligence and organic controls. In A. G. Kaczman & J. C. Eccks (Eds.), *Brain and human behavior* (pp. 221–250). New York: Springer-Verlag.

Prechtl, H. F. R. (1982). Regressions and transformations during neurological development. In T. B. Bever (Ed.), *Regressions in mental development: Basic phenomena and theories* (pp. 103–116). Hillsdale, NJ: Erlbaum.

Prutting, C. A., & Kirchner, D. M. (1983). Applied pragmatics. In T. Gallagher & C. Prutting (Eds.), *Pragmatic assessment and intervention issues in language* (pp. 29–64). San Diego: College-Hill Press.

Prutting, C. A., & Kirchner, D. M. (1987). A clinical appraisal of the pragmatic aspects of language. *Journal of Speech and Hearing Disorders, 52*, 105–119.

Ritvo, E. R., Freeman, B. J., Mason-Brothers, A., Jorde, L. B., Jenson, W. R., McMahon, W. M., Petersen, P. B., Mo, A., & Ritvo, A. (1985). Concordance of the syndrome of autism in 40 pairs of afflicted twins, *American Journal of Psychiatry, 142*, 74–77.

Ritvo, E. R., Freeman, B. J., Pingree, C., Mason-Brothers, A., Jorde, L. B., Jensen, W. R., McMahon, W. M., Peterson, P. B., Mo, A., & Ritvo, A. (1990). The UCLA-University of Utah epidemiologic survey of autism: prevalence. *American Journal of Psychiatry, 146*, 194–199.

Rosenbloom, S., Campbell, M., George, A., Kricheff, I., Taleporos, E., Anderson, L., Reuben, R., & Korein, J. (1984). High-resolution CT scanning in infantile autism: A quantitative approach. *Journal of the American Academy of Child Psychiatry, 23*, 72–77.

Rourke, B. P. (1989). *Nonverbal learning disabilities: The syndrome and the model.* New York: Guilford.

Rumsey, J. M. (1985). Conceptual problem-solving in highly verbal, non-retarded autistic men. *Journal of Autism and Developmental Disorders, 15*, 23–36.

Rumsey, J. M., & Hamburger, S. D. (1988). Neuropsychological findings in high functioning men with infantile autism, residual state. *Journal of Clinical and Experimental Neuropsychology, 10*, 201–221.

Rutter, M. & Schopler, E. (1992). Classification of pervasive developmental disorders: Some concepts and practical considerations. *Journal of Autism and Developmental Disorders, 22*(4), 459–482.

Sameroff, A. S., & Chandler, M. J. (1975). Reproductive risk and the continum of caretaking causality. In F. D. Horowitz (Ed.), *Review of child development research* (Vol. 4, pp. 291–313). Chicago: University of Chicago Press.

Schaefer, C. G., Gitlin, K., & Sandgrund, A. (1991). *Play diagnosis and assessment.* New York: Wiley.

Schopler, E. (1985). Editorial: Convergence of learning disability, higher-level autism, and Asperger's diagnostic issues. *Journal of Autism and Developmental Disorders, 15*, 359.

Schopler, E., Short, A., & Mesibov, G. (1989). Relation of behavioral treatment to "normal functioning": Comment on Lovaas. *Journal of Consulting and Clinical Psychology, 57*, 162–164.

Shapiro, T., & Hertzig, M. E. (1991). Social deviance in autism: A central in tegrative failure as a model for social nonengagement. *Psychiatric Clinics of North America: Pervasive Developmental Disorders, 14*(1), 19–32.

Siegel, B. (1991). Toward DSM-IV: A developmental approach to autistic disorder. *Psychiatric Clinics of North America: Pervasive Developmental Disorders 14*(1), 53–68.

Smalley, S. L. (1991). Genetic influences in autism. *Psychiatric Clinics of North America: Pervasive Developmental Disorders, 14*(1), 125–139.

Snow, C., Perlman, R., & Nathan, D. (1987). Why routines are different: Toward a multiple-factors model of the relation between input and language acquisition. In K. E. Nelson & A. van Kleeck (Eds), *Children's language* (Vol. 6, pp. 65–97). Hillsdale, NJ: Erlbaum.

Sperber, D., & Wilson, D. (1988). *Relevance: Communication and cognition.* Cambridge, MA: Harvard University Press.

Steffenburg, S., Gillberg, C., Hellgren, L, Andersson, L, Gillberg, I., Jakobsson, G., & Bohman, M. (1989). A twin study of autism in Denmark, Finland, Iceland, Norway, and Sweden. *Journal of Child Psychology and Psychiatry, 30*, 405–410.

Stiles, J., & Nass, R. (1991). Spatial grouping activity in young children with congenital right or left hemisphere brain injury. *Brain and Cognition, 15*, 201–222.

Stiles-Davis, J. (1988). Developmental change in young children's spatial grouping activity. *Developmental Psychology, 24*(4), 522–531.

Stiles-Davis, J., Janowksy, P., Engel, M., & Nass, R. (1988). Drawing ability in four young children with congenital unilateral brain lesions. *Neuropsychologia, 26*(3), 359–371.

Stiles-Davis, J., Sugarman, S., & Nass, R. (1985). The development of spatial and class relations in four young children with right-cerebral-hemisphere damage: Evidence for an early spatial constructive deficit. *Brain and Cognition, 4*, 388–412.

Stubbs, M. (1983). *Discourse analysis.* Oxford, UK: Blackwell.

Szatmari, P. (1991). Asperger's syndrome: Diagnosis, treatment, and outcome. *Psychiatric Clinics of North America, 14*(11), 81–94.

Szatmari, P. (1992a). A review of the DSM-III-R criteria for autistic disorder. *Journal of Autism and Developmental Disorders, 22*, 507–523.

Szatmari, P. (1992b). The validity of autistic spectrum disorders: A literature review. *Journal of Autism and Developmental Disorders, 22*, 583–600.

Szatmari, P., Bartolucci, G., Bremner, R., Bond, S., & Rich, S. (1989). A follow-up study of high-functioning autistic children. *Journal of Autism and Developmental Disorders, 11*, 45–56.

Szatmari, P., Bremner, R., & Nagy, J. (1989). Asperger's syndrome: A review of clinical features. *Canadian Journal of Psychiatry, 34*, 554–560.

Szatmari, P., Tuff, L., & Finlayson, M. A. J. (1990). Asperger's syndrome and autism: Neurocognitive aspects. *Journal of the American Academy of Child and Adolescent Psychiatry, 20,* 130–136.

Thal, D., & Bates, E. (1988). Language and gesture in late talkers. *Journal of Speech and Hearing Research, 31,* 115–123.

Thal, D., & Tobias, S. (1992). Communicative gestures in children with delayed onset of expressive vocabulary. *Journal of Speech and Hearing Research, 35,* 1281–1289.

Thal, D., Tobias, S., & Morrison, D. (1991). Language and gesture in later talkers: A one year follow-up. *Journal of Speech and Hearing Disorders, 34,* 604–612.

Thomas, A., & Chess, S. (1977). *Temperament and development.* New York: Brunner-Mazel.

Thomas, A., & Chess, S. (1980). *Dynamics of psychological development.* New York: Brunner-Mazel.

Torrey, E. F., Hersch, S. P., & McCabe, K. D. (1975). Early childhood psychosis and bleeding during pregnancy. *Journal of Autism and Childhood Schizophrenia, 5,* 287–297.

Tsai, L. Y. (1992). Is Rett syndrome a subtype of pervasive developmental disorders? *Journal of Autism and Developmental Disorders, 22,* 551–561.

Tunnell, C. (1977). Three dimensions of naturalness: An expanded definition of field research. *Psychological Bulletin, 84,* 426–437.

VanAcker, R. (1991). Rett syndrome: A review of current knowledge. *Journal of Autism and Developmental Disorders, 21*(4), 381–406.

Van Bourgondien, M. E., Marcus, L. M., & Schopler, E. (1992). Comparison of DSM-III-R and childhood autism rating scale diagnoses of autism. *Journal of Autism and Developmental Disorders, 22*(4), 493–506.

Volkmar F. R., (1992) Childhood disintegrative disorder: Issues for DSM-IV. *Journal of Autism and Developmental Disorders, 22,* 625–642.

Volkmar, F., Cicchetti, D., Cohen, D., & Bregman, J. (1992). Brief report: Developmental aspects of DSM-III-R criteria for autism. *Journal of Autism and Developmental Disorders, 22*(4), 1992, 657–662.

Volkmar, F., Domenic, V., Cicchetti, V., Bregman, J., & Cohen, D. J. (1992). Three diagnostic systems for autism: DSM-III, DSM-III-R, and ICD-10. *Journal of Autism and Developmental Disorders, 22*(4), 483–492.

Vygotsky, L. (1962). *Thought and language* (E. Harfmann & G. Vakar, trans.). Cambridge, MA: MIT Press. (Original work published 1934.)

Vygotsky, L. (1978). *Mind in society: The development of higher psychological processes* (M. Cole, V. John-Steiner, S. Scribner, & E. Souberman, Eds. & Trans.). Cambridge, MA: Harvard University Press.

Vygotsky, L. (1986). Thinking and speech. In R. W. Rieber & A. S. Carton (Eds.), *The collected works of L.S. Vygotsky: I. Problems of General psychology* (pp. 39–285). New York: Plenum. (Original work published 1934)

Waddington, C. H. (1962). *New patterns in genetic development.* New York: Columbia University Press.

Waterhouse, L., Wing, L., Spitzer, R., & Siegel, B. (1992). Pervasive developmental disorders: From DSM-III to DSM-III-R. *Journal of Autism and Developmental Disorders, 22*(4), 525–549.

Weatherby, A., & Prizant, B. (1992). *Communication and symbolic behavior scales.* Chicago: The Riverside Publishing Company.

Wellman, H. H., & Estes, D. (1986). Early understanding of mental entities: A re-examination of childhood realism. *Child Development, 57,* 910–923.

Werry, J. (1992). Child and adolescent (early onset) schizophrenia: A review in light of DSM-III-R. *Journal of Autism and Developmental Disorders, 22*(4), 601–618.

Wertsch, J. W. (1985a). *Culture, communication, and cognition: Vygotskian perspectives.* New York: Cambridge University Press.

Wertsch, J. W. (1985b). *Vygotsky and the social formation of mind.* Cambridge, MA: Harvard University Press.

Wieder, S. (1992). Opening the door: Approaches to engage children with multisystem developmental disorders. *Zero to Three: National Center for Clinical Infant Programs, 13*(2), 10–15.

Wimmer, H., & Perner, J. (1983). Beliefs about beliefs: Representation and constraining function of wrong beliefs in young children's understanding of deception. *Cognition, 13,* 103–128.

Wing, L. (1981a). Asperger's syndrome: A clinical account. *Psychological Medicine, 11,* 115–130.

Wing, L. (1981b). Language, social and cognitive impairments in autism and severe mental retardation. *Journal of Autism and Developmental Disorders, 11,* 31–33.

Wing, L. (1988). The continum of autistic characteristics. In E. Schopler & G. Mesibov (Eds.), *Diagnosis and assessment in autism* (pp. 3–19). New York: Plenum.

Wing, L., & Gould, J. (1979). Severe impairments of social in teraction and associated abnormalities in children: Epidemiology and classification. *Journal of Autism and Developmental Disorders, 9,* 11–30.

Wolff, P. H. (1981). Normal variations in human maturation. In K. J. Connolly & H. F. R. Precht (Eds.), *Maturation and development: Biological and psychological perspectives* (pp. 96–115). Philadelphia: Lippincott.

Woodyatt, G., & Ozanne, A. (1992). Communication abilities and Rett Syndrome. *Journal of Autism and Developmental Disorders, 22*(2), 155–173.

World Health Organization. (1990). *International classification of diseases: Tenth revision. Mental and behavioral disorders.* [May 1990 draft for field trials, unpublished.] Geneva: WHO.

9

Acquired Childhood Language Disorders

MICHAEL W. CASBY, PH.D.

Introduction

In the 1960s, attempts were made to define a group of children who for no obvious reasons had great difficulty acquiring language (cf. Benton, 1964; Eisenson, 1968; West, 1962). Due to the presumption of maldevelopment, damage, or dysfunction of the central nervous system, these children were described as possessing congenital, developmental, primary, childhood, or idiopathic aphasia, although no discernable neurological complications were identified in the children. An early example of this comes from the 1962 *Proceedings of the Institute on Childhood Aphasia* (West, 1962) wherein it was stated that childhood language disorders are an

> impairment of language function (receptive and expressive) resulting from *maldevelopment or injury to the central nervous system* [italics added], prenatally, perinatally, or postnatally (not later . . . than the normal time for the development of speech . . .). . . . Excluded are language problems associated primarily with: 1) mental deficiency, 2) hearing impairment, 3) central nervous system damage affecting the peripheral speech mechanism, 4) emotional disturbance, and 5) delayed maturation in language development resulting from social and emotional factors or physical factors not primarily due to central nervous system involvement. (p. 1)

Eisenson stated in 1968 that "an aphasic child is one with *central nervous system dysfunction* [italics added] . . . associated with severe difficulty in the normal acquisition of language." (p. 3)

Another interesting example, although without pointedly attributing the cause to neurological deficits, comes from Benton (1964), who offered the following:

> In order to avoid possible confusion, a definition of developmental aphasia should be offered. We use the term to designate the condition in which a child shows a relatively specific failure of normal growth of language functions [sic]. The failure can manifest itself either in disability in speaking with near normal speech understanding or in a disability in both understanding and expression of speech. The disability is called a "specific" one because it cannot readily be ascribed to those factors . . . in which failure of language

development is usually observed, namely, deafness, mental deficiency, motor disability or severe personality disorder. (p. 41)

Benton goes on to offer that

> many names have been given to the condition . . . *congenital* or *developmental aphasia*. . . . This large number of terms suggests that the clinical picture has many facets (which indeed it has) and also raises the question of whether we may be dealing here with a number of essentially different conditions which have in common only the fact that one aspect of the end-results of each is a failure in language development.
>
> It is well known that the clinical picture varies from one case to case; in fact, so markedly that some workers feel that the only general statement which can be made with any assurance is that all have a serious language disability. There is certainly no such thing as a "typical case." (p. 41)

Benton's reflections in particular may be as true today as they were in the 1960s—especially those concerning the unknown origin, specific language disability, and diversity of performance. They also bear an interesting and timely similarity to contemporary views of children with developmental language disorders or those labeled "specifically language impaired" (cf. Kamhi, 1991; Leonard, 1982, 1987; Tallal, 1988).

Why would a chapter on acquired childhood language disorders begin with such historic examples of definitions intended to describe developmental language disorders? One reason is that few attempts have been made to define truly acquired childhood language disorders, and we shall attempt one here. Further, the earlier definitions of developmental language disorders used the term *aphasia,* which led to the presumption (and, in some cases, the explicit statement) that the language impairment observed was the direct result of some neurological complications. Yet the definitions were tendered as ones of developmental language disorders. This has led to some confusion and speculation about definitions, etiology, and characteristics of children who experience language disorders, whether developmental or acquired.

It might be argued that the use of the term *aphasia* should be limited to those cases of language impairment in which the language deficit is secondary to known neurological disorders. Alajouanine and Lhermitte proposed in 1965 that children with acquired aphasia are those that have language disorders resulting from focal cerebral lesions. They stated that "acquired aphasia in children is entirely different from retarded speech often unfortunately labeled congenital aphasia" (p. 644); however, they did not cite any evidence for this position, nor did they describe what the "entirely different" aspects are. We will come to see that their strong stance about the magnitude of difference between the language abilities of children with developmental language disorders and those with acquired language disorders is not entirely justified.

Acquired childhood language disorders are those language disorders that occur secondary to some central nervous system disorder—there is a known neurological basis for the disruption in the child's acquisition of language. Children with acquired childhood language disorders are those who demonstrate linguistic deficits in either expressive and/or receptive aspects of linguistic content, form, and/or use which are secondary to some form of cerebral insult occurring pre-, peri-, or postnatally. The language impairment is the result of neurological complications and not sensory impairments (such as hearing disorders), or other central impairments (such as mental retardation), or psychosocial impairments (such as autism), although it may occur in concert with any of them. As stated, the phrase *acquired childhood language disorders* is used broadly here to mean those childhood language disorders that are acquired secondarily to some form of brain damage. Because of the wide range of neurological complications that can result in acquired childhood language disorder, its definition is broader than that which might historically be applied to (acquired) aphasia in children (wherein it might be claimed that the neurological insult is limited to more focal lesions). Acquired childhood language disorders may be secondary, for example, to such pathogenic conditions as infantile or childhood cerebral vascular accidents, seizure disorders, cerebral vascular maldevelopment or malformation, disease, closed-head injury, or surgical intervention, and they may have a variety of etiologies (e.g., maldevelopment, anoxia, toxin or drug exposure, trauma). In so arguing for a broad perspective of acquired childhood language disorders, it is proposed that children who compose the population form a heterogeneous group with regard to cause and effect. Further, in so arguing for a broad perspective, it is proposed that acquired childhood language disorders be described as occurring secondarily to the contributing neurological condition (e.g., acquired childhood language disorder secondary to hemispherectomy, acquired childhood language disorder secondary to focal brain lesion, acquired childhood language disorder secondary to closed-head injury, etc.).

An issue that arises when considering acquired childhood language disorders is the age at which the child may have incurred the cerebral damage. This is particularly true when one considers the use of the term *aphasia* in some of the earlier literature. For example, it is not unusual to encounter the argument that the term *aphasia* should be limited to those children who have acquired childhood language disorders after a period of some normal language development, because aphasia may be viewed as the loss or reduction of previously existing linguistic abilities. Continuing with a broad perspective of acquired childhood language disorders, it is argued here that the term *acquired childhood language disorder* suggests that the cerebral damage may have occurred sometime during the prenatal, perinatal, or postnatal period of development in addition to having a number of potential neurological contributors. Postnatally, the lesion may have occurred between infancy and adolescence. The effect of early versus late-occurring lesions will be taken up later. Language disorders resulting from neurological insult occurring after age 18 would be considered acquired adulthood language disorders.

Pathogeneses and Characteristics of Acquired Childhood Language Disorders

A number of neurologically based pathogenic conditions may give rise to acquired childhood language disorders. In general, the literature has followed along those lines. The literature on acquired childhood language disorders may be divided according to the following neurological conditions: (1) children with cerebrovascular disorders leading to brain lesions, (2) children who have undergone hemispherectomies and therefore continue to function with one remaining hemisphere (right or left), (3) children who have seizure disorders, (4) children with closed-head injury, (5) children with brain tumors and the following effects of surgery and/or central nervous system prophylaxis, and (6) children who suffer such maladies as metabolic disorders, neural tube disorders, and acute cerebral anoxia (cf. Aram, 1988; Aram & Whitaker, 1988; Murdoch, 1990; Weiner, Urion, & Levitt, 1988). All of these conditions may also vary along the variable of age such that they may have occurred prior to a period of presumably normal language development, or they may have occurred during or after such a period.

Despite the many neurological conditions which are involved with acquired childhood language disorders, there is little available evidence of any particular profile of linguistic deficits characteristic of any particular pathogenesis (Cooper & Flowers, 1987). However, some research shows that children suffering from traumatic brain injury show better recovery of linguistic abilities than do either children with cerebrovascular accidents or seizure disorders (Loonen & Van Dongen, 1990). Furthermore, children with bilateral lesions and/or seizure disorders have more severe and/or pervasive language impairment than those with unilateral damage.

This lack of characteristic linguistic deficit profiles related to any particular neurological pathogenesis of acquired childhood language disorders is not surprising. Although research investigating the existence of patterns of linguistic deficits for the large heterogeneous population of children with language disorders has indeed found profiles of deficits (e.g., comprehension deficit, production deficit, comprehension and production deficit) (cf. Aram & Nation, 1975; Wolfus, Moscovitch, & Kinsbourne, 1980), none of these patterns have been found to be related to any particular contributing-disabling condition. Rosenthal, Eisenson, and Luckau (1972) found no validation of the concept that children from different pathogenic conditions demonstrate similar patterns of language impairment relative to their related disability. Results of their discriminant analysis revealed that children from the same handicapping condition (e.g., hearing impairment, mental retardation, neurological impairment, maturational lag) could not be grouped on the basis of the similarity of their oral language performances. Likewise, Waterhouse and Fein (1982) found no significant language differences between various groups of developmentally disabled children.

Children with Cerebrovascular Disorders Leading to Brain Lesions and Acquired Language Disorders

Although it has been proposed that neurological conditions with the potential to cause acquired childhood language disorders are varied and that the term itself may have broad application, this chapter will be limited primarily to that literature on acquired childhood language disorders secondary to cerebrovascular disorders, along with pertinent evidence from research on children with acquired language disorders secondary to hemispherectomy.

Children may suffer from cerebrovascular disorders leading to unilateral or bilateral brain lesions and brain lesions accompanied by seizure disorders. The lesions may occur pre-, peri-, or postnatally. If postnatal, they may occur in infancy or later. The cerebrovascular lesions that young children experience result from a number of neurological complications (Weiner et al., 1988). One prominent condition is that of cerebral vascular accident (CVA) in childhood. Cerebral vascular accidents in childhood are often associated with pediatric cardiac disorders, primarily thromboses or cardiac emboli associated with congenital heart disease and its surgical management risks (Weiner et al., 1988). For example, in Aram and Ekelman (1987), the majority of their 28 subjects with either left- or right-hemisphere lesions had suffered CVA sustained after cardiac catheterization or surgery, and the second most frequent lesion etiology was arterial venous malformation. Another likely cause of cerebrovascular disorders in children is occlusive cerebrovascular disease (cf. Casby, 1992; Weiner et al., 1988). In addition to those children with cerebrovascular complications, children with systemic diseases such as sickle-cell disease are at risk for CVAs. Hariman, Griffith, Hurtig, and Keehn (1991, p. 498) have reported that although CVAs are relatively rare in childhood, they are a major complication in children with sickle-cell disease. Notably, the cause of many cerebrovascular disorders in childhood remains idiopathic.

Impact of Infantile Cerebrovascular Disorders

This section will concentrate on research which has addressed the impact of cerebrovascular lesions during approximately the first 2 years of life. The impact of later acquired lesions will be discussed in a later section.

An example of early research addressing the impact of infantile brain lesions on children's language development is Aicardi, Amsili, and Chevrie (1969). They reviewed patient medical records of infants and young children who sustained sudden onset of hemiplegia prior to 2 years of age. They reported that aphasia was present at the onset of the neurological difficulties in a remarkably few 22 out of 122 children and that 20 of these 22 children had left-hemisphere lesions, as evidenced by right hemiplegia. Aicardi, Amsili, and Chevrie further noted that the language difficulties demonstrated by the children were predominantly expressive difficulties and that the language difficulties were reported to be transitory, lasting only a few months. However, "persistence of verbal disability was evident on formal testing in some of these patients months or years later" (Aicardi et al., 1969, p. 164). Exacting details of the assessment or the children's actual linguistic performance were not reported.

In 1973, Annett reported the results of a retrospective study of children who had incurred brain lesions prior to 13 months of age. They ranged in age from 5 to 18 years at the time of the testing. The available measure of language abilities in the study was the scores on the Wechsler Intelligence Scale for Children (WISC) verbal IQ. Annett noted that the language deficit was associated with left-hemisphere lesions significantly more so than with right-hemisphere ones and that the children with right-hemisphere lesions performed slightly better than did the children with left lesions, but the difference was not significant.

Kershner and King (1974) assessed the WISC verbal IQ of children who had right- or left-hemisphere lesions prior to 15 months of age and who ranged in age from 6 to 9 years at the time of testing. They found that the children with infantile left-hemisphere lesions performed significantly below control children and those with early right-hemisphere damage. The verbal IQs of the children with right-hemisphere damage were not significantly below that of the controls. Similar results have been reported by Rudel, Teuber, and Twitchell (1974) and Riva and Cazzaniga (1986). Children who had suffered infantile left-hemisphere injury had lower verbal IQs upon follow-up assessment, whereas those who experienced early right-hemisphere damage did not display such a verbal deficit.

In summary, infantile cerebral insult to the left hemisphere has a significant effect on language abilities as assessed generally by verbal IQ upon follow-up assessment. Early brain damage to the right hemisphere does not appear to have the same effect. Furthermore, although the verbal IQ of children with left-hemisphere damage is reportedly less than that of controls, the verbal deficit itself does not appear to be severe.

The early research conducted on the effects of brain lesions on children's language development (e.g., Aicardi et al., 1969; Annett, 1973; Kershner & King, 1974) has not been as exacting as some of the more contemporary work (cf. Aram & Ekelman, 1987; Aram, Ekelman, & Whitaker, 1986, 1987; Feldman, Holland, Kemp, & Janosky, 1992; Thal et al., 1991). In particular, this early research lacked specificity related to subjects' characteristics—experimental and control—such as lesion lateralization, localization, and the dependent language measures employed. Therefore, it has been difficult to determine with a high degree of exactness the effects of brain lesions on young children's language development.

Aram and her collaborators have conducted a series of studies on the effects of known focal unilateral brain lesions on young children's language acquisition. In one of their earlier studies (Rankin, Aram, & Horwitz, 1981), they examined the language abilities of children between the ages of 6 and 8 who demonstrated either right or left hemiplegia. All of the children studied had pre- or perinatal acquired unilateral lesions confirmed by computed tomography (CT) scan. Results showed that the linguistic abilities of the children with left-hemisphere damage were inferior to those of the children with right-hemisphere injury. The children with left-hemisphere damage had lower performances on speech articulation, vocabulary comprehension, and syntactic comprehension. It was also noted that, developmentally, the children with left lesions produced single-word and two-word utterances later than did the children with right lesions. The syntactic measures (i.e., The Northwestern Syntax Screening Test and The Token Test) showed the most difference between the two samples of children.

Aram, Ekelman, Rose, and Whitaker (1985) further studied the impact of unilateral lesions on children's language development with samples of eight children with left-hemisphere lesions and eight children with right-hemisphere lesions. For all of the experimental subjects, the neurological complications were associated with congenital heart disorders. Following from this, Aram et al.'s control subjects were selected from children who also had congenital heart disorders but no neurological involvement; further, they were matched for age, sex, and ethnicity. Significant differences were found between the experimental children with left lesions and their controls for all language measures: Peabody Picture Vocabulary Test (PPVT), Expressive One-Word Picture Vocabulary Test (EOWPVT), mean length of utterance (MLU), Developmental Sentence Scoring (DSS), and Northwestern Syntax Screening Test—Receptive and Expressive

(NSST-R and NSST-E). The exception was speech articulation (i.e., Photo Articulation Test, or PAT). Significant differences in language performance between children with right lesions and their controls were found only for the areas of receptive vocabulary and MLU, although no such statistical difference was found between experimental right-lesioned children and their controls for the variable of DSS.

Although it was found that both experimental groups performed significantly below their control groups for receptive vocabulary, a closer inspection of the data revealed that all but one of the left-lesioned children and all but one of the right-lesioned children, however, scored within normal limits on the PPVT. Similarly, all but one left-lesioned child and all but two right-lesioned children scored within normal limits on the EOWPVT. Furthermore, despite the noted group differences, there were individual experimental children (left- or right-lesioned) who scored as well or better on receptive vocabulary than did some of the nonlesioned control children. The inspection of the individual data and the noting of individual performance and differences over the group trends are important regarding the wide range of individual differences and heterogeneity among this as well as other populations of children with language disorders.

As noted, both left-lesioned and right-lesioned children performed more poorly than their controls did on vocabulary measures in the Aram et al. (1985) research. Age differences between the two experimental groups of children did not allow simple direct comparison of raw score data between the two. However, because the two vocabulary measures employed (i.e., PPVT and EOWPVT) generate standard scores (e.g., deviation IQs), a comparison between the two experimental groups based on the standard scores was possible. In comparing the performance of children with left- versus right-hemisphere lesions, as a group the children with left-hemisphere lesions scored better than did the children with right-hemisphere lesions for both receptive and expressive single-word vocabulary. Interesting findings such as this point out the right cerebral hemisphere's contribution to linguistic functioning (e.g., lexical aspects).

In a more detailed investigation of the spoken syntax of these children, Aram, Ekelman, and Whitaker (1986) reported that those children with left-hemisphere lesions performed more poorly on most measures of simple and complex expressive syntax (i.e., MLU, DSS, percentage of simple sentences attempted and produced correctly, percentage of complex sentences attempted and produced correctly, and grammatical markers) than did their nonlesioned control subjects. However, significant differences between children with right-hemisphere lesions and their control counterparts were not found.

The comprehension of syntax by children with unilateral brain lesions was the focus of a study conducted by Aram and Ekelman (1987). The receptive language measure employed was the Revised Token Test (RTT). Seventeen children with left-hemisphere lesions and 11 children with right-hemisphere lesions, as well as their age, sex, ethnicity, and social class matched controls, served as subjects. As in previous studies conducted under Aram et al.'s research protocol, the control subjects were normally developing pediatric cardiology patients who possessed no hemispheric lesions. The results showed that the children with left-hemisphere lesions performed lower than their matched controls on certain subtests of the RTT. Further analyses of the left-hemisphere lesioned children's performance showed that they had notably lower performance than their controls for all 11 linguistic aspects assessed by the RTT (e.g., color, shape, size adjectives, prepositions). Although the performance of the children with right-hemisphere damage was generally and consistently below that of their matched controls for all of the subtests of the RTT, the differences did not reach statistical significance.

Again, in 1987, Aram, Ekelman and Whitaker presented results of an investigation of lexical retrieval of left- and right-hemisphere lesioned children who ranged in age from approximately 6 to 14 years at the time of testing. The subjects of this study were 19 left- and 13 right-lesioned children whose brain injury had occurred at an age of less than 1 month to an age of approximately 11 years. In general, it was found that children with left lesions had significantly slower naming latencies and were significantly less accurate in naming than were their matched control subjects. Children with right-hemisphere lesions had faster naming latencies (albeit not statistically significant); however, like the left-lesioned subjects, the children with right-hemisphere lesions were significantly less accurate in naming than were their controls.

The aforementioned studies have all been retrospective in nature in that the assessment of language abilities came some time following the cerebral neurological complications that occurred in infancy. Recently, results from prospective, developmental, and longitudinal studies of children with infantile brain injury have become available.

Thal et al. (1991) reported on the results of a prospective longitudinal study of the lexical development of infants who incurred either a right- or left-hemisphere lesion within the first 6 months of life. Data were obtained from infants between the ages of 12 to 35 months. Using the experimental version of the MacArthur Communicative Development Inventory, a significant delay in expressive vocabulary was noted for both groups of children. The longitudinal nature of the research provided an interesting insight into a differential effect of the early left- versus right-hemisphere lesions on lexical development. As mentioned earlier, both groups of children demonstrated lexical delay when compared to the norms of the MacArthur Inventory. Interestingly, no differences between the children with left lesions and those with right lesions were noted during the early period of development (i.e., 12 to 17 months), but children with right lesions did perform better than did children with left lesions during the later period of lexical development (i.e., 17 to 35 months). Significant delay in receptive vocabulary was noted for both groups of children throughout the entire time period of development observed (i.e., 12 to 35 months), with no differences noted between the children with left- versus right-hemisphere lesion.

Feldman et al. (1992) presented results of their longitudinal study of syntactic and lexical development of nine children with unilateral pre- and perinatal brain injury. Five of the children had left-hemisphere damage, and four had right-hemisphere damage. Based on data from spontaneous language samples collected across the age span of 15 to 48 months, growth curves for MLU, Index of Productive Syntax, and number of different words were generated. Feldman et al. (1992) reported that seven of the nine children demonstrated early delays in initial word use and that five were delayed in their onset of multiword utterances.

Yet by 24 months of age, six of the nine youngsters (four with left-hemisphere lesion and two with right-hemisphere lesion) had syntactic abilities comparable to children without brain injuries. Laterality of lesion was not considered to have markedly influenced the children's language performances.

Age at Onset of Lesion

In her 1973 study, Annett reported that early acquired lesions (i.e., prior to 13 months of age) had more of an impact on linguistic abilities than did those acquired later for both left- and right-hemisphere lesions. Woods (1980) found that age at onset of lesion only had an impact on children with right-hemisphere lesions. He reported that right-hemisphere lesions occurring before 12 months of age resulted in both low verbal and performance WISC IQ scores and that later childhood right-hemisphere lesions led only to lower performance IQ scores. However, both infantile and childhood left-hemisphere lesions led to significantly low WISC verbal and performance IQ scores. Woods (1980) and Woods and Teuber (1978) also found that age at onset of lesion significantly affected children with right-hemisphere lesions. They reported that lesions occurring within the first year of life (whether right- or left-hemisphere) lowered both verbal and performance scores. The impact of later occurring left-hemisphere lesions was the same as infantile ones, but the impact of later occurring right-hemisphere lesions affected only performance scores.

Riva and Cazzaniga (1986) reported that early left-hemisphere lesions (prior to 1 year of age) equally affected verbal and performance scores; whereas later left-hemisphere lesions (after 1 year of age) did not affect either verbal or performance scores of their subjects as much as early lesions did. As for right-hemisphere lesions, Riva and Cazzaniga reported that early and late lesions only significantly affected performance scores.

Loonen and Van Dongen (1990), reporting on a group of children who suffered their neurological insults across an age span later in development than that of Woods's (1980) subjects (i.e., 3 years 9 months to 13 years 6 months), found no evidence of an age-at-onset effect. For either early or later lesions, most of the children had not recovered 1 year after onset, regardless of age at onset.

In an attempt to sort out the effects of early versus later brain lesions, an analysis of Aram and colleagues' data reveals the following with regard to age at which lesions occur and their ensuing effects on language acquisition: Children with left-hemisphere lesions acquired prior to 6 months of age consistently performed below their controls, as did those children who acquired their lesions between 6 and 12 months of age; those children who acquired their lesions between 12 and 24 months of age; those children who acquired their lesions between 24 and 36 months of age; and those children who suffered their brain lesions sometime after 3 years of age.

In summary, the preponderance of research shows that children with acquired childhood language disorder secondary to cerebrovascular disorders occurring during infancy or childhood demonstrate language impairment with receptive and expressive aspects of syntax, morphology, lexical semantics, and naming/word-finding difficulties. Little is known about these children's pragmatic abilities, such as communication functions and discourse skills. Nonetheless, some results show that later acquired lesions may have less of an impact (Annett, 1973; Riva & Cazzaniga, 1986). When it has been reported that later lesions have not caused a significant language deficit (i.e., Riva & Cazzaniga, 1986), the question of localization and severity of the lesion needs to be addressed. Perhaps it is reasonable to argue that for either early or late brain lesions, the laterality and localization are as important if not more important as age in determining impact on linguistic abilities.

Site of Lesion

The impact of the site of lesion (i.e., lateralization and localization of lesion within a hemisphere) has been difficult to determine from research on young children with brain lesions until recent research, which has been able to obtain data from cerebral imaging techniques (cf. Aram et al., 1985, 1986, 1987; Feldman et al., 1992; Thal et al., 1991). Prior to this, site of lesion was more speculative and was based on behavioral data, such as presence of hemiplegia, with the presumption that site of lesion would be contralateral to the side of the hemiplegia.

LATERALIZATION OF LESION

One often invoked generality about acquired childhood language disorders is that if a child is to encounter some neurological insult which will affect language development, such damage is better sustained early in life versus at a later point in development. This perspective is often attributed to Lennenberg's (1967, 1969) early notions on the equipotentiality of the right and left cerebral hemispheres regarding language abilities. This viewpoint posited that as a result of a lack of cerebral lateralization and specialization and the presence of neurodevelopmental plasticity during the early part of one's life, if one cerebral hemisphere was incapacitated then the other healthy hemisphere would compensate and take on the added functioning of the damaged hemisphere (cf. Basser, 1962; Lennenberg, 1967, 1969). These assumptions were based on an earlier view of neurological development, which proposed that hemispheric specialization developed over the course of infancy and early childhood.

Research has demonstrated, however, that both anatomic and functional asymmetry already exist in infancy (cf. Chi, Dooling, & Gilles, 1977; Molfese, 1977; Wada, Clarke, & Hamm, 1975; Witelson & Pallie, 1973). However, there is diversity with regard to this finding of early cerebral asymmetry, and it is not in fact found in all cases. For example, although Chi et al. (1977) did find that 54% of their sample of fetal brains had a more extensive left- than right-hemisphere temporal plane, they also found that such asymmetry was not the case for the remaining 46% of the sample. (See also Wada et al., 1975, for further evidence of the lack of totality of cerebral asymmetry in infants and adults, and see Galaburda, LeMay, Kemper, and Geschwind, 1978, who reported that the left planum temporale was larger than the right for 65% of the cases. But Galaburda et al., 1978, additionally reported that the right planum temporale was larger in 11% of the cases and that there was no size difference between the left and right in 24% of the cases studied.)

The strong equipotential view of the cerebral hemispheres was driven by an interpretation of data available during Lennenberg's life, which reported that young children who sustained left-hemisphere lesions early in life recovered language abilities rapidly throughout the course of their recovery (Alajouanine & Lhermitte, 1965; Basser, 1962; Byers & McLean, 1962). Although these early reports tended to emphasize the equipotentiality of right- and left-hemisphere contributions to language acquisition following early brain lesions, the landmark work of Dennis and colleagues on children undergoing early hemispherectomies provided considerable insight into the issue of the differential impact of early damage to the left versus the right cerebral hemisphere (cf. Dennis, 1980; Dennis & Kohn, 1975; Dennis & Whitaker, 1976, 1977). This line of research showed that although youngsters who underwent a left-hemisphere hemispherectomy recovered considerable language functioning, they also continued to demonstrate linguistic difficulties, primarily with syntax—albeit subtle difficulties. Those youngsters who underwent early removal of their right hemisphere and hence had a remaining healthy, but single, left hemisphere showed remarkable recovery and essentially normal linguistic functioning. Day and Ulatowska (1979) also reported that subjects who had undergone a left hemispherectomy demonstrated relatively weak syntactic skills but that expressive semantics was a strength; and that the linguistic abilities of subjects who had undergone a right hemispherectomy remained basically intact. This work, which employed more detailed assessment of linguistic ability, is in contrast to the earlier report of Basser (1962), wherein it was reported that linguistic abilities developed and maintained in the lone remaining intact hemisphere (irrespective of whether it was the right or left hemisphere).

These children do recovery language abilities, and in many cases remarkably. But the language abilities of children with left-hemisphere lesions are significantly delayed when compared to controls or to children with right-hemisphere lesions—there is a differential effect of lateralization of lesion in acquired childhood language disorders (cf. Annett, 1973; Aram & Ekelman, 1987; Aram et al., 1985, 1986, 1987; Feldman et al., 1992; Kershner & King, 1974; Kiessling, Denckla, & Carlton, 1983; McFie, 1961; Rankin et al., 1981; Riva & Cazzaniga, 1986; Rudel et al., 1974; Woods, 1980, 1983; Woods & Carey, 1979; Woods & Teuber, 1978). Characteristic of these findings are the results of Kiessling et al. (1983), in which children with left-hemisphere lesions performed significantly less well than did children with right-hemisphere lesions and controls on linguistic measures, although the actual linguistic deficits were not relatively severe.

The equipotentiality position was also fueled by the early proposition that children who suffered right-hemisphere lesions were as likely as those who suffered left-hemisphere lesions to have resultant language deficits (Basser, 1962). The likelihood of a language disorder resulting from a focal right-hemisphere lesion has been strongly contested in the more contemporary literature. However, early on Annett (1973, p. 10) reported that when laterality of lesion was examined for association with language deficit, some 40% of 59 cases with left-hemisphere damage and only 15% of 47 children with right-hemisphere damage demonstrated language disorders. Further, Aram and colleagues have demonstrated that in many cases of right-hemisphere damage the children's language abilities are not significantly below that of matched controls. In a meta-analysis of the literature, Carter, Hohenegger, and Satz (1982) reported that the probability of a language deficit resulting from right-hemisphere damage during childhood was in the range of zero to .06, and it was .94 for left hemisphere damage when such variables as evidence of known focal lesion and handedness were accounted for (see also Woods, 1983).

The preceding insights indicate that the two hemispheres are not entirely equipotential with regard to linguistic abilities and, in particular, syntax. Research has consistently shown that the right hemisphere does not compensate completely for an early damaged left hemisphere vis-à-vis language abilities. Those children who suffer an early left-hemisphere lesion continue to demonstrate lowered language abilities than matched controls, whereas children with early right-hemisphere lesions do not suffer the same degree of language disorder (but see Feldman et al., 1992). Such findings do not strongly support a homologous view of neuroplasticity of the brain for the development of linguistic abilities. However, the plasticity of the developing cerebral cortex and the collateral responsibility of the paired cerebral hemispheres should not be denied. As noted in much of the previous research on the impact of brain lesions in children's language acquisition, the language recovery of these children is remarkable. The relatively rapid and exceptional recovery of language abilities by children with brain lesions itself is significant evidence of the neuroplasticity of the developing central nervous system (versus the lessened and protracted recovery from aphasia in adults). Although it is questionable if the right hemisphere plays a homologous equipotential role to the left in developing language, this should not rule out the process of developmental neuroplasticity. It is arguable that the neuroplasticity of the linguistically dominant hemisphere itself (i.e., left hemisphere) may largely be involved in the recovery seen in acquired childhood language disorders resulting from focal lesions. Although I am unaware of any studies utilizing dynamic cerebral imagining/functioning techniques (e.g., positron-emission tomography [PET], single photon emission computer tomography [SPECT], regional cerebral blood flow [RCBF]) of children with acquired language disorders to ascertain which areas of the brain are active during linguistic processing, such studies may provide significant evidence about the contribution of either hemisphere during the recovery from acquired childhood language disorders. Papanicolaou, DiScenna, Gillespie, and Aram (1990) employed an evoked-potential paradigm to ascertain differential activity between the right and left hemisphere in a group of children with acquired language disorders secondary to focal left-hemisphere lesion. They found that the left hemispheres of these children continued to respond differentially to linguistic stimuli and that the right hemispheres did not. This is evidence of the potential recruitment of adjacent neurological areas and reorganization of language functioning within the same preincident language-dominant hemisphere during the recovery/development of linguistic abilities in acquired childhood disorders.

LOCATION OF LESION

Compared to what is known about the age of onset and lateralization of lesion and acquired childhood language disorders, relatively little is known about the effects of location of lesions within a hemisphere and acquired childhood language disorders. However, work by Aram and Ekelman (1987), Hecaen (1983), Thal et al. (1991), Feldman et al. (1992), and Van Dongen, Loonen, and Van Dongen (1985) has begun to address location of lesions within hemispheres through cerebral imaging technology.

For example, Aram and Ekelman (1987) reported that there was a trend in their data for children with left-hemisphere lesions posterior to the Rolandic fissure to perform more poorly on receptive syntax than did children with left-hemisphere pre-Rolandic lesions. No such differences were reported for children with right-hemisphere lesions in different locations or for children with left cortical versus left subcortical lesions. However, Aram et al. (1987) offer the caveat that because of the small number of subjects available with only pre- or post-Rolandic fissure and only subcortical lesions, it is difficult to sort out the effects of location of lesion. They observe further that diverse lesion sites within the left hemisphere may cause linguistic deficits in young children. Expressive difficulties resulted from pre-Rolandic lesions in 63% of the cases reported and from temporal lesions in 10% of the cases in a report by Hecaen (1983).

In contrast to Aram et al. (1987) and Hecaen (1983), Thal et al. (1991) reported that left-hemisphere lesions that were located posterior to the Rolandic fissure were associated with greater delays in expressive language and that delays were more protracted in children with this left posterior damage. The significant expressive delay resulting from posterior lesions in Thal et al.'s subjects is in some contrast to the effect of posterior lesions in adults, wherein the most likely impact would be reduced receptive abilities. Likewise, Van Dongen et al. (1985) also reported that expressive deficits may not always result from pre-Rolandic lesions in children based on a case of expressive language difficulties for a child who had suffered a posterior temporal lobe lesion. Age was one difference between the subjects of Thal et al. and Hecaen and those of Aram, Eckelman, and Whitaker. Thal et al.'s subjects were age 15 to 37 months at the time of observation, whereas the children in Hecaen's report were age 3 to 14 years at the time of testing.

Feldman et al. (1992) reported no such location of lesion effects. In their sample of nine children with either left- or right-hemisphere lesions, they found that location of lesion (e.g., parietal, frontal, temporal) had no significant impact on the children's acquisition of language within their first 48 months of life. However, recall that Feldman et al.'s subjects showed little linguistic deficit and no particular lateralization-of-lesion effect. This may be evidence of the relative mild cerebrovascular disorders possessed by the Feldman et al. subjects. Clearly future research needs to address and account for severity of lesion.

In summary, research on acquired childhood language disorder indicates that a language impairment can result from brain injury to either of the cerebral hemispheres, although left lesions lead to more significant language deficits. Early or late left-hemisphere brain damage appears to lessen both syntax and lexical aspects, whereas early right-hemisphere injury appears to affect lexical development more selectively, with late right-hemisphere lesions having little, if any, effects. Recovery for children with early left-hemisphere damage is not as complete as it is for those with right-hemisphere injury. The data on localization of lesion within a hemisphere are sparse, and the available data show diverse effects and some that are unlike those observed in adults with acquired language disorders.

Acquired Childhood Language Disorders and Developmental Language Disorders

One reason for a comparison of acquired childhood language disorders with developmental language disorders is the often cited presumed neurological basis of developmental language impairment. The term *developmental language disorder* (DLO) will be used in this discussion rather than the term *specific language impairment.* Although the term *specific language impairment* is used to refer to children who possess developmental as opposed to acquired language disorders, children with acquired language disorders also demonstrate specific language impairments. That is, the language deficit is apparently the primary disability. There is some compelling evidence that questions the typicality of the central nervous system of children assessed as developmental language disordered. The focus of these investigations has been the presence or absence of functional asymmetry and the presence or absence of anatomic asymmetry of the cerebral cortex. Although the combined literature is too massive and complex to discuss here, the data are interesting and mount an argument for neurological bases of developmental language disorders (cf. Caparulo et al., 1981; Cohen, Campbell, & Yaghmai, 1989; Denays et al., 1989; Harcherik et al., 1985; Hier & Rosenberger, 1980; Jernigan, Hesselink, Sowell, & Tallal, 1991; Plante, 1991; Plante, Swisher, Vance, & Rapcsak, 1991; Rapcsak, 1991; Rosenberger & Heir, 1980; Stefanatos, Green, & Ratcliff, 1989).

If the bases of developmental and acquired childhood language disorders are the same (i.e., neurological damage to the language-dominant hemisphere), then one might expect to see striking similarities in the linguistic abilities and disabilities of these two populations. An admittedly liberal integration of available data from research on acquired childhood language disorders secondary to focal left-hemisphere lesions or left hemispherectomy and developmental language disorders seems to lead to the position that there are some generally notable similarities and yet some narrow differences. No direct comparisons of the two populations of children's language performances have been accomplished, but see Miller, Campbell, Chapman, and Weismer (1984) for a brief look at correspondences in language performance of children with acquired and those with developmental language disorders.

Nonetheless, one likely similarity between children with acquired language disorders and those with developmental language disorders are patterns of language impairment or, more specifically, the diversity of language impairments observed in either population of children. Children with developmental and acquired language disorders have been reported to demonstrate receptive and expressive difficulties. Available research has also demonstrated that children with acquired and developmental language disorders also demonstrate difficulties with syntax, semantics, phonology, and morphology; there has not been much research on the pragmatic abilities of acquired childhood language disorders as yet.

It could be argued that children with acquired language disorders secondary to focal left-hemisphere cerebrovascular disorders have difficulty primarily with syntax. For example, the area of syntax has repeatedly been shown to be an area of difficulty for children with acquired language disorders (cf. Aram et al., 1985,

1986, 1987; Dennis et al., 1975, 1976, 1977). Language structure is arguably the component of language that children with developmental language disorders have the most difficulty in acquiring as well (cf. Leonard, 1989).

As for the narrow differences between children with acquired and those with developmental language disorders, we need to look at level of severity and the protracted nature of the development of language. The research on children with known focal unilateral brain lesions and hemispherectomies has generally reported that the impact of these on language abilities is relatively mild and subtle. For example, although research has demonstrated that children with left-hemisphere lesions have language abilities below that of matched controls, they often score within normal limits on norm-based tests of language. Even a casual look at the literature on developmental language disorders reveals that subjects are repeatedly considerably below the norms on standardized language measures as well as significantly below their experimental controls for language performance.

In addition, as reported in the literature, the recovery observed in language abilities of children with acquired language disorders resulting from focal left-hemisphere brain lesions is sweeping, but not complete. Byers and McLean (1962) reported that all 10 of the children they were following recovered language abilities "spontaneously" 3 to 7 years following onset of lesion and language disorder. Alajouanine and Lhermitte (1965) reported that 24 out of 32 of their subjects with left-hemisphere lesion acquired language disorder regained normal or nearly normal language abilities 1 year post-onset. Although this was generally reported, it is indicative of the relatively nonsevere language disorder of children with acquired language disorders due to focal cerebral lesions. Much of the contemporary work on acquired childhood language disorders has also made it clear that the initial language impairment might be relatively mild and that most of these children do remarkably well with postincident language acquisition. Interestingly, Aram (1991a, pp. 315–316) stated that it is rare for a child with a focal left- or right-hemisphere lesion to present a severe language disorder compared to some of the more prevalent severe cases of developmental language disorders; furthermore, for those children requiring language intervention, abilities typically improve sufficiently that the language intervention "is relatively short lived and long-standing clinically significant language disorders are not present" (p. 316). Follow-up studies of children with developmental language disorders do not come anywhere near these types of findings or statements on the prognosis of normal language functioning for those children (cf. Aram & Nation, 1980; Aram et al., 1984; Hall & Tomblin, 1978).

This may advance the view that the language impairment demonstrated by children with acquired language disorders may not be of the same magnitude as that demonstrated by children with developmental language disorders; however, again, no studies have been completed that have made direct comparisons of the severity of linguistic deficit in children with developmental versus acquired language disorders. One might logically think that this recovery would be significantly influenced by the severity of the lesion, a perspective endorsed by Feldman et al. (1992). Nonetheless, such a size-of-lesion effect was not found by Loonen and Van Dongen (1990) or by Thal et al. (1991).

As noted earlier, neurological complications have often been proposed to be causally linked to specific language impairment. The lack of close specific similarity in severity of language impairment between acquired childhood language disorders and developmental language disorders/specific language impairment does not strongly support the viewpoint that both share a neurological or a similar neurological basis. One hypothesis arising from the review of acquired childhood language disorders that are a result of focal cerebrovascular disorders is that if the developmental language disorder's (DLD's) suspected origin is neurological, then such neurological components must be much more diffuse and pervasive than in unilateral focal lesions, given the DLD's reported severity of linguistic impairment beyond that reported for acquired childhood language disorders; and DLD's protracted period of language acquisition. The severity of language impairment seen in developmental language disorder may be more similar to that observed in children with acquired language disorders secondary to seizure disorders (e.g., less focal neurological impairment) (cf. Miller et al., 1984).

In an attempt to compare and contrast and look for similarities and differences between children with acquired and those with developmental language disorders, perhaps Aram's (1991b) thoughts are of particular relevance. She insightfully proposed that the population of young children with language disorders has clusters or subcategories that have some degree of overlap and significant heterogeneity with regard to causation and linguistic deficit.

Intervention Issues

Few data are available which purposefully address the issue of language intervention directly related to any one of the potential pathogeneses of acquired childhood language disorders. This is not the case for acquired aphasia in adults. The question of effectiveness of intervention vis-à-vis aphasia in adults has been addressed in a number of investigations (cf. LaPointe, 1990; Prins & Schoonen, 1989; Rosenbeck, LaPointe, & Wertz, 1989). Although substantial and significant work has been done on intervention for child language disorders generally, little research has addressed the effectiveness or appropriateness of various intervention approaches for the population of children with acquired language disorders. General comments and precautions have been offered with regard to special consideration of these children's state of alertness, distractibility, emotion, and memory as contributory to difficulty in remediation attempts. Yet, little data exist to support or refute such considerations.

Perhaps a reasonable statement on intervention practices for acquired childhood language disorders is that the prevailing treatment philosophy is to intervene as one might for other childhood language disorders, for which a wide range of strategies and tactics are available (Leonard, 1981). Perhaps the most prevailing strategy in language intervention is to focus on the aspect(s) of communication that the child has difficulty with—that is, focus on the content of intervention (i.e., syntax, semantic, morphology, phonology, pragmatics). Along with the focus on content, one must also focus on a particular process of intervention (i.e., child initiated, clinician initiated, comprehension based, production based, etc.). An interesting perspective on language intervention discussed by Leonard (1983) may have some particular merit as a hypothesis for language intervention with children with acquired language disorders as well. Leonard (1983) discussed an "intervention linked" model in which children are sorted according to characteristics that have a potential bearing on the choice of language intervention procedure regardless of presumed etiology. One of these possible characteristics may be level of severity of language disorder. Friedman and Friedman (1980) found that language-impaired children's linguistic characteristics did interact with the type of intervention that was successful. They reported that children with low pretreatment scores on syntax gained more from a highly structured, programmed intervention approach. Their study also showed that a less structured, more interactive approach worked best with those children who had less severe pretreatment syntactic deficits.

Casby (1992) demonstrated the effectiveness of a semantic concept elaboration intervention scheme based on the Craik and Lockhart (1972) levels-of-processing memory framework for the remediation of naming problems in a young boy who had a history of infantile and childhood occlusive cerebrovascular disorder. The child's language deficit was characterized by significantly delayed expressive language abilities, including word-finding/naming difficulties; his receptive language was assessed as within normal limits. The levels-of-processing based semantic concept elaboration intervention required the child to use words which he demonstrated naming difficulties proactively in an elaborated paradigmatic and syntagmatic fashion. Results showed that he had improved his naming speed and reduced his naming errors as a result of the treatment. The intervention approach used by Casby (1992) was not selected based on the etiology of the child's language disorder, but rather it was based on the pattern of language impairment the child demonstrated (in particular the word-finding/naming difficulty).

Conclusion

This chapter has been confined primarily to acquired childhood language disorders secondary to cerebrovascular disorders and hemispherectomy, although acquired childhood language disorders may result from other neurological complications. As critiqued by Aram (1988) and Aram and Whitaker (1988), research on the effects of brain lesions in children's language and cognitive development suffers from the following shortcomings, which we are offered as a final caveat: Many studies fail to specify the location and level of laterality of the lesion reliably and validly. Related to this is a lack of clear demonstration of the exact location or extent of the lesion. It is often not clear whether the lesion is entirely unilateral or if some degree of bilateral damage may exist, or whether the lesion is anterior or posterior. Furthermore, children with suspected focal brain lesions are included with children suffering from more global effects of such conditions, such as accompanying seizure disorders. All of this points to problems that arise with highly variable heterogeneous subjects. In addition to these subject description variables, Aram and Whitaker (1988) advise that at least three other areas of subject specification need to be considered in work with children with brain lesions. The first deals with measurement of subjects' premorbid linguistic and cognitive abilities. In most of the research on the impact of brain lesions on children's language development, little systematic information is available about the children's language prior to the insult. The second concerns the level of specificity/description of the language measure. More specific and descriptive data reports are needed rather than general summary or overall test scores. The subjects' language needs to be described at the level of performance with the various components of language (i.e., syntax, morphology, phonology, semantics, and pragmatics) as well as with the processes of language (i.e., production, comprehension, and imitation). Third, more detail with regard to individual differences and diversity in subjects' performance on dependent measures is called for. Fundamental needs and issues such as these in the evaluation of research on acquired childhood language disorders indicate that although there is much information available about the disorder, we are merely on the threshold of comprehending it.

References

Aicardi, J., Amsili, J., & Chevrie J. J. (1969). Acute hemiplegia in infancy and childhood. *Developmental Medicine and Child Neurology, 11,* 162–173.

Alajouanine, T. H., & Lhermitte, F. (1965). Acquired aphasia in children. *Brain, 88,* 653–662.

Annett, M. (1973). Laterality of childhood hemiplegia and the growth of speech and intelligence. *Cortex, 9,* 4–33.

Aram, D. M. (1988). Language sequelae of unilateral brain lesions in children. In F. Plum (Ed.), *Language, Communication, and the brain* (pp. 171–197). New York: Raven Press.

Aram, D. M. (1991a). Brain lesions in children: Implications for developmental language disorders. In J. Miller (Ed.), *Research on child language disorders: A decade of progress* (pp. 309–320). Austin, TX: Pro-ed.

Aram, D. M. (1991b). Comments on specific language impairment as a clinical category. *Language, Speech, and Hearing Services in Schools, 22,* 84–87.

Aram, D., & Ekelman, B. (1987). Unilateral brain lesions in childhood: Performance on the revised token test. *Brain and Language, 32,* 137–158.

Aram, D., et al. (1984). Preschoolers with language disorders: 10 years later. *Journal of Speech and Hearing Research, 27,* 232–244.

Aram, D., Ekelman, B., Rose, D., & Whitaker, H. (1985). Verbal and cognitive sequelae following unilateral lesions acquired in early childhood. *Journal of Clinical and Experimental Neuropsychology, 7,* 55–78.

Aram, D., Ekelman, B., & Whitaker, H. (1986). Spoken syntax in children with acquired unilateral hemisphere lesions. *Brain and Language, 27,* 75–100.

Aram, D., Ekelman, B., & Whitaker, H. (1987). Lexical retrieval in left and right brain lesioned children. *Brain and Language, 31,* 61–87.

Aram, D., Ekelman, B., & Nation, J. (1975). Patterns of language behavior in children with developmental language disorders. *Journal of Speech and Hearing Research, 18,* 229–214.

Aram, D., & Nation, J. (1980). Preschool language disorders and subsequent language and academic difficulties. *Journal of Communication Disorders, 13,* 159–170.

Aram, D., & Whitaker, H. (1988). Cognitive sequelae of unilateral lesions acquired in early childhood. In D. L. Molfese & S. J. Segalowitz (Eds.), *The developmental implications of brain lateralization* (pp. 417–436). New York: Guilford.

Basser, L. (1962). Hemiplegia of early onset and the faculty of speech with special reference to the effects of hemispherectomy. *Brain, 85,* 427–460.

Benton, A. (1964). Developmental aphasia and brain damage. *Cortex, 1,* 40–52.

Byers, R. K., & McLean, W. T. (1962). Etiology and course of certain hemiplegias with aphasia in childhood. *Pediatrics,* March, 376–383.

Caparulo, B., Cohen, D., Rothman, S., Young, J., Katz, J., Shaywitz, S., & Shaywitz, B. (1981). Computed tomographic brain scanning in children with developmental neuropsychiatric disorders. *Journal of the American Academy of Child Psychiatry, 20,* 338–357.

Carter, R., Hohenegger, M., & Satz, P. (1982). Aphasia and speech organization in children. *Science, 218,* 797–799.

Casby, M. (1992). An intervention approach for naming problems in children. *American Journal of Speech-Language Pathology, 1,* 35–42.
Chi, J., Dooling, E., & Gilles, F. (1977). Gyral development of the human brain. *Annals of Neurology, 1,* 86–93.
Cohen, M., Campbell, R., & Yaghmai, F. (1989). Neuropathological abnormalities in developmental dysphasia. *Annals of Neurology, 25,* 567–570.
Cooper, J., & Flowers, C. (1987). Children with a history of acquired aphasia: Residual language and academic impairments. *Journal of Speech and Hearing Disorders, 52,* 251–252.
Craik, F., & Lockhart, R. (1972). Levels of processing: A framework for memory research. *Journal of Verbal Learning and Verbal Behavior, 11,* 671–684.
Day, P. S., & Ulatowska, H. K. (1979). Perceptual, cognitive, and linguistic development after early hemispherectomy: Two case studies. *Brain and Language, 7,* 17–33.
Denays, R., Tondeur, M., Foulon, M., Verstraeten, F., Ham, H., Piepsz, A., & Noel, P. (1989). Regional brain blood flow in congenital dysphasia: Studies with Technetium-99m HM-PAO SPECT. *The Journal of Nuclear Medicine, 30,* 1825–1829.
Dennis, M. (1980). Capacity and strategy for syntactic comprehension after left or right hemidecortication. *Brain and Language, 10,* 287–317.
Dennis, M., & Kohn, B. (1975). Comprehension of syntax in infantile hemiplegics after cerebral hemidecortication: Left hemisphere superiority. *Brain and Language, 2,* 472–482.
Dennis, M., & Whitaker, H. (1976). Language acquisition following hemidecortication: Linguistic superiority of the left over the right hemisphere. *Brain and Language, 3,* 404–433.
Dennis, M., & Whitaker, H. (1977). Hemispheric equipotentiality and language acquisition. In S. Segalowitz & F. Gruber (Eds.), *Language development and neurological theory* (pp. 93–106). New York: Academic Press.
Eisenson, J. (1968). Developmental aphasia: A speculative view with therapeutic implications. *Journal of Speech and Hearing Disorders, 33,* 3–13.
Feldman, H. M., Holland, A. L., Kemp, S. S., & Janosky, J. E. (1992). Language development after unilateral brain injury. *Brain and Language, 42,* 89–102.
Friedman, P., & Friedman, K. (1980). Accounting for individual differences when comparing the effectiveness of remedial language teaching methods. *Applied Psycholinguistics, 1,* 151–170.
Galaburda, A., LeMay, M., Kemper, T., & Geschwind, N. (1978). Right-left asymmetries in the brain. *Science, 199,* 852–856.
Hall, P., & Tomblin, B. (1978). A follow-up study of children with articulation and language disorders. *Journal of Speech and Hearing Disorders, 43,* 227–241.
Harcherik, D., Cohen, D., Ort, S., Paul, R., Shaywitz, B., Volkmar, F., Rothman, S., & Leckman, J. (1985). Computed tomographic brain scanning in four neuropsychiatric disorders of childhood. *American Journal of Psychiatry, 142,* 731–734.
Hariman, L., Griffith, E., Hurtig, A., & Keehn, M. (1991). Functional outcomes of children with sickle-cell disease affected by stroke. *Archives of Physical Medicine and Rehabilitation, 72.*
Hecaen, H. (1983). Acquired aphasia in children: Revisited. *Neuropsychologia, 21,* 581–587.
Hier, D. B., & Rosenberger, P. B. (1980). Focal left temporal lobe lesions and delayed speech acquisition. *Developmental and Behavioral Pediatrics, 1,* 54–57.
Jernigan, T., Hesselink, J., Sowell, E., & Tallal, P. (1991). Cerebral structure on magnetic resonance imaging in language- and learning-impaired children. *Archives of Neurology, 48,* 539–545.
Kamhi, A. (1991). Specific language impairment as a clinical category—an introduction. *Language, Speech, and Hearing Services in Schools, 22,* 65.
Kershner, J., & King, A. (1974). Laterality of cognitive functions in achieving hemiplegic children. *Perceptual and Motor Skills, 39,* 1283–1289.
Kiessling, L., Denckla, M., & Carlton, M. (1983). Evidence for differential hemispheric function in children with hemiplegic cerebral palsy. *Developmental Medicine and Child Neurology, 25,* 727–734.
LaPointe, L. (Ed.) (1990). *Aphasia and related neurogenic language disorders.* New York: Thieme Medical Publishers.
Lennenberg, E. (1967). *Biological foundations of language.* New York: Wiley.
Lennenberg, E. (1969). On explaining language. *Science, 164,* 635–643.
Leonard, L. (1981). Facilitating linguistic skills in children with specific language impairment. *Applied Psycholinguistics, 2,* 89–118.
Leonard, L. (1982). Specific language impairment. In S. Rosenberg (Ed.), *Handbook of applied psycholinguistics* (pp. 295–328). Hillsdale, NJ: Erlbaum.
Leonard, L. (1983). Defining the boundaries of language disorders in children. In J. Miller, D. Yoder, & R. Schiefelbusch (Eds.) *ASHA reports 12: Contemporary issues in language intervention* (pp. 107–112). Rockville, MD: The American Speech-Language-Hearing Association.
Leonard, L. (1987). Is specific language impairment a useful construct? In S. Rosenberg (Ed.),

Advances in applied psycholinguistics: Volume 1—Disorders of first-language development (pp. 1–39). New York: Cambridge University Press, 1987.

Leonard, L. (1989). Language learnability and specific language impairment in children. *Applied Psycholinguistics, 10,* 179–292.

Loonen, M. C. B. & Van Dongen, H. R. (1990). Acquired childhood aphasia. *Archives of Neurology, 47,* 1324–1328.

McFie, J. (1961). Intellectual impairment in children with localized post-infantile cerebral lesions. *Journal of Neurology, Neurosurgery and Psychiatry, 24,* 361.

Miller, J., Campbell, T., Chapman, R., & Weismer, S. (1984). Language behavior in acquired childhood aphasia. In A. Holland (Ed.), *Language disorders in children* (pp. 57–100). San Diego, CA: College-Hill Press.

Molfese, D. (1977). Infant cerebral asymmetry. In S. Segalowitz & F. Gruber (Eds.), *Language development and neurological theory* (pp. 21–35). New York: Academic Press.

Murdoch, B. (1990). *Acquired neurological speech/language disorders in childhood.* Hillsdale, NJ: Erlbaum.

Papanicolaou, A., DiScenna, A., Gillespie, L., & Aram, D. (1990). Probe-evoked potential findings following unilateral left-hemisphere lesions in children. *Archives of Neurology, 47,* 562–566.

Plante, E. (1991). MRI findings in the parents and siblings of specifically language-impaired boys. *Brain and Language, 41,* 67–80.

Plante, E., Swisher, L., Vance, R., & Rapcsak, S. (1991). MRI findings in boys with specific language impairment. *Brain and Language, 41,* 52–66.

Prins, R., & Schoonen, R. (1989). Efficacy of two different types of speech therapy for aphasic stroke patients. *Applied Psycholinguistics, 10,* 85–123.

Rankin, J., Aram, D., & Horwitz, S. (1981). Language ability in right and left hemiplegic children. *Brain and Language, 14,* 292–306.

Rapcsak, S. (1991). MRI findings in boys with specific language impairment. *Brain and Language, 41,* 52–66.

Riva, D., & Cazzaniga, L. (1986). Late effects of unilateral brain lesions sustained before and after age one. *Neuropsychologia, 3,* 423–428.

Rosenbeck, J., LaPointe, L., & Wertz, R. (1989). *Aphasia: A clinical approach.* San Diego: College-Hill Press.

Rosenberger, P. B., & Hier, D. B. (1980). Cerebral asymmetry and verbal intellectual deficits. *Annals of Neurology, 8,* 300–304.

Rosenthal, W., Eisenson, J., & Luckau, J. (1972). A statistical test of the validity of diagnostic categories used in childhood language disorders. *Papers and Reports on Child Language Development,* 121–143.

Rudel, R. G., Teuber, H-L., & Twitchell, T. E. (1974). Levels of impairment of sensori-motor functions in children with early brain damage. *Neuropsychologia, 12,* 95–108.

Stefanatos, G., Green, G., & Ratcliff, G. (1989). Neurophysiological evidence of auditory channel anomalies in developmental dysphasia. *Archives of Neurology, 46,* 871–875.

Tallal, P. (1988). Developmental language disorders. In J. Kavanagh & T. Truss (Eds.), *Learning disabilities: Proceedings of the national conference,* (pp. 181–272). Parkton, MD: York Press.

Thal, D., Marchman, V., Stiles, J., Aram, D., Trauner, D., Nass, R., & Bates, E. (1991). Early lexical development in children with focal brain injury. *Brain and Language, 40,* 491–527.

Van Dongen, H. R., Loonen, M. C. B., & Van Dongen, K. J. (1985). Anatomical basis for acquired fluent aphasia in children. *Annals of Neurology, 17,* 306–309.

Wada, J., Clarke, R., & Hamm, A. (1975). Cerebral hemispheric asymmetry in humans. *Archives of Neurology, 32,* 239–246.

Waterhouse, L., & Fein, D. (1982). Language skills in developmentally disabled children. *Brain and Language, 15,* 307–333.

Weiner, H., Urion, D., & Levitt, L. (1988). *Pediatric neurology for the house officer* (3rd ed.). Baltimore: Williams & Wilkins.

West, R. (1962). Childhood aphasia: Proceedings of the institute on childhood aphasia. San Francisco: California Society of Crippled Children and Adults.

Witelson, S., & Pallie, S. (1973). Left hemisphere specialization for language in the newborn. *Brain, 96,* 641–646.

Wolfus, B., Moscovitch, M., & Kinsbourne, M. (1980). Subgroups of developmental language impairment. *Brain and Language, 9,* 152–171.

Woods, B. T. (1980). The restricted effects of right-hemisphere lesions after age one; Wechsler test data. *Neuropsychologia, 18,* 65–70.

Woods, B. T. (1983). Is the left hemisphere specialized for language at birth? *Topics in Neurosciences, 6,* 115–117.

Woods, B., & Carey, S. (1979). Language deficits after apparent clinical recovery from childhood aphasia. *Annals of Neurology, 6,* 405–409.

Woods, B., & Teuber, H. (1978). Changing patterns of childhood aphasia. *Annals of Neurology, 3,* 273–280.

10

Communicative Development of Children with Severe Disabilities

MARY ANN ROMSKI, PH.D., AND
ROSE A. SEVCIK, PH.D.

Introduction

The communication development of children with severe disabilities has been a focus of research and practice for over 2 decades (e.g., McLean, Yoder, & Schiefelbusch, 1970; Schiefelbusch, 1980; Schiefelbusch & Hollis, 1979; Schiefelbusch & Lloyd, 1974; Warren & Reichle, 1992). Their communication skills can range from speaking in sentences to using augmentative forms of communication to compensate for limited spoken language skills (Romski & Sevcik, 1988a; Rosenberg, 1982). Historically, however, children with severe disabilities have been an underserved population by speech-language pathologists and other professionals. A number of factors contributed to the underserved status of children with severe disabilities, ranging from philosophies that excluded them from speech-language treatment to a lack of available communication instructional strategies to meet their unique needs. The purpose of this chapter is to provide an overview of the assessment and treatment issues related to the communication development of children with severe disabilities within the broader context of childhood language disorders.

Profiles of Children with Severe Disabilities

By definition, children with severe disabilities, across all ages, have significant intellectual impairments as evidenced by extremely low scores on intelligence tests (Snell, 1993). Although children with severe disabilities are often grouped together because of their cognitive disabilities, they typically exhibit a range of accompanying disabilities, which may include (but are not limited to) cerebral palsy, sensory impairments, seizure disorders, other medical conditions, and maladaptive behaviors (Guess & Horner, 1978; Snell, 1993). Such children require extensive ongoing support in more than one major life activity to participate in their communities and to enjoy a quality of life that is available to children with fewer or no disabilities.

One area of life activity which frequently requires support is communication (American Association on Mental Retardation [AAMR], 1993). The heterogeneous profiles of children with severe disabilities result in diverse communication patterns. At one end of the continuum are children who acquire oral communication skills, albeit slowly and often incompletely, and exhibit varying degrees of impairment in the comprehension and production of the semantics, syntax, pragmatics, and/or phonology of language. At the other end of the continuum are children who fail to develop functional spoken communication skills sometimes even after considerable speech and language instruction directed toward that goal. Exclusionary criteria coupled with a shortage of appropriate output modes and instructional strategies have limited the communicative achievements of children at this end of the continuum. Relatively recently, changes in educational philosophies and programs as well as access to assistive technology have permitted children with severe disabilities to have a greater participatory role in home, school, community, and work settings. As such participation becomes attainable, society's perceptions of this group of children are slowly being radically altered as well.

Social Policy and Philosophy for Service Delivery

Broad changes in social policy have played an important role in increasing the delivery of speech-language pathology services to children with severe disabilities and, as a result, in clarifying their communication development. Federal legislation has addressed issues related to education, assistive technology devices and services, and, most recently, civil rights.

In 1975, the passage of Public Law (P.L.) 94-142 guaranteed all children from 5 to 21 years of age (regardless of the degree of their disability) the right to a free and appropriate public education, including the related services (e.g., speech and language) that they needed to obtain that education. In 1986, P.L. 99-457 amended P.L. 94-142 to include children as young as 3 years of age and, in some states, children at birth. In addition, it included educational planning for young children within the family system. In 1990, P.L. 94-142 was reauthorized as the Individuals with Disabilities Education Act (IDEA; P.L. 101-476). It continues to entitle all children to a free and appropriate education and now includes planning the transition from the educational environment to postschool living environments including work, community/residence, and leisure and recreation.

In 1988, the Technology-Related Assistance Act (P.L. 100-407) was passed by Congress and highlighted the role that assistive technology devices and services can play in ensuring that people with disabilities are able to participate in society. An assistive technology device is defined as any item, piece of equipment, or product system (whether commercially off the shelf, modified, or customized) that is used to increase, maintain, or improve functional capabilities of individuals with disabilities (e.g., an augmentative communication device). Under Title I of this act, funding was provided to states for the development of consumer-driven assistive technology programs whose goal is the comprehensive incorporation of assistive technology devices and services into extant public and private service delivery systems (e.g., education, rehabilitation).

Most recently, the Americans with Disabilities Act of 1990 (P.L. 101-336) was signed into law. This landmark piece of legislation guarantees the basic civil rights of persons with disabilities and addresses the employment and educational access needs they encounter. Although the effects of this legislation have only just begun to be implemented, it promises to enhance the participation of people with disabilities in our society.

The impact of 2 decades of federal legislation is that children with severe disabilities now have a basic right to be included in all aspects of our society and be provided with the supports needed to do so. A fundamental support for the successful implementation of any and all of this legislation is one that is often overlooked: communication. Without the ability to communicate, education, employment and inclusion are clearly compromised.

Recently, the National Joint Committee on the Communication Needs of Persons with Severe Disabilities proposed a set of 12 communication rights that all persons, regardless of the degree or severity of their disabilities, must possess (National Joint Committee for the Communication Needs of Persons with Severe Disabilities, 1992). These rights, shown in Table 10–1, provide a clear and specific perspective on which current speech-language service delivery systems, including evaluation and treatment, must be built.

Evaluation

In the past, children with severe disabilities were frequently excluded from speech and language treatment because their assessed levels of intelligence and their sensorimotor development were not commensurate with cognitive/sensorimotor skills that had been linked to early typical language development (Romski & Sevcik, 1988a; Sheehan, Martyn, & Kilburn, 1968). Although one may argue that some basic cognitive skills are essential for language to develop, the interactions between the domains of cognition and language are complex (see Rice, 1983, and Rice & Kemper, 1984, for reviews). Communication and language skills are of critical importance if the child is to make functional gains in all areas of development and function successfully in society. From the time typical children utter their first words, language is used to meet wants and needs, to maintain social contact with others, and to gain knowledge about the world (Berko-Gleason, 1988; Berko-Gleason, Hay, & Cain, 1989; Bruner, 1983). There is no question that a language impairment, especially one of significant magnitude, can affect children's development (especially their cognitive knowledge base and their social interactional skills). Given the impact language can exert on cognitive development, a lack of productive spoken language skills may put a child at a distinct developmental disadvantage (Rice & Kemper, 1984). Thus, more recently, investigators have argued against excluding children from language instruction based solely on intellectual performance and/or prerequisite sensorimotor skills (Kangas & Lloyd, 1988; Reichle & Karlan, 1985; Romski & Sevcik, 1988a).

Table 10–1. Communication Bill of Rights

1. The right to request desired objects, actions, events, and persons and to express personal preferences or feelings.
2. The right to be offered choices and alternatives.
3. The right to reject or refuse undesired objects, events, or actions, including the right to decline or reject all proffered choices.
4. The right to request, and be given, attention from and interaction with another person.
5. The right to request feedback or information about a state, an object, a person, or an event of interest.
6. The right to active treatment and intervention efforts that will enable people with severe disabilities to communicate messages in whatever modes and as effectively and efficiently as their specific abilities will allow.
7. The right to have communication acts acknowledged and responded to, even when the intent of these acts cannot be fulfilled by the responder.
8. The right to have access at all times to any needed augmentative and alternative communication devices and other assistive devices, and to have those devices in good working order.
9. The right to environmental contexts, interactions, and opportunities that expect and encourage persons with disabilities to participate as full communicative partners with other people, including peers.
10. The right to be informed about the people, things, and events in one's immediate environment.
11. The right to be communicated with in a manner that recognizes and acknowledges the inherent dignity of the person being addressed, including the right to be part of communication exchanges about individuals that are conducted in his or her presence.
12. The right to be communicated with in ways that are meaningful, understandable, and culturally and linguistically appropriate.

Source: Guidelines for meeting the communication needs of persons with severe disabilities (National Joint Committee for the Communicative Needs of Persons with Severe Disabilities, 1992).

Other children with severe disabilities have been excluded from speech-language services because there was little or no discrepancy between their mental ages and their language ages, as measured by standardized tests. The rationale was that because cognition was the base from which language emerged, children with this profile could not advance their language and communication skills beyond their intellectual skills (American Speech-Language-Hearing Association [ASHA], 1989b); thus, they could not benefit from speech and language intervention services. The rationale for this exclusionary criterion has also been questioned given the role language can play in development. A 1989b ASHA report advises that the exclusionary criterion must be avoided.

Not surprisingly, then, standardized speech and language assessment batteries (as well as standardized psychological tests) are difficult to employ with children with severe disabilities because of the severity of their oral language impairments. Often, the children are unable to obtain basal scores on tests or their scores are so far below those of their chronological age peers that converting a raw score into a standard score is not possible. Some of the factors that may influence these outcomes include unfamiliar examiners, lack of a communication output mode, difficulty understanding the requirements of the task, stimuli that are too complex (e.g., line drawings), and stimuli that are configured in a difficult manner (e.g., 2 x 2 display).

For children with severe disabilities, speech and language evaluation usually does not focus on determining whether there is a delay in speech and language development. The answer to that question is obvious. First and foremost, the purpose of evaluation is to assess functional language and communication skills regardless of whether the child has any extant spoken words, phrases, or sentences. Specifically, the intent is to characterize the extent of the delays within a functional context and the children's communicative strengths and weaknesses and to set goals for a course of treatment that will permit the child to communicate, at the least, basic wants and needs. It is, therefore, more typical to employ informal measures and systematic behavioral observation within usual environments than standardized tests within isolated settings with this group of children.

Evaluation of Functional Communication

Communication can be defined in the broadest sense as "any act by which one person gives to or receives from another person information about that person's needs, desires, perceptions, knowledge, or affective states" (National Joint Committee, 1992, p. 2). The modes by which children can communicate range along a representational continuum from symbolic (e.g., spoken words, manual signs, arbitrary visual-graphic symbols) to iconic (e.g., real objects, photographs, line drawings, pictographic visual-graphic symbols) to nonsymbolic (e.g., signals such as crying or physical movement; see Sevcik, Romski, & Wilkinson, 1991, for a discussion of visual-graphic representational systems). Some children with severe disabilities who have no conventional way to communicate may express their communicative wants and needs in socially unacceptable ways, such as through aggressive or destructive means (e.g., Donnellan, Mirenda, Mesaros, & Fassbender, 1984; Doss & Reichle, 1991).

Functional communication assessment includes two primary components: the child's current communication development (i.e., comprehension skills, communication mode, extant skills) and the child's environments (i.e., partners, opportunities; see Reichle, Mirenda, Locke, Piche, & Johnson, 1992). Relevant assessment begins with systematic behavioral observations in everyday environments and informal measures that inventory and describe these two components.

Young typical children learn to comprehend spoken language before they begin to speak (Golinkoff & Hirsh-Pasek, 1990; Huttenlocher, 1974). For children with severe disabilities, it is important to ascertain the level of speech comprehension they currently exhibit. If standardized language comprehension tests, such as the Peabody Picture Vocabulary Test—Revised (Dunn & Dunn, 1981), are not appropriate, informal measures may provide an indication of the child's receptive abilities in context.

The children's ability to act intentionally on partners in their environments and to affect the behaviors of those partners plays an important role in language and communication development. Communicative intentions vary along a continuum from perlocutionary to locutionary (McLean & Snyder-McLean, 1988). As shown in Table 10–2, the modes the child uses to make his or her wants and needs

Table 10–2. Continuum of Communicative/Linguistic Skills

Communicative Intentionality	*Communicative Role*		*Communicative Form*
	Child	*Partner*	
Perlocutionary			
Reactive	Passive	Active	Cry, eye gaze, laugh, movement "fussing"
Proactive	Active	Active	Reach
Illocutionary			
Primitive	Active	Active	Physical manipulation
Conventional	Active	Active	Point, vocalization with inflection
Locutionary			
Emerging	Active	Active	Words, signs, graphic symbols combined with gesture and vocalization
Conventional	Active	Active	Words, signs, graphic symbols

Source: Adapted from McLean and Snyder-McLean (1988).

known to partners and the role the partner plays in the interaction will vary with the child's status along the continuum. For children who exhibit conventional communicative modes, the functions served by those modes must be specified. For example, does the child make requests, answer questions, or direct another's attention? How varied are these functions across environments and partners? Romski and Sevcik (1988b) described a four-part coding scheme, the Communication Coding Scheme, that characterized the conventional communications of school-age children with severe disabilities in terms of partner and type, mode, function, and outcome (i.e., the success of the communication with respect to the partner's response). This real-time coding scheme can be employed reliably in a variety of environments and subsequently incorporated within a language sample to provide a systematic means for measuring meaningful dimensions of communication for children with severe disabilities.

If the child does not exhibit conventional communicative modes, there are three main areas to consider. First, the child may not have physical access to a mode by which to communicate. If physical access is an issue, an evaluation for alternative forms of access may be appropriate. A range of microswitches and eye-gaze techniques are available to interface with computer-based technology and permit the child to make a response and access a mode by which to communicate (see Beukelman & Mirenda, 1992, pp. 49–67, and York & Weimann, 1991, for detailed descriptions of alternative access issues). Second, all of the child's environments may not support communication. What types of opportunities does each environment provide to promote communication? Sometimes the opportunities vary across environments and even across partners within environments. Table 10–3 lists suggested components for an assessment of environments

Table 10–3. Assessment of the Environment

1. Identify the familiar and unfamiliar partners for communication in each environment.
2. Describe the opportunities (frequency and type) for communication typically observed in each environment.
3. Compare the opportunities for communication among the different environments and partners within each environment.
4. Determine the proportion of communications that are responded to appropriately and inappropriately in each environment.
5. Identify the specific communicative modes and functions that might be useful in each environment.
6. Identify the partners in each environment who have relatively high rates of permitting, accepting, and responding to the communications of the children.

Source: Guidelines for meeting the communication needs of persons with severe disabilities (National Joint Committee for the Communicative Needs of Persons with Severe Disabilities, 1992).

(National Joint Committee, 1992). Third, when no everyday environment appears to provide opportunities for communications, the practitioner can set up a situation in which to elicit intentional communication from the child (see Cirrin & Rowland, 1985, for an example). Finally, it may be that the child is at an earlier point along the continuum of communication development and does not exhibit intentional communication. In this case, the environment should be configured to support communication by, for example, setting up routines (see Siegel-Causey & Guess, 1989, for a detailed discussion of nonsymbolic assessment and treatment strategies).

Even though some children exhibit conventional modes of communication, such as vocalizations and gestures, these modes may limit the breadth of function their communications can convey to familiar and unfamiliar partners across multiple environments (Romski, Sevcik, Reumann, & Pate, 1989). It is most often the case that augmentative and alternative communication (AAC) approaches will provide the most effective mode by which children with severe disabilities can communicate (Beukelman & Mirenda, 1992; Reichle, York, & Sigafoos, 1991; Romski & Sevcik 1988a). AAC is an area of clinical practice that attempts to compensate (either temporarily or permanently) for the impairment and disability patterns of individuals with severe expressive communication disorders (i.e., the severely speech-language and writing impaired) (ASHA, 1989a, p. 107). Manual signs, communication boards, and electronic communication devices that speak all provide avenues by which children with severe disabilities develop communication skills. These approaches augment what extant communication skills the children bring to the language-learning task and compensate for the limited spoken communication skills they have developed (Bjorklund & Schwartz, this volume).

In summary, for children with severe disabilities, speech and language evaluation requires an assessment of the children and their environments. Such assessment usually includes augmentative and alternative communication. Finally, it is important to remember that assessment is an ongoing process that continues throughout the course of treatment. Change must be measured on an ongoing basis and serve as a foundation for the reassessment of treatment approaches.

Treatment Issues

Similar to conventional speech and language evaluation approaches, traditional speech and language treatment approaches have not adequately facilitated the communication development of most children with severe disabilities. The obvious explanation for their failure is that the content of traditional treatment approaches focuses on oral language production skills, which typically are lacking in children with severe disabilities. Consequently, a range of language intervention approaches that incorporate AAC (i.e., manual signs, visual-graphic symbols) to facilitate communication development are usually the choice for children with severe disabilities. There are some children with severe disabilities, however, who do develop spoken language skills. It is essential that their spoken language treatment programs focus on developing those skills within a functional communication context (e.g., asking questions in class, ordering food at a restaurant, carrying on conversations with classmates).

A number of treatment issues related to the communication development of children with severe disabilities have emerged in the literature. Among these issues are the choice of augmentative and alternative communication systems; initial communication teaching strategies, including the role of comprehension, the available lexicon, and generalization; service delivery models; and early intervention.

Choice of Augmentative and Alternative Communication Systems

Manual sign systems and communication boards have been the historic choice for able-bodied children with severe disabilities (Romski & Sevcik, 1988a). With the exception of a few early studies that explored the use of electronic communication devices for able-bodied children with severe disabilities (Locke & Mirenda, 1988; Romski, Sevcik, & Pate, 1988; Romski, White, Millen, & Rumbaugh, 1984), electronic communication devices were usually reserved for youth with substantial physical disabilities who could not generate manual signs or point to symbols on a communication board.

There appear to be two main reasons for this distinction. First, the sophisticated operational demands of early technology appeared to influence their availability to children with severe disabilities. The electronic devices that were available 10 to 15 years ago often relied on advanced modes (such as spelling or printed English words) for access. The studies by Romski and her colleagues and Locke and Mirenda adapted computers to permit their subjects to communicate via large symbols that represented individual words. Second, Turner (1986) suggested that economics were a major reason for this distinction. He argued that professionals typically did not think that these children would benefit from electronic devices because of the degree of their cognitive disability.

Recently, however, there has been an increase in the scope of reasonably priced speech-output communication systems that are manufactured and marketed specifically for this group of children (e.g., MEGA WOLF, IntroTalker, Speak Easy, MaCaw, Message Mate, to name a few). These devices provide access to a range of vocabulary from as little as two large-sized symbols to 36 one-inch symbols on a single display page. With these devices now available specifically for this group, more children with severe disabilities may gain access to assistive technology devices for communication.

Families and practitioners must make a choice, however, about which type of augmentative communication system (manual signs, communication boards, electronic devices) to employ with children with severe disabilities. Although nonelectronic systems serve some of the children's needs, there are disadvantages. First, for manual signs there are some production demands that may make their intelligibility difficult. Second, partners must be knowledgeable in manual signs to interpret the children's communications. Third, with respect to manual signs and communication boards, the visual modality, a well-established strength of these systems (Fristoe & Lloyd, 1979), simultaneously may place the children at a communicative disadvantage. This disadvantage occurs because the modality requires the partner to monitor visually and then attend visually to the child as the communication is produced.

Alternatively, speech-output communication devices also afford the opportunity for distal communicative exchanges by easing the visual demands on communicative partners. The synthetic auditory signal permits partners to hear the "speech" feedback produced when a symbol is activated and immediately comprehend the message. This feature is particularly important when children are integrated within the general community and interact with unfamiliar communicative partners.

The speech-output feature of electronic computer devices also permits the child to compensate for the use of a visual communication system by automatically linking the child's visual communication with the more familiar auditory/spoken modality in social interactional contexts. It can provide the child with a multimodal system of communication, including a "voice" (albeit artificial), yet it retains the visual modality that may be helpful to the child (Romski & Sevcik, 1993). Romski and her colleagues (Romski, Sevcik, Robinson, & Bakeman, 1994; Romski, Sevcik, & Wilkinson, 1994) reported that school-age youth with severe disabilities and little or no functional speech used their speech-output communication devices, in concert with extant forms of communication (i.e., vocalizations, gestures), to communicate effectively with both adults and peers. The choice of speech-output communication devices over manual signs and communication boards can permit children with little or no functional speech to follow a course of language development that is more similar to that of children who speak, because synthetic speech technology empowers them to speak through computerized means.

Initial Communicative Teaching Strategies

Regardless of the specific AAC system selected, its use must be coupled with teaching strategies to facilitate the communicative development of words, signs, or symbols. Until fairly recently, the dominant theme reflected in the literature has been that children with severe cognitive disabilities require continuous prompting and structured practice to learn to communicate (Reichle, York, & Sigafoos, 1991). Some current research, however, suggests that children with severe disabilities can learn through observation and use in an environment carefully arranged to support communication (Romski & Sevcik, 1992, 1993).

A number of strategies, which vary in the amount of direct instruction and structure they require, have been developed to teach the initial productive use of words, signs, or symbols to children with severe disabilities. Through a highly motivating learning situation, children learn that they can use words, signs, or symbols to effect changes in their environments. Of all the communicative functions of language, request is the one most directly tied to function (Bruner, 1983). It is also the earliest function to develop in young typical children (Bruner, 1983). Strategies that facilitate requesting may take a range of forms. Reichle and his colleagues (Reichle et al., 1991) have espoused the use of a generalized requesting procedure. This approach begins with a single consistent symbol, such as "want," and is used in multiple situations to initiate requesting. Once a request is initiated, the child is given a choice of items (e.g., cookie, drink). After the child learns to make generalized requests, differentiated requests for specific referents, such as "want cookie" versus "want drink," are incorporated into the child's communicative repertoire. Another approach is to begin with requests that specify each item being requested using words, signs, or symbols (Romski et al., 1988). Using this approach, children must establish conditional discriminations between the item being requested and the word, sign, or symbol used to request the item. Mirenda and Santogrossi (1985) have used verbal, prompt-free procedures to teach requesting. This strategy requires that the facilitator refrain from using any verbal prompt from the outset of instruction so that there is no need to fade the prompt later in the teaching process. The mand-model teaching strategy, a component of milieu teaching strategies, can also be employed to teach initial requesting skills. This procedure uses teacher-initiated instructions to generate opportunities for the child to request in the natural environment.

Another early developing communicative function is rejecting (i.e., "no"): the ability to refuse an undesired item or to cease an activity. Reichle et al. (1991) also developed specific structured instructional strategies for teaching this communicative function. Once the children learn to use basic communicative functions, like requesting and rejecting, more complex communicative skills must be incorporated into their repertoires. With one exception (Romski & Sevcik, 1992, 1993), we know little about the long-term process of communication development in children with severe disabilities.

Romski and Sevcik (1992, 1993) took a longitudinal approach to symbol learning and use. They introduced the System for Augmenting Language (SAL) to 13 school-age youth with severe disabilities and little or no functional speech. The SAL included five components: a speech-output communication system; an appropriate vocabulary; naturalistic communicative experiences during which the child is encouraged, but not required, to communicate; partners who were taught how to use the device and how to provide input via speech and symbols to the youth; and a resource and feedback mechanism to monitor progress across the study. During naturalistic communicative experiences, the youth had opportunities to employ a range of communicative functions from greeting, requesting, and attention directing to answering and questioning. Romski and Sevcik found that the 13 youth integrated their use of the SAL with extant vocalizations and gestures, which resulted in a rich, multimodal form of communication. Some of these youth went on to develop combinatorial symbol skills as well as intelligible spoken words.

THE ROLE OF SPEECH COMPREHENSION

Traditionally, the focus of most language intervention programs for children with severe disabilities has been on production. Although this focus is essential and permits children to have an immediate and visible communicative effect on their environment, it does not exist in isolation (Romski & Sevcik, 1993). Teaching communication skills also demands that the children assume the role of listener or message receiver. To assume this role flexibly, children must comprehend the information that is being conveyed to them by their communicative partners.

It is well documented that spoken language comprehension skills play an extremely important role in early language learning for typical children (Golinkoff & Hirsh-Pasek, 1990; Huttenlocher, 1974). For children with severe disabilities who do not talk, however, one pathway for a child's early language development can be through the comprehension of language (Romski & Sevcik, 1992). The extent of children's productive language achievement may be influenced by the receptive language skills they bring to the language-learning task. Some children have already established a relationship between spoken words and their referents during their life experience. When a viable AAC route becomes accessible to them, these extant receptive skills may serve as a basis for expressive language development. For children who evidence little comprehension of speech, there is no preexisting base of word understanding with which to link the new words they are being exposed to expressively. Thus, they must begin the acquisition process by first establishing the relationship between signs or symbols and their referents. Because they do not understand the meanings of spoken words, they must rely on the cues inherent in the communicative context to extract meaning. Language comprehension, then, is an essential foundation on which children can build productive language competence. It is critical to include a receptive component (i.e., having the child take the listener's role) as part of communication teaching strategies for this group of children.

AVAILABLE LEXICON

Another important component for early word learning through AAC is the lexicon available to the child for understanding and expression. Children who speak hear many more words spoken in context than they can ever produce at any one time. Production of words, however, is dependent on the children's physical abilities (i.e., oral-motor mechanism). Although children with little or no functional speech are often exposed to a spoken input vocabulary comparable to that of a speaking child, their output is likely externally constrained by the number of manual signs they are exposed to or the visual-graphic symbol vocabulary items available on their communication board. One of the features that has been proposed to facilitate their learning via AAC is the use of recognition rather than recall memory (Fristoe & Lloyd, 1979). This feature, however, may also constrain their symbol use capabilities because there are a limited number of vocabulary items available simultaneously.[1] A wide range of vocabulary items, which is updated or changed as needed by environmental transitions (e.g., preschool to elementary school, school to work), can facilitate vocabulary learning.

The signs and symbols children use are based on the lexicon that is available to them (Beukelman, McGinnis, & Morrow, 1991). Often, referential, easily depictable, lexical items are chosen for children with severe disabilities. The rationale has been that referential words are concrete and more easily learned than action or social-regulative words. Adamson, Romski, Deffebach, and Sevcik (1992) found that when social-regulative symbols (such as "please," "thank you," "help") were available for use on a speech-output communication system along with referential symbols, youth with severe disabilities acquired them rapidly and employed them during well over half of the communicative turns with a social focus. Moreover, their availability immediately and continually shifted the focus of the participants' conversational turns from referential to social. When these social-regulative symbols were available, the youth often combined them with other symbols to form more semantically complex utterances (e.g., "more milk please") (Wilkinson, Romski, & Sevcik, 1994). Social-regulative words, then, may play an important role in facilitating the interactive dimension of communication development.

The lexicon made available to children can shape their social interactions as well as the content of their communications. If these children can also master action and social-regulative terms (e.g., "please," "more," "help"), their ability to regulate interpersonal exchanges using culturally appropriate ways of communicating may be greatly enhanced. The use of a broad lexicon influences the children's ability to engage in communication with multiple partners in varied social contexts. It can also influence the partners' perceptions of the children's social competence.

GENERALIZATION

Generalization has always been a critical language intervention issue for children with severe disabilities (Reichle & Sigafoos, 1991; Stokes & Baer, 1977; Warren & Rogers-Warren, 1985). If an intervention program is to be considered successful, its goal must be the generalized use of communication skills across a range of communicative environments as well as familiar and unfamiliar partners.

One approach to generalization is to transfer language learning from its instructional environment to the natural environment using milieu teaching strategies. Milieu teaching strategies (Hart & Rogers-Warren, 1978) encompass a range of naturalistic procedures and include incidental teaching (Warren & Kaiser, 1986), mand-model (Warren, McQuarter, & Rogers-Warren, 1984), time delay (Halle, Marshall, & Spradlin, 1979), and child-cued modeling (Alpert & Kaiser, 1992) (see Kaiser, Yoder, & Keetz, 1992, for a review of milieu teaching studies). A study of manual sign use by children with severe cognitive disabilities who did not speak suggested that incidental teaching strategies may function as well as structured teaching approaches (Oliver & Halle, 1982). Yoder, Kaiser, and Alpert (1991) clearly indicated that speaking children acquiring early vocabulary learned better from an incidental teaching approach than from a direct instruction

[1] As technology advances, dynamic computer displays that permit the availability of multiple pages of vocabulary are becoming available.

approach. As Halle (1982) has noted, however, no single milieu procedure alone can facilitate functional communication. Taken as an instructional package, however, he has suggested that these procedures may promote generalization to a range of natural settings. Another approach to generalization is for the intervention itself to take place in everyday environments, where the children may have a strong motivation to communicate (Romski & Sevcik, 1992). Transfer is then not necessary. Regardless of the approach, generalization is a critical component of the treatment process and must be considered from the onset of intervention.

SUMMARY

Facilitating the development of communication is a complex process. It includes focusing on teaching communicative functions, the role of comprehension, and generalization. One procedure will not, by itself, make the child communicatively competent. Practitioners must consider not only the immediate task but also the long-term perspective on communication as they plan intervention for children with severe disabilities.

Service Delivery

The delivery of communication intervention services to children with severe disabilities requires the collaboration and competence of families, professionals, and paraprofessionals (National Joint Committee, 1992). Conventional pull-out therapy approaches have not successfully accommodated the communication development of this group of children. A broad-based communication treatment plan is best implemented in all contexts of the child's daily life and coordinated by a team of people who can manage the many and varied components of the plan. A collaborative team approach to service delivery incorporates families and a range of professional disciplines, including (though not limited to) speech-language pathologists, regular and special educators, physical and occupational therapists, and psychologists (see Catlett, 1993, for a discussion of teams).

Early Intervention

Perhaps the most critical long-term issue related to the communication development of children with severe disabilities is the age at which intervention begins. Even though federal legislation has made early intervention the norm rather than the exception, we have been inclined, at least to date, to focus these early intervention efforts on the development of spoken language skills exclusively. It is not until children are school aged and these intervention efforts have failed that AAC approaches have been considered. The reason for this outcome appears to be related to beliefs about speech development. Many speech-language pathologists, as well as parents, still believe that if there is an early focus on augmentative communication, the children will have no desire or motivation to talk because they have another "easier" means by which to communicate. The empirical literature suggests that this is not the case. A number of empirical studies suggest that children who employ AAC systems may develop vocal and spoken language skills after experience with an AAC system (Romski, Sevcik, Robinson, & Wilkinson, 1990; Yoder & Layton, 1988).

If the children have a conventional way to communicate early in childhood, perhaps their overall communicative interaction skills and adaptive behavior skills might not lag as far behind other children. In a recent review of the general early intervention literature, Shonkoff, Hauser-Cram, Krauss, and Upshur (1992) suggested that the more significant the developmental delay, the more important it may be to initiate intervention early in childhood to ensure steady developmental progress. The role AAC experience might play in the early intervention process has not been investigated systematically. In a pilot study, Romski, Sevcik, and Adamson (1992) introduced the use of an AAC approach that combined naturalistic teaching strategies with a speech-output communication system for a 4-year-old child with severe developmental disabilities. They observed an immediate positive shift in the child's receptiveness for communication. That is, the child spent significantly more time engaged in tasks that included communicative opportunities than before the approach was employed. The child's frequency of communicative attempts also increased after he had access to the AAC system.

The earlier children's language and communication development is augmented, in the truest sense of the word, the earlier the children will have a means by which to communicate with their parents, siblings, and significant others in their environments. The introduction of an AAC system should not be viewed as "giving up speech" but instead as another approach to the development of speech and language skills for young children with severe disabilities.

Conclusion

This chapter provided an overview of issues related to the communication development of children with severe disabilities. Over the last 5 to 10 years, significant advances have been made in social policy, research, and practice. Children with severe disabilities have demonstrated communication achievements far beyond our historically pessimistic clinical expectations. Practitioners have an ethical responsibility to provide children with severe disabilities with the supports they need to develop functional communication. Research and best practices are continuing to develop, and the communication future is finally optimistic for children with severe disabilities.

Acknowledgments

Preparation of this chapter was supported in part by NICHD-06016, which sustains the Language Research Center of Georgia State University. Additional support was provided by the Department of Communication and the College of Arts and Sciences, Georgia State University. The authors wish to thank Paul Alberto for comments on portions of this manuscript.

References

Adamson, L. B., Romski, M. A., Deffebach, K., & Sevcik, R. A. (1992). Symbol vocabulary and the focus of conversations: Augmenting language development for youth with mental retardation. *Journal of Speech and Hearing Research, 35,* 1333–1344.

Alpert, K., & Kaiser, A. (1992). Training parents as milieu language teachers. *Journal of Early Intervention, 16,* 31–52.

American Association on Mental Retardation (1993). *Mental retardation: Definition, classification, and systems of supports* (9th ed.). Washington, DC: American Association on Mental Retardation.

American Speech-Language-Hearing Association (1989a). Competencies for speech-language pathologists providing services in augmentative communication. *ASHA, 31,* 107–110.

American Speech-Language-Hearing Association (1989b). Issues in determining eligibility for language intervention. *ASHA, 31,* 113–118.

Berko-Gleason, J. (1988). Language and socialization. In F. Kessel (Ed.), *The development of language and language researchers* (pp. 269–280). Hillsdale, NJ: Erlbaum.

Berko-Gleason, J., Hay, D., & Cain, L. (1989). Social and affective determinants of language acquisition. In M. Rice & R. L. Schiefelbusch (Eds.), *The teachability of language* (pp. 171–186). Baltimore: Paul H. Brookes.

Beukelman, D., McGinnis, J., & Morrow, D. (1991). Vocabulary selection in augmentative and alternative communication. *Augmentative and Alternative Communication, 7,* 171–185.

Beukelman, D., & Mirenda, P. (1992). *Augmentative and alternative communication.* Baltimore: Paul H. Brookes.

Bjorklund, D. F., & Schwartz, R. (this volume). The adaptive nature of developmental immaturity: Implications for language acquisition and language disabilities.

Bruner, J. (1983). *Child's talk: Learning to use language.* Oxford, UK: Oxford University Press.

Catlett, C. (1993). Teams and teamwork. *ASHA, 35,* 30–31.

Cirrin, F., & Rowland, C. (1985). Communicative assessment of nonverbal youths with severe/profound mental retardation. *Mental Retardation, 23,* 52–62.

Donnellan, A., Mirenda, P., Mesaros, R., & Fassbender, L. (1984). Analyzing the communicative functions of aberrant behavior. *Journal of the Association for the Severely Handicapped, 9,* 201–212.

Doss, S., & Reichle, J. (1991). Replacing excess behavior with an initial communicative repertoire. In J. Reichle, J. York, & J. Sigafoos (Eds.), *Implementing augmentative and alternative communication: Strategies for learners with severe disabilities* (pp. 215–238). Baltimore: Paul H. Brookes.

Dunn, L. M., & Dunn, L. M. (1981). *Peabody Picture Vocabulary Test–Revised.* Circle Pines, MN: American Guidance Service.

Fristoe, M., & Lloyd, L. L. (1979). Nonspeech communication. In N. R. Ellis (Ed.), *Handbook of mental deficiency: Psychological theory and research* (pp. 401–430). Hillsdale, NJ: Erlbaum.

Golinkoff, R. M., & Hirsh-Pasek, K. (1990). Let the mute speak: What infants can tell us about language acquisition. *Merrill-Palmer Quarterly, 36,* 67–91.

Guess, D., & Horner, R. (1978). The severely and profoundly handicapped. In E. L. Meyen (Eds.), *Exceptional children and youth: An introduction* (pp. 218–268). Denver: Love Publishing.

Halle, J. (1982). Teaching functional language to the handicapped: An integrative model of natural environment teaching techniques. *Journal of the Association for the Severely Handicapped, 7,* 29–37.

Halle, J., Marshall, A., & Spradlin, J. (1979). Time delay: A technique to increase language use and facilitate generalization in retarded children. *Journal of Applied Behavior Analysis, 12,* 431–439.

Hart, B., & Rogers-Warren, A. P. (1978). A milieu approach to teaching language. In R. L. Schiefelbusch (Ed.), *Language intervention strategies* (pp. 193–235). Baltimore: University Park Press.

Huttenlocher, J. (1974). The origins of language comprehension. In R. L. Solso (Ed.), *Theories in cognitive psychology: The Loyola Symposium* (pp. 331–368). Hillsdale, NJ: Erlbaum.

Kaiser, A., Yoder, P., & Keetz, A. (1992). Evaluating milieu teaching. In S. Warren & J. Reichle (Eds.), *Causes and effects of communication and language intervention* (pp. 9–47). Baltimore: Paul H. Brookes.

Kangas, C., & Lloyd, L. L. (1988). Early cognitive skill prerequisites to augmentative and alternative communication use: What are we waiting for? *Augmentative and Alternative Communication, 4,* 211–221.

Locke, P., & Mirenda, P. (1988). A computer-supported communication approach for a nonspeaking child with severe visual and cognitive impairments. *Augmentative and Alternative Communication, 4,* 15–22.

McLean, J., & Snyder-McLean, L. (1988). Applications of pragmatics to severely mentally retarded children and youth. In R. L. Schiefelbusch & L. L. Lloyd (Eds.), *Language perspective: Acquisition, retardation, and intervention* (2nd ed., pp. 255–288). Austin, TX: Pro-ed.

McLean, J., Yoder, D., & Schiefelbusch, R. L. (1970). *Language intervention with the retarded.* Baltimore: University Park Press.

Mirenda, P., & Santogrossi, J. (1985). A prompt-free strategy to teach pictorial communication system use. *Augmentative and Alternative Communication, 1,* 143–150.

National Joint Committee for the Communication Needs of Persons with Severe Disabilities. (1992). Guidelines for meeting the communication needs of persons with severe disabilities. *ASHA, 34* (Suppl. 7), 1–8.

Oliver, C., & Halle, J. (1982). Language training in the everyday environments. Teaching functional signs to a retarded child. *Journal of the Association for the Severely Handicapped, 7,* 50–62.

Reichle, J., & Karlan, G. (1985). The selection of an augmentative system in communication intervention: A critique of decision rules. *Journal of the Association for the Severely Handicapped, 10,* 146–156.

Reichle, J., Mirenda, P., Locke, P., Piche, L., & Johnson, S. (1992). Beginning augmentative communication systems. In S. Warren & J. Reichle (Eds.), *Causes and effects in communication and language intervention* (pp. 131–156). Baltimore: Paul H. Brookes.

Reichle, J., & Sigafoos, J. (1991). Establishing spontaneity and generalization. In J. Reichle, J. York, & J. Sigafoos (Eds.), *Implementing augmentative and alternative communication: Strategies for learners with severe disabilities* (pp. 157–172). Baltimore: Paul H. Brookes.

Reichle, J., York, J., & Sigafoos, J. (1991). *Implementing augmentative and alternative communication: Strategies for learners with severe disabilities.* Baltimore: Paul H. Brookes.

Rice, M. (1983). Contemporary accounts of the cognition/language relationship: Implications for language clinicians. *Journal of Speech and Hearing Disorders, 48,* 347–359.

Rice, M., & Kemper, S. (1984). *Child language and cognition.* Baltimore: University Park Press.

Romski, M. A., & Sevcik, R. A. (1988a). Augmentative and alternative communication systems: Considerations for individuals with severe intellectual disabilities. *Augmentative and Alternative Communication, 4,* 83–93.

Romski, M. A., & Sevcik, R. A. (1988b). Augmentative communication system acquisition and use: A model for teaching and assessing progress. *NSSLHA Journal, 16,* 61–75.

Romski, M. A., & Sevcik, R. A. (1992). Developing augmented language in children with severe mental retardation. In S. Warren & J. Reichle (Eds.), *Causes and effects in communication and language intervention* (pp. 113–130). Baltimore: Paul H. Brookes.

Romski, M. A., & Sevcik, R. A. (1993). Language learning through augmented means: The process and its products. In A. Kaiser & D. Gray (Eds.), *Enhancing children's communication: Research foundations for intervention* (pp. 85–104). Baltimore: Paul H. Brookes.

Romski, M. A., & Sevcik, R. A. (1993). Language comprehension: Considerations for augmentative and alternative communication. *Augmentative and Alternative Communication, 9,* 281–285.

Romski, M. A., Sevcik, R. A., & Adamson, L. B. (1992, November). *Augmentative communication development in a preschool child with severe disabilities.* Poster presented at the annual meeting of the American Speech-Language-Hearing Association, San Antonio, TX.

Romski, M. A., Sevcik, R. A., & Pate, J. (1988). The establishment of symbolic communication in persons with severe retardation. *Journal of Speech and Hearing Disorders, 53,* 94–107.

Romski, M. A., Sevcik, R. A., Reumann, R., & Pate, J. (1989). Youngsters with moderate or severe retardation and severe spoken language impairments I: Extant communicative patterns. *Journal of Speech and Hearing Disorders, 54,* 366–373.

Romski, M. A., Sevcik, R. A., Robinson, B. F., & Bakeman, R. (1994). Adult-directed communications of youth with mental retardation using the system for augmenting language. *Journal of Speech and Hearing Research, 37,* 617–628.

Romski, M. A., Sevcik, R. A., Robinson, B. F., & Wilkinson, K. (1990, November). *Intelligibility and form changes in the vocalizations of augmented language learners.* Paper presented at the annual meeting of the American Speech-Language-Hearing Association, Seattle, WA.

Romski, M. A., Sevcik, R. A., & Wilkinson, K. (1994). Peer-directed communicative interactions of augmented language learners with mental retardation. *American Journal on Mental Retardation, 98,* 527–538.

Romski, M. A., White, R., Millen, C., & Rumbaugh, D. M. (1984). Effects of computer-keyboard teaching on the symbolic communication of severely retarded persons: Five case studies. *The Psychological Record, 34,* 39–54.

Rosenberg, S. (1982). The language of the mentally retarded: Development, processes, and intervention. In S. Rosenberg (Ed.), *Handbook of applied psycholinguistics* (pp. 329–392). Hillsdale, NJ: Erlbaum.

Schiefelbusch, R. L. (1980). *Nonspeech language and communication: Analysis and intervention.* Baltimore: University Park Press.

Schiefelbusch, R. L., & Hollis, J. (1979). *Language intervention from ape to child.* Baltimore: University Park Press.

Schiefelbusch, R. L., & Lloyd, L. L. (1974). *Language perspective: Acquisition, retardation, and intervention.* Baltimore: University Park Press.

Sevcik, R. A., Romski, M. A., & Wilkinson, K. (1991). Roles of graphic symbols in the language acquisition process for persons with severe cognitive disabilities. *Augmentative and Alternative Communication, 7,* 161–170.

Sheehan, J., Martyn, M., & Kilburn, K. (1968). Speech disorders in retardation. *American Journal of Mental Deficiency, 73,* 251–256.

Shonkoff, J., Hauser-Cram, P., Krauss, M., & Upshur, C. (1992). Development of infants with disabilities and their families: Implications for theory and service delivery. *Monographs of the Society for Research in Child Development, 57* (6, Serial No. 230). Chicago: University of Chicago Press.

Siegel-Causey, E., & Guess, D. (1989). *Enhancing nonsymbolic communication interactions among learners with severe disabilities.* Baltimore: Paul H. Brookes.

Snell, M. (1993). *Instruction of students with severe disabilities.* Columbus, OH: Charles Merrill.

Stokes, T., & Baer, D. (1977). An implicit technology of generalization. *Journal of Applied Behavior Analysis, 10,* 349–367.

Turner, G. (1986). Funding VOCAS for the lower cognitive functioning population. *Closing the Gap, 5,* 26.

Warren, S., & Kaiser, A. (1986). Incidental language teaching: A critical review. *Journal of Speech and Hearing Disorders, 51,* 291–299.

Warren, S., McQuarter, R., & Rogers-Warren, A. (1984). The effects of teacher mands and models on the speech of unresponsive language-delayed children. *Journal of Speech and Hearing Research, 51,* 291–299.

Warren, S., & Rogers-Warren, A. P. (1985). *Teaching functional language.* Baltimore: University Park Press.

Warren, S., & Reichle, J. (1992). *Causes and effects of communication and language intervention.* Baltimore: Paul H. Brookes.

Wilkinson, K. M., Romski, M. A., & Sevcik, R. A. (1994). Emergence of visual-graphic symbol combinations by youth with moderate or severe mental retardation. *Journal of Speech and Hearing Research, 37,* 883–895.

Yoder, D., Kaiser, A. P., & Alpert, K. (1991). An exploratory study of the interaction between language teaching methods and child characteristics. *Journal of Speech and Hearing Research, 34,* 155–167.

Yoder, P., & Layton, T. (1988). Speech following sign language training in autistic children with minimal verbal language. *Journal of Autism and Developmental Disorders, 18,* 217–229.

York, J., & Weimann, G. (1991). Accommodating severe physical disabilities. In J. Reichle, J. York, & J. Sigafoos (Eds.), *Implementing augmentative and alternative communication: Strategies for learners with severe disabilities* (pp. 239–256). Baltimore: Paul H. Brookes.

11

Substance Abuse Risk Factors and Childhood Language Disorders

LESLEY A. MAXWELL, M.S., AND
JILL GESCHWINT-RABIN, M.S.

Introduction

The study of alterations in the biologic development of organisms is called teratology. Researchers examining pre- and postnatal exposure to drugs are concerned with identifying their teratogenic effects. The word *teratogen* stems from the Greek root *teras* or *monster* and, in literal translation, refers to the "production of monstrosities."

The arrival of crack cocaine in this country was accompanied by a sensationalist rush to judgment by the media. Given the implications of the word *teratogen,* this misguided Worfian leap from label to belief was perhaps predictable. Without a body of research data to substantiate its conclusions, the media heralded the creation of a "biological underclass" (*Washington Post,* 1989) and suggested that children prenatally exposed to cocaine might develop into "adults unable to develop basic employment skills and unable to form human attachments" (*New York Times,* 1989).

The truth is that we are a nation of drug users. Alcohol is a bigger threat to larger numbers of children than any illegal drug known to humans, including cocaine (Streissguth, 1992). Alcohol's use during pregnancy can cause permanent physical and intellectual impairments in the children of drinking mothers (Abel, 1980). Cigarette smoking during pregnancy can result in babies with low birth weights and toddlers with developmental delays (Fried & Watkinson, 1990). Recent research has revealed that the exposure of nonsmokers to the legal cigarette smoke of others has dangerous implications for children and for pregnant women (Martin & Bracken, 1986).

As a compassionate society, we have an obligation to avoid pointing culturally biased fingers of blame. The formalized result of this impulse has been a movement toward legalized retribution in the form of state laws aimed at women who use illegal substances during their pregnancies. These laws have been proposed at a time when most drug rehabilitation programs do not accept pregnant women and the methodology of drug use identification is inconsistent at best (Gittler & McPherson, 1990). Research has demonstrated that human development is a complex process, an enterprise which involves the interplay of individual genetic endowments and environmental interactions. Because of this, the study of the effects of prenatal exposure to drugs, alcohol, and cigarettes is fraught with methodological difficulties (Myer, Olson, & Kallenback, 1992). Group trends are obscured by the wide ranges of individual outcomes. It is precisely the complex interaction of variables which confounds researchers that challenges clinicians. Rooted within the multiple factors which influence the development of human communicative abilities is the potential for adaptation. Our success as clinicians lies in our ability to facilitate adaptation and in our ability to guide the development of human potential by treating it as more robust than fragile, more adaptive than vulnerable.

As clinicians, we approach this chapter from a perspective grounded in the application of information gleaned from research and current practice. Given the recent emergence of interest in cocaine and its effects, we will review the specifics of research on cocaine use more extensively than that of other teratogens.

Cocaine

Prevalence

Crack cocaine use was first reported in New York City in 1983, and its use became widespread there in late 1985 (Department of the Treasury, 1988). Presently, crack is sold across the country, not only in major cities but in rural areas as well. The arrival of this cheap form of cocaine on the market resulted in a flood of media attention, much of it directed at the effects of cocaine on the children of addicted mothers. Early reports in the popular press frequently had sensationalist with titles like "Crack's Toll Among Babies: A Joyless View of Even Toys" (*New York Times*, 1989). Fortunately, the number of scientific research projects in the area of substance abuse during pregnancy and its effects on child development have increased dramatically in the past 10 years, most notably in reference to cocaine.

It has been reported that 20 million people in the United States have tried cocaine at least once and that 5 million use it regularly (Chasnoff, 1987). In the 1990 *National Household Survey*, over 6 million Americans reported using cocaine in the previous year (National Institute on Drug Abuse, 1991). Given that this survey assumes that drug users will admit to illegal substance use over the phone to a person identified as working for the U.S. government, it appears that the actual numbers may be much higher.

The incidence of cocaine use among pregnant women is difficult to assess due to methodological issues inherent in the identification procedures used to ascertain substance abuse. Reviews of the prevalence estimates from individual hospitals have reported cocaine exposure percentages ranging from 3% to 50% of live births (Sparks, 1993). In 1988, 11% of all women delivering at 36 U.S. hospitals were identified as positive for ingestion of one or more illegal substances during pregnancy (Chasnoff, 1989). In a study conducted in Pinellas County, Florida, urine screening for alcohol, opiates, cocaine, and cannaboids was performed on all pregnant women. Of the 715 pregnant women screened within the 6-month study period, 14.8% had a positive urine screen for cocaine, marijuana, or heroin (Chasnoff, 1990). An important finding of this study was that the frequency of positive result for illicit drug use was similar among white women (15.4%) and black women (14.1%). During that same time period, 133 women in Pinellas County were reported to health authorities after delivery for substance abuse during pregnancy. Black women were reported 10 times more frequently than white women, and poor women were more likely than others to be reported. Given the growing body of objective medical evidence that illicit drug use is common among pregnant women across socioeconomic and racial groups, patterns and procedures for legally mandated reporting must be reexamined.

Methodological Issues in Examining Usage Patterns

One of the central problematic issues in the study of cocaine exposure and its effects is the polydrug nature of substance abuse patterns in people who use cocaine. Few cocaine users abuse only one substance. The majority of cocaine users also use marijuana, alcohol, benzodiazephines, or cigarettes, if not all of them (Frank et al., 1988). These drugs exert differential effects on the fetus. They may be used in any combination, with varying amounts, frequency, and durations of use. Studies of possible teratogens require accurate identification of gestational timing of exposure as well as frequency and intensity (Zuckerman, 1991).

Urine assays are the most commonly used form of identification procedure in research and clinical practice. Urine screenings are highly dependent on the time of drug ingestion in relation to when the urine sample is obtained. The duration of positive urine findings for cocaine or marijuana varies with the amount, mode, and chronicity of use as well as fluid intake and renal function (Zuckerman & Frank, 1992). Benzoylecgonine, a metabolite of cocaine, may be detected in the urine of adults for only 24 to 72 hours after last use (Hamilton et al., 1977). Urine assays do not accurately identify patterns of usage. Many infrequent users are missed regardless of the amount of drug ingested. Discrepancies in findings of cocaine metabolites in both mothers and newborns immediately following delivery (MacDonald, 1992) suggest that the urine of both mother and child should be screened. The short duration of cocaine metabolite excretion in urine following last use results in a bias toward women who use cocaine late in their pregnancies when urine assays are obtained upon delivery (Fulroth, Phillips, & Durand, 1989). Urine screens positive at delivery may identify frequent heavy users and underrepresent those who use cocaine early in their pregnancies (Frank et al., 1988).

Radioimmunoassay of meconium (the first neonatal stools) is a promising technique for the analysis of exposure to cocaine, marijuana, and opiate metabolites (Ostrea, Brady, Gause, Raymundo, & Steven, 1992). Meconium is produced by the fetus from about 18 to 20 weeks gestation until delivery. Meconium assays may eventually be able to quantify cumulative dosages to the fetus, however; issues regarding the number of samples required and the distribution of drug metabolites in the samples diminish the reliability of meconium sampling at this time. Analysis of maternal and neonatal hair is another procedure that is under study (Baily, 1989). Questions regarding the effect on hair of passive exposure, chemical cosmetic processing, and the tendency of black coarse hair to retain the drug longer than blonde and fine hair bring up issues of accuracy and racial testing biases.

Self-report is another form of identification frequently utilized. Obtaining reliable historic information is understandably difficult given the illegal nature of cocaine use. A study done at Mercy Catholic Medical Center in Pennsylvania in 1990 utilized meconium testing of 500 consecutively born infants; 59 or 11.8% of the babies tested positive for cocaine. Of the 316 mothers returning the written anonymous questionnaire, only five admitted prenatal drug use (Shutzman, Frankenfield-Chernicoff, Clatterbaugh, & Singer, 1991). In a similar study of 670 pregnant women in an urban setting using urine assay and self-report, 17% were found to have used cocaine at least once during their pregnancy, and 24% of the cocaine users identified through urine screening denied use at the time of the interview (Frank et al., 1988). From a clinical perspective, Shirley Sparks has postulated that history taking within the context of a long-term clinical relationship yields more accurate and comprehensive information than interview techniques used in research (Sparks, 1993). Regardless of the technique, identification continues to be problematic, and many researchers have conjectured that current incidence percentages represent low estimates of actual prevalence.

Action of the Drug

Cocaine is the most potent stimulant of natural origin. It is extracted from the leaves of the coca plant, which has been cultivated in the Andean highlands of South America since prehistoric times. Cocaine may be inhaled nasally in a powder form, smoked in its volatilized form, or injected intravenously in combination with other substances or alone. Cocaine acts on neurotransmitter systems in the central nervous system (specifically in the mesolimbic or mesocortical dopaminergic tracts), blocking the presynaptic reuptake of the neurotransmitters dopamine, serotonin, and norepinephrine following their release. The blocking of reabsorption produces a prolonged and exaggerated period of stimulation and excitability, associated with pleasure and reward. With repeated use, cocaine depletes dopamine in the central nervous system, which is believed to cause depressive symptoms and result in withdrawal symptoms and a form of addiction (Gawin, 1991).

When cocaine is inhaled in smoke form, it rapidly diffuses across the lungs, resulting in a high blood level followed by rapid metabolism and clearance. The euphoric state is achieved more rapidly than with "snorting," which results in a slower uptake and delayed clearance due to vasoconstriction in the nasal mucosa (MacDonald, 1992). Women smoking crack or injecting the drug must administer higher amounts of the drug to achieve and maintain the desired effect, and thus their fetuses may experience more toxicity. Cocaine crosses the placenta and the blood-brain barrier freely (Wang, Rudolph, & Benet, 1980). Most drugs taken by pregnant women have a longer half-life in the fetus than the adult because the fetal liver is incompletely developed and cannot excrete the drugs quickly (Chasnoff, 1987). As discussed in the previous section, the route and form of administration are variables which complicate research findings on the effects of prenatal exposure to cocaine. In addition, the frequently polydrug nature of substance abuse must be considered when specific single-drug effects are reviewed.

Effects of Cocaine on the Fetus and Newborn

Evidence is accumulating linking patterns of adverse pregnancy outcomes to prenatal cocaine exposure. Findings of fetal growth retardation, microcephaly, and low birth weight have been reported in a number of studies (Fulroth et al., 1989; Little & Snell, 1991; Pettiti & Coleman, 1990). The pattern of microcephaly in these cases is opposite to the typical growth retardation pattern caused by undernutrition. Reduced head circumference in the absence of catch-up growth by age 2 has been associated with poor developmental outcomes (Eckerman, Lynne, & Gross, 1985). Cocaine has been linked to prematurity in some studies (Chasnoff et al., 1989; Handler, Kistin, Davis, & Ferre, 1991; Phibbs, Bateman, & Schwartz, 1991). Other studies have disputed this finding (Hadeed & Siegal, 1989; Ryan, Ehrlich, & Finnegan, 1987). Increased incidence of spontaneous first-trimester abortion and abruptio placenta have been reported, findings which are consistent with placental vasoconstriction induced by cocaine (Chasnoff et al., 1989).

An increased risk of intracerebral hemorrhage and cerebral infarction has been noted in cocaine-exposed infants, associated with cocaine's ability to produce sudden changes in cerebral blood flow (Dixon & Bejar, 1989; Dominguez, Vila-Coro, Slopes, & Bohan, 1991). These findings of the direct effects of cocaine on the developing fetal brain are of great concern and warrant more study. Structural abnormalities, including distal limb reduction, urogenital abnormalities, cardiac lesions, and ocular malformations, have been noted in the research (Dominguez et al., 1991; Hannig & Phillips, 1991; Hayme et al., 1990; Lipschultz, Frassica, & Orav, 1991). Although it has not been proven that cocaine causes congenital abnormalities, cocaine's ability to disrupt blood flow to developing structures through its vasoconstrictive action strongly suggests that it is an etiologic factor. Other complications often displayed in infants prenatally exposed to cocaine include hypertonia, hyperactive moro reflex, abnormal rapidity of respiration, cardiorespiratory abnormalities, loose stools, and nasal stuffiness (Fulroth et al., 1989; MacGregor et al., 1987).

Ototoxic effects of cocaine exposure have been suggested (Shih, Cone-Wesson, & Reddix, 1988). Auditory brain stem response studies have shown no increased risk of hearing impairment among full-term cocaine exposed infants (Carzoli, Murphy, Hammer-Knisely, & Houy, 1991). However, auditory brain stem response (ABR) studies have revealed abnormal findings in central auditory nervous system function (Salamy, Eldredge, Anderson, & Bull, 1990; Shih et al., 1988). Postnatal exposure to cocaine has been reported via breast feeding, passive inhalation, and direct ingestion (Chasnoff, Lewis, & Squires, 1987; Kharasch; Glotzer, Vinci, Weitzman, & Sargent, 1991). The percentages of exposure and the long-term risk to development for children postnatally cocaine exposed are unknown at this time.

In summary, evidence is accumulating that prenatal exposure to cocaine is associated with a number of adverse pregnancy and fetal/neonatal outcomes, including intrauterine growth retardation, placental abruption, low birth weight, prematurity, reduced head circumference, intracerebral hemorrhage, cerebral infarction, limb reduction, urinary tract abnormalities, ocular malformations, and cardiac lesions. Specific outcomes are tied closely to multiple risk factors, making the isolation of cocaine's specific effects methodologically difficult. A clinical rush to judgment should not be made based on identification of prenatal drug exposure because many cocaine-exposed infants show none of the adverse effects cited in the literature.

Neurobehavioral and Language Effects

It is important that a risk model rather than a deficit model be applied when evaluating the effects of prenatal exposure to cocaine on developmental outcomes. Neonatal neurobehavioral abnormalities have been found in some but not all studies, and multiple confounding variables are present in the clinical population. A deficit model, assuming that the infant has experienced specific damage resulting in developmental problems, is therefore inappropriate.

At this time, the findings of most of the research into developmental outcomes for children prenatally exposed to cocaine have involved neonates and infants. A number of studies have assumed that termination of exposure to cocaine would result in withdrawal syndrome and have utilized the Neonatal Abstinence Scale (NAS) as an assessment tool. The NAS was designed to study opiate withdrawal and is not an appropriate tool for cocaine-exposed infants who do not demonstrate systematic signs of withdrawal (Zuckerman & Frank, 1992). Studies utilizing scales such as the Brazelton Neonatal Behavioral Assessment Scale (NBAS) have many of the methodological problems discussed previously but reveal some consistencies in neurobehavioral findings. Difficulties with state control are a significant factor for cocaine- and polydrug-exposed infants during the first few weeks following birth (Chasnoff, Burns, Schnoll, & Burns, 1985). Cocaine-exposed infants tend to display disorganized nervous systems that interfere with their ability to regulate their own states of arousal. They tend to be irritable, poorly responsive, and easily overstimulated when awake. When confronted with even minimal environmental stimuli, they may cry inconsolably or return to a deep sleep state (Schneider, Griffith, & Chasnoff, 1989).

A distinctive high-pitched cry has been associated with cocaine-exposed infants (Lester et al., 1991). It has been postulated that the characteristics of this cry in the first few weeks after birth have a deleterious effect on parent-child interactions. A number of studies have looked at cocaine-exposed infants and their early dyadic interactions with their mothers. Consistent positive relationships have been found between the level of alertness and responsiveness of the infants and the sensitivity of mothers (Osofsky, 1976). Dyadic disturbances appear to be exacerbated by the drug-exposed infant's reduced responsiveness, poor state regulation, and feeding difficulties. These infants have specific difficulty maintaining the "quiet alert" state from which most reciprocal parent-infant interactions spring. Contributing to the infant's neurobehavioral problems is the tendency of drug-abusing mothers to be rigid and overcontrolling in their parenting and to exhibit a limited range of emotional involvement and responsivity in their interactions (Burns, Chetnik, Burns, & Clark, 1991). The findings in the area of early parent-infant interactions suggest that many cocaine-exposed infants are at risk for developmental delay and strongly support family-focused early intervention.

Initial information from longitudinal studies evaluating development outcomes for children prenatally exposed to cocaine has only recently begun to be published. At the National Association for Perinatal Addiction Research and Education (NAPARE), Ira Chasnoff and his researchers are following a group of 300 cocaine/polydrug-exposed children. Major risk factors have been eliminated by recruiting cocaine/polydrug-abusing women into the program during the early phases of pregnancy and providing them with prenatal care, nutritional counseling, and therapy for chemical dependence. At age 2, the infants exposed to cocaine and usually marijuana and/or alcohol at birth had caught up with the control group in mean length and weight. They continued to demonstrate significantly smaller head circumference. On the Bayley Scales of Infant Development, the mean developmental scores of the drug-exposed children did not vary significantly from the control group, although an increased proportion scored greater than two standard deviations below the mean on both the mental and psychomotor indexes than in the control group. A correlation between small head size and developmental scores was found across infants. This study suggests that prenatal drug exposure does not result in poor developmental outcomes at age 2 across children but that these children are at significant risk and that head growth after birth may be an important biological marker (Chasnoff, Griffith, Freir, & Murray, 1992).

Findings from studies utilizing global developmental scales do not always present a clear picture of developmental behavior. Researchers, clinicians, and teachers frequently report that the low thresholds for overstimulation and self-regulatory difficulties evidenced in the neonatal period persist over time for some children. The structured nature of standardized testing may actually mask attentional difficulties exhibited in more naturalistic environments. Evaluators report that these children are difficult to test and require a high level of examiner provided regulation.

Rodnig, Beckwith, and Howard (1990) compared drug-exposed 18-month-old toddlers to a control group of high-risk toddlers in a structured free-play setting. The drug-exposed children demonstrated significant deficits in their play, with decreased representational and combinatorial play and increased throwing, scattering, and batting of toys. Drug-exposed children have also been shown to demonstrate flat affect, unclear affective cues, and insecure disorganized attachments to their caregivers. These characteristics are more marked in children raised by biologic mothers who continue to abuse drugs. (Howard, Beckwith, Rodnig, & Kropenske, 1989).

A group of eight speech and language pathologists working with children maternally exposed to cocaine in hospital, school, and private clinic settings were surveyed in a 1992 study based in Orlando, Florida. In the birth to age 2 category, delayed expressive language, attention deficits, decreased problem-solving skills, low muscle tone, rapid mood swings, and difficulties in being consoled were reported. At ages 2 to 4, word retrieval difficulties, poor syntactic sequencing, reduced mean length of utterance (MLU), difficulties acquiring number and color concepts, and poor pragmatic skills were reported to be common problems. At ages 4 to 6, reduced vocabulary skills, difficulties with abstract concepts (multiple-meaning words, temporal/spatial concepts), reduced attention spans, and impulsivity were observed. Trouble with task transitions was described across age groups. The children prenatally exposed to cocaine described in this study exhibited few behaviors that were typical across children. Variability and individuality of developmental outcome must be considered to be a central clinical factor for cocaine-exposed children. The findings of this study must be viewed with great caution given the subjective nature of the survey, its restricted sample size (eight clinicians, 50 children), the sampling bias, and the lack of a control group. However, preliminary results in ongoing studies suggest that cocaine- and polydrug-exposed children are at significant risk for speech and language delays (Rivers & Hedrick, 1992).

In two studies of 21 cocaine/polydrug-exposed preschoolers which were controlled for stable home environment, a consistent pattern of mild to moderate language delays was found (Johnson, Foose, Seikel, & Madison, 1992; Johnson, Gettles, Seikel, & Madison, 1992). In an ongoing study of children and adolescents at an acute care psychiatric facility at UCLA, preliminary findings suggest links between prenatal substance abuse exposure and disruptive behavior disorders. A highly variable communication ability profile characterized the subjects in the group prenatally exposed to illicit drugs (Baltaxe, D'Angiola, & Simmons, 1992).

Summary

There is a great need for further large-sample longitudinal studies of developmental outcomes for children prenatally exposed to cocaine. Given cocaine's alteration of neurotransmitter levels, concern has been raised regarding the long-term impact on the attention and self-regulation capacities of prenatally exposed children. These issues highlight the need for controlled studies of effects in cocaine-exposed school-age children, who may theoretically be at risk for language and learning disabilities. The good news is that initial findings from studies of prenatally exposed toddlers and preschoolers indicate that, for the majority, cognitive skills fall within normal limits on standardized developmental measures. However, preliminary findings in ongoing studies suggest that cocaine-exposed infants are at risk for receptive and expressive language delay. In addition, evaluator reports of reduced abilities in the areas of play, pragmatic, organizational, and self-regulatory skills in cocaine-exposed children emphasize the importance of utilizing observational methods within functional communication settings to supplement standardized measures of evaluation.

Marijuana

Prevalence

Information regarding the effects of marijuana use during pregnancy is limited, although marijuana is one of the most widely used illegal substances in this country. Societal and cultural attitudes toward the use of marijuana appear to be reflected in the behavior of women who use the drug during pregnancy. In one study of illicit drug use during pregnancy, white women were shown to have a higher incidence of cannaboid use than black women (Chasnoff, 1990). Prevalence estimates of marijuana use during pregnancy range from 5% to 34% (Zuckerman, 1988).

Action of the Drug

Cannabis sativa L., the hemp plant, has been used as a drug for centuries. Cannabis products are usually smoked in the form of loosely rolled cigarettes called joints. The isomer delta-9-tetrahydrocannabinol (THC) is the chemical component of marijuana responsible for its psychoactive effects (Department of the Treasury, 1988). THC is stored in the fatty tissues of the body and may take up to 30 days to be completely excreted (Nahas, 1976). Marijuana crosses the placenta easily during the early stages of pregnancy. Inhalation of marijuana places fetuses at risk for hypoxia due to decreased oxygenation (Clapp, Wesley, Cooke, Pekals, & Holstein, 1986).

Effects on the Fetus and Newborn

As in studies of cocaine, confounding variables, including issues involving identification, cloud the results of studies involving marijuana use during pregnancy. Lower birth weight and shorter length have been reported for infants born to women with positive urine assays for marijuana (Zuckerman et al., 1989). Lower sleep efficiency on electroencephalogram (EEG) studies conducted on prenatally exposed 3-year-olds has been cited recently (Day & Richardson, 1991). Postnatal exposure through passive smoke inhalation and breast milk is a risk factor for infants of mothers who use the drug following delivery (Astley & Little, 1990).

Neurobehavioral and Language Effects

Neurobehavioral effects, including tremors, decreased responsiveness to visual stimuli, and high-pitched cries, have been associated with moderate to heavy marijuana use during pregnancy (Fried & Makin, 1987). Few studies have examined developmental outcomes for children prenatally exposed to marijuana. In a group of children examined longitudinally, no association between prenatal exposure to marijuana and developmental scores was seen at 12 or 24 months; however, at 4 years heavy prenatal marijuana use (more than six joints per week) was associated with poor memory and verbal scores on the McCarthy Test (Fried & Watkinson, 1988, 1990). A study by another group found no IQ differences at age 4 (Streissguth et al., 1989). There is a need for further longitudinal studies involving older children prenatally exposed to marijuana.

Cigarettes

Prevalence

Smoking is one of the most highly researched areas in the study of teratology. Because the use of cigarettes is not illegal, information on use is more easily collected and prenatal exposure more widespread. The percentage of women using cigarettes during pregnancy has been reported to be between 22% and 28%

(Williamson, Serdula, Kendrick, & Binkin, 1989). Some estimates indicate that one third to one half of all pregnant women are passively exposed to smoke (Karakostav, 1985; Smith, Austen, & Rolles, 1982). Levels of nicotine and carbon monoxide, which are judged to be the components of smoke most dangerous to offspring of smokers, are present in higher levels in sidestream smoke, placing passive smokers and their offspring at great risk.

Action of the Drug

Negative pregnancy outcomes and neurobehavioral effects are attributable to nicotine in combination with hypoxia/ischemia resulting from the act of smoking. The anoretic effects of nicotine contribute to poor maternal nutritional intake, which has been linked to adverse pregnancy outcomes. The primary components of tobacco attributed with producing negative fetal outcomes are nicotine, cyanide, and carbon monoxide. Direct infusion of nicotine into pregnant animals has demonstrated negative effects, including cellular damage, impairment of the acquisition of cells throughout the central nervous system, suppressed synapse formation, and deficits in impulse activity (Slotkin, 1992).

Effects of Smoking on the Fetus and Newborn

A number of adverse pregnancy effects have been associated with maternal smoking, including sudden infant death syndrome (Haglund & Cnattingus, 1990), spontaneous abortions (Risch, Weiss, Clarke, & Miller, 1988), and perinatal death (Cnattingus, Haglund, & Meirik, 1988). Low birth weight has been consistently linked with maternal smoking, with lower weights associated with heavier dosages (Meyer, Jonas, & Tonascia, 1976). Use in the third trimester has been found to be significantly related to low birth weights, although negative effects have been found across trimesters (Fried & O'Connell, 1987).

Neurobehavioral and Language Effects

Decreased auditory habituation and responsiveness has been noted in neonates born to smoking mothers, suggesting reduced nervous system integrity (Fried & Makin, 1987). Maternal use of cigarettes has been associated with increased tremors, a delayed onset of crying, and poorer autonomic regulation (Fried & Makin, 1987; Picone, Allen, Olsen, & Ferris, 1982). At 30 days of age, maternal smoking has been associated with increased tonicity, heightened motoric reflexivity, and continued incidence of tremor (Fried & Makin, 1987; Picone et al., 1982). At 1 year of age, the children of heavy maternal smokers have been shown to do more poorly on the mental developmental index (MDI) of the Bayley Scales (Ernhart et al., 1985). At 2 years of age, no significant differences were found for the same children on the MDI or on the Reynell Developmental Language Scale (Reynell & Huntley, 1989), which looks at receptive and expressive language. Although prenatal exposure to cigarettes may not have an effect on language and cognition at 2 years, it has been postulated that postnatal environment may act as an intervening variable (Fried, 1992). Decreased maternal involvement has been cited as a possible risk factor for children of heavy smokers (Fried, 1992), but evidence in the research is conflicting.

A relationship between lowered cognitive skills and maternal smoking has been found in a number of studies (Rush & Callahan, 1989). Significantly lower scores on the verbal components of the McCarthy Scales of Children's Abilities (McCarthy, 1972) have been obtained at age 3 by children of heavy smokers. Means on each of the six McCarthy subscales as well as the expressive portion of the Reynell were lower than for children of light smokers, which were lower in turn than those of children of nonsmokers. At age 4, the children's scores continued to be significantly lower on all six subscales of the McCarthy, the expressive portion of the Reynell, and the receptive vocabulary measure of the Peabody Picture Vocabulary Test-Revised (1981). Findings of increased incidence of hyperactivity and reduced attentional vigilance have been reported in 4-year-olds maternally exposed to smoking (Streissguth et al., 1984). Problems with information processing and attention have been identified in school-age children of smokers (Kristjansson, Fried, & Watkinson, 1989). Maternal passive exposure to cigarette smoke appears to have similar long-term negative effects on child development, but to a milder degree than for children prenatally exposed by an active smoker (Makin, Fried, & Watkinson, 1991). The specific effect of postnatal passive exposure to cigarette smoke upon cognitive and linguistic development is unclear, but the risk appears to be significant (Makin et al., 1991).

Alcohol

Prevalence

Maternal alcohol use during pregnancy is the leading known cause of mental retardation in the United States (Abel & Sokol, 1987). Alcohol's teratogenic effects were identified over 20 years ago and are now widely recognized (Lemoine, Harrousseau, Borteyru, & Menuet, 1968). Given alcohol's widespread usage, there has been a surprisingly limited amount of clinical research aimed at developing public policy, intervention, and treatment for affected children. In North America, 9 out of 10 women of child-bearing age drink occasionally, and statistics indicate that as many as 7 out of 10 of these drink regularly, on an average of one drink per day, with 5% to 10% of the women in this category being characterized as alcoholics (Hilton, 1988). Younger and unmarried women drink more than older and married women. Women of higher social class are more likely to be alcohol users than women of lower social class, and white women are more likely to be drinkers and heavier drinkers than black women (Herd, 1988). The incidence of fetal alcohol syndrome (FAS) in the general population has been estimated to be 0.33 cases per 1000 (Abel & Sokol, 1991), but FAS is judged to be widely underdiagnosed, indicating that incidence may be much higher (Little, Snell, Rosenfeld, Gilstrap, & Gant, 1990). FAS is the most severe end of a continuum of fetal alcohol effects resulting from prenatal exposure to alcohol, effects which are much more difficult to diagnose and are not reflected in these prevalence numbers.

Action of the Drug

Alcohol is a sedative hypnotic drug, and its effects on neurotransmitters can have both excitatory and inhibitory actions. Alcohol, called ethanol in the form that we drink, passes into the blood from the digestive tract and is distributed evenly through the body. Alcohol passes freely across the placental barrier as well as the blood-brain barrier and is eventually metabolized in the liver. Because the human fetus has a reduced capacity to eliminate alcohol, levels are higher and effects are more long lasting in utero. The specific actions of alcohol on the fetus are unknown. Alcohol interferes with biologic processes at the molecular, cellular, and physiological levels; thus it is unlikely that the multifaceted effects of alcohol on development can be accounted for by one mechanism or action. The development of the central nervous system begins early in the life of the fetus and undergoes a series of sequential developmental stages. As with other teratogenic substances, exposure to alcohol at different stages will affect different developmental processes, and so the effects on the brain will be a function of its stage of development at exposure (Goodlett & West, 1992).

Effects of Alcohol on the Fetus and Newborn

Fetal alcohol syndrome was first described in 1973 (Jones & Smith, 1973). FAS is a clinical diagnosis which does not include all individuals affected by alcohol in utero but which classifies the extreme end of a continuum of disabilities caused by maternal use of alcohol during pregnancy. FAS is a medical diagnosis usually given by a dysmorphologist, a geneticist, or a specially trained pediatrician. Because many physicians have not been trained to identify syndromes, many children with FAS go undiagnosed. Fetal alcohol syndrome is diagnosed when there is a positive history of maternal alcohol use during pregnancy and the following features: (1) growth deficiency in height or weight of a prenatal origin; (2) facial anomalies, generally including short palpebral fissures, midface hypoplasia (a long or smooth philtrum, thin upper lip); and (3) central nervous system manifestations, which can include microcephaly, delayed development, attention deficits, hyperactivity, learning deficits, intellectual impairment, and seizures (Clarren & Smith, 1978; Smith, 1982; Streissguth, 1992). At puberty, many of the characteristic features of the faces of children with FAS become less distinctive, so a diagnosis is more easily made in childhood, specifically between 8 months and 8 years of age (Streissguth et al., 1991). Children exposed to alcohol in utero presenting with some of the characteristics of the syndrome, but without sufficient features to confirm a diagnosis of FAS, are identified to be possible victims of fetal alcohol effects (FAEs) (Clarren & Smith, 1978). It is important to use the words *probable* or *possible FAE* to reflect the fact that many of the features of FAS are present in populations not prenatally exposed to alcohol; thus in absence of the full syndrome there is some uncertainty in the attribution of causation to alcohol. Often, children without typical facial characteristics who exhibit more subtle cognitive and behavioral deficits miss early diagnosis, escaping detection until they exhibit learning problems in school (Shaywitz, Cohen, & Shaywitz, 1980). Among siblings of drinking mothers, younger children are more likely to be impaired than older ones because the severity of alcohol embryopathy is linked to heavy exposure and chronicity of maternal use (Majewski & Majewski, 1988).

Neurobehavioral and Language Effects

As with other substances, the amount and timing of alcohol use interacts with maternal and child genetic and biologic factors to result in multiple outcomes for neonates. Environmental factors can exacerbate the neurobehavioral manifestations of FAS/FAE. The often unstable and chaotic environment of the alcohol-abusing mother may place the child at increased risk for developmental delay and behavioral problems. For these reasons, studies of the neurobehavioral effects of maternal alcohol use on newborns have been divergent in their findings. Although some studies have not found specific neurobehavioral effects on neonates using the Neonatal Behavioral Assessment Scale (Enhart et al., 1985), in others, alcohol-exposed infants have been reported to be less able to habituate to aversive stimuli (Streissguth, Barr, & Martin, 1983), demonstrate increased irritability (Fried & Makin, 1987), and show depressed range of state (Jacobson, Fein, Jacobson, Schwartz, & Dowler, 1984). Clinical reports include increased incidence of feeding difficulties, erratic sleep patterns, failure to thrive, heart defects, pneumonia, hip dysplasia, and developmental delays (Sparks, 1993).

Delays in language and cognitive development have been reported in alcohol-exposed infants and toddlers by a number of studies. Significantly lower than average scores on the mental and motor indexes of the Bayley Scales have been found at 6 and 8 months of age (Coles, Smith, Lancaster, & Falek, 1987; Streissguth, Barr, Martin, & Herman, 1980). At 13 months, reduced scores on the mental index and the verbal comprehension and spoken language clusters of the Bayley Scales have been reported (Gusella & Fried, 1984).

Long-term growth deficits result in children appearing small for their age (Day et al., 1991). Due to their short stature, developmental delays are often overlooked by parents and teachers, who adjust their expectations to fit the child's small size. Hyperactivity, attention deficits, and impulsivity have been associated with prenatal exposure to alcohol in longitudinal research across ages and time, with initial manifestations occurring in infancy and early childhood (Brown et al., 1991; Streissguth et al., 1984). Clinically, FAS children have been described as outgoing, excessively friendly, indiscriminate in their reactions to friends and strangers, more interested in people than objects, fearless, poorly responsive to limit setting, and needy of bodily contact (Sparks, 1993). Language delays in early childhood are more notable in the expressive domain, with an increased incidence of articulation disorders related to deviations in structure and function of the oral motor mechanism (Hill, Hegemier, & Tennyson, 1989). Malformations of the mouth can consist of prominent lateral palatine ridges, cleft lip and palate, a thin upper lip and indistinct philtrum, retrognathia (a receding chin), and dental problems, such as malalignment or malocclusion of the teeth (Clarren & Smith, 1978; Hill et al., 1989).

Children prenatally exposed to alcohol are at an increased risk for hearing loss. Congenital malformations of the ears can result in a poorly formed concha, posterior rotation of the ears, and malformation of the external ear (Clarren & Smith, 1978). A high incidence of bilateral serous otitis media and bilateral sensorineural hearing loss has been found in FAS populations. FAS children may also exhibit hyperacusis (Hill et al., 1989).

At school age, hyperactivity and distractibility continue to be two significant handicapping conditions present in the majority of alcohol-exposed children (Spohr & Steinhausen, 1987). In addition to hyperactivity and attentional deficits, neuropsychological symptoms such as short memory span, perceptual difficulties, difficulties with concentration, impulsivity, and perservation have been reported into adolescence (Aronson, Sandin, Sabel, Kyllerman, & Olegard, 1984). Academically, FAS and FAE children have more difficulty with math and higher level reading comprehension than with spelling and decoding (Streissguth, Clarren, & Jones, 1985).

A direct relationship between the severity of dysmorphology in infancy and lowered IQ has been reported (Streissguth, Herman, & Smith, 1978). It is important to note that the IQ scores of FAS/FAE children cover a broad range from severely retarded to normal. The greatest increases in IQ scores for FAS/FAE children take place between the preschool and early school-age years (Streissguth, Randels, & Smith, 1991), which has important implications for early intervention. Perhaps a more significant cognitive measure than IQ for FAS/FAE is that of adaptive functioning. Adaptive skills of daily living, socialization, and communication are severely reduced in comparison to chronological age in adolescents, and adults classified as FAS are severely reduced in comparison to chronological age. FAS and FAE adolescents who are not technically retarded frequently fail to develop adaptive behaviors. They fail to consider and understand the consequences of actions, are unable to respond to subtle social language cues, and lack reciprocity in communication and thus friendships (Streissguth, Randels, & Smith, 1991).

Language-based deficits have been clinically described as falling into two categories: those related to intellectual impairments such as problems with abstraction and memory, and those distinctively related to pragmatic issues associated with poor adaptive skills. Typical language deficits can include receptive processing difficulties complicated by attention deficits and reduced expressive skills such as poor descriptive narrative abilities. Pragmatically, FAS/FAE individuals are often superficially talkative, speaking too quickly and frequently with little content or intent in their utterances. They have difficulties with perseveration on topics, turn-taking with listeners, and choosing appropriate conversational topics. They may exhibit an inability to understand appropriate physical boundaries and be described as touchy or inappropriately curious (Sparks, 1993).

Summary

The effects of prenatal alcohol exposure fall along a continuum of severity which is related to the amount of alcohol that the fetus was exposed to prenatally. Although individuals diagnosed with FAS or FAE span a wide range of intellectual abilities, the majority of identified cases fall within the borders of a mentally retarded range of abilities and have specific difficulties with adaptive skills. A diagnosis of FAS does not specify any inevitable limits to academic performance or achievement levels, but it does mean that some degree of brain damage has occurred and that the ramifications are lifelong in nature, with probable expression in adaptive behaviors. Alcohol continues to be a larger threat to children in this country than any illicit drug.

Assessment and Intervention

Introduction

Under the service guidelines of Public Law (P.L.) 99-457, it is inevitable that speech and language pathologists will be providing services to children prenatally exposed to drugs and alcohol. P.L. 99-457 mandates services for children who are exhibiting developmental delays or who are at risk for developmental delay secondary to a mental or physical condition (Lesar, 1992). P.L. 99-457 also emphasizes the role of the family in the assessment and intervention process by requiring the development of an Individual Family Service Plan (IFSP). It is crucial that the family be viewed as an integral part of the treatment plan if our efforts in the areas of prevention, assessment, and intervention are to be successful.

Services for drug- and alcohol-exposed children should utilize an interdisciplinary approach (Crites, Fischer, Stengel, & Siegel, 1992) which is parent centered in nature (Freeman & Mayo, 1992). Medical, social, and educational agencies need to provide collaborative and coordinated services, with one agency serving as the designated case manager (Lesar, 1992). Comprehensive treatment programs that allow mothers to receive treatment for chemical dependence, while their children receive early intervention services at the same facility, are the most highly recommended treatment models (Sparks, 1993).

Intervention programs should be based on the theoretical framework of a risk (Lesar, 1992) or transactional model (Chapman, Worthington, Cook, & Mayfield, 1992) versus a deficit (Lesar, 1992) or main-effects model (Kaplan-Saroff Rice, 1992). The transactional model recognizes that the effects of drug exposure are not functionally independent of multiple environmental variables, and it focuses on patterns of mutual regulation between the caregiver and child. On the other hand, the deficit model attributes the child's developmental difficulties solely to drug exposure, deeming the scope of the influence of drugs on the family and the child as possibly beyond professional assistance. It is imperative that we avoid labels which create low expectations. Each child should be viewed as an individual with unique needs whose primary caregivers are a vital part of the treatment plan.

The following sections will briefly review some of the behaviors exhibited by children prenatally exposed to drugs and alcohol and suggest assessment and intervention strategies. The scope of clinical practice with this population is broad, encompassing the vast topic of assessment and intervention with developmentally delayed populations from birth to adulthood. Given the recent influx of crack cocaine in this country and the concomitant increase in the number of cocaine/polydrug-exposed children, specific intervention strategies focusing on this population will be outlined in detail.

Cocaine/Polydrug Exposure Assessment and Intervention

Premature Infants

As discussed previously, cocaine use during pregnancy may result in placental abruption (MacDonald, 1992), cerebral infarction (Chasnoff, 1988), increased risk for fetal death in utero, intrauterine growth, retardation, small-for-gestation infants, and premature labor and delivery (Krug, 1989). Premature infants prenatally exposed to drugs may exhibit tremulousness and a high-pitched cry (Chasnoff, 1988) or irritability and poor self-regulation (Poulsen, 1989). In addition, these effects are further complicated by many of the typical medical problems associated with prematurity. Medical complications may include respiratory distress syndrome, low birth weight, and feeding difficulties (Harrison, 1983). This section will focus on the areas to assess in the preterm, prenatally drug exposed infant; possible assessment tools; and intervention strategies.

A positive urine screen, a previous history of drug use, or other children exposed to drugs and born to the same mother serve as indicators that prenatal drug exposure may have occurred. Many neonatal intensive care units (NICUs) already have physical and occupational therapists, speech-language pathologists, and developmental therapists present. The assessment and intervention process can and should begin immediately within the context of the NICU.

Motor abnormalities such as hyperextension, or fluctuating muscle tone, can be assessed by a physical or occupational therapist with the neonatal neurological examination (Dubowitz & Dubowitz, 1981). The various subsystems of preterm behavior can be assessed through the Neonatal Individualized Developmental Care and Assessment Program (NIDCAP; Als et al., 1982) or the Assessment of Preterm Infant Behavior (APIB; Als, Lester, Tronick, & Brazelton, 1982). The APIB focuses on the interplay of the autonomic, motor, state, attention-interaction, and self-regulatory systems as the infant deals with a variety of tactile, sensory, and postural inputs and demands.

Premature infants often exhibit feeding problems, such as poor coordination of suck/swallow with breathing, poor ability to initiate suck, and immature oral motor musculature (Vandenberg, 1990). These children may require gavage feedings in order to receive nutrition (Morris, 1987). Feeding difficulties may be further complicated by abnormal feeding patterns exhibited by the drug-exposed infant (Schneider et al., 1989) and difficulties in state control. The Neonatal Oral Motor Assessment Scale (NOMAS) (Palmer, 1991) evaluates jaw and tongue function during nutritive and non-nutritive sucking (Vandenberg, 1990). The NOMAS can be used to distinguish between normal and disorganized or dysfunctional feeding patterns and to quantify oral motor skills (Braun & Palmer, 1985).

With premature prenatally drug-exposed infants, mother-infant interactions should be a central focus of intervention. The intimidating environment of the NICU in combination with infant state control difficulties and frequently poor feeding abilities puts mother-infant attachment at risk (Lewis, Bennett, & Schmeder, 1989). Mothers should be aided in reading their infant's distress cues and be educated about the types of behaviors frequently exhibited by drug-exposed infants (Sparks, 1993).

Hearing assessment through ABR should be considered if the infant meets the risk criteria for audiological screening. Premature infants may be at risk for sensorineural hearing loss due to birth weight less than 1500 grams, prolonged mechanical ventilation, ototoxic medications, and so on (American Speech, Language, and Hearing Association, 1993).

Goals for the prenatally drug-exposed, premature infant may include enhancing the infant's ability to self-console and organize state, enhancing the infant's toleration of stimulation and handling, developing visually organized attention, reducing irritability, and preventing and managing agitation. These goals can be accomplished through proper positioning and handling of the preterm infant and manipulation of the NICU environment, through reducing noise levels, dimming lights, and so on (Vandenberg, 1991). Intervention strategies for improving motor and state control, feeding, and mother-infant interaction are listed in Table 11–1.

Newborn Stage

Full-term newborns exhibit many behaviors secondary to prenatal cocaine exposure, including jitteriness, irritability, increased muscle tone (MacDonald, 1992), frequent startles, irregular sleeping patterns, and poor feeding abilities (Lewis et al., 1989). The newborn may move rapidly from one extreme state to another (Schneider et al., 1989). These infants require proper positioning and handling and appropriate sensory stimulation to decrease irritability and poor self-regulation (Lesar, 1992). The Neonatal Behavior Assessment Scale (NBAS; Brazelton, 1984), which assesses organization in the full-term infant (Sparks, 1993), is often used with newborns prenatally exposed to drugs. The drug-exposed newborn may exhibit tremors, hyperextension, and overshooting, and thus positioning to improve posture and movement patterns is extremely important (Schneider & Chasnoff, 1987). Handling techniques such as swaddling (Sparks, 1993), reducing environmental stimuli, and vertical rocking (Schneider et al., 1989) may help calm the drug-exposed newborn.

Full-term prenatally exposed newborns also demonstrate poor state control and depressed interactive abilities (Schneider et al., 1989). The newborn's reduced responsiveness to caregivers may create a negative cycle, inhibiting the mother-infant bonding process (Lesar, 1992). To facilitate mother-infant interactions, caregivers should be taught proper positioning and handling techniques. The caregivers need to be instructed in how to read stress cues, such as gaze aversion and hiccoughing, and learn to adapt their interactions accordingly (Sparks, 1993). Techniques such as limiting input to one sensory modality may prevent the newborn from becoming overstimulated and improve the caregiver-child interaction. For example, caregivers might be encouraged to use eye contact initially when holding their baby, without any auditory input, and to combine both as the newborn's tolerance increases. It is important that caregiver-regulated calming and soothing techniques be gradually withdrawn from the drug-exposed newborn so that the newborn can learn to regulate his or her own state (Schneider & Chasnoff, 1987).

The drug-exposed newborn may exhibit feeding difficulties in the form of immature sucking/swallowing patterns, poor oral motor control (Schneider et al., 1989), and gastrointestinal problems such as regurgitation and vomiting (Lewis et al., 1989). Proper positioning and handling techniques; shorter, more frequent feedings; and experimentation with different bottle nipple temperatures may improve the newborn's feeding abilities. These infants may exhibit oral hypersensitivity (Schneider & Chasnoff, 1987), which may be decreased with

Table 11–1. Premature Stage

Goals:
1. Increase infant's ability to self-console and organize states
2. Improve infant's toleration of stimulation and handling
3. Develop visually organized attention
4. Reduce irritability

Behaviors	**Possible assessment tools**	**Intervention strategies**
I. Motor a. Abnormal muscle tone b. Fluctuating muscle tone c. Hyperextension	I. The Neonatal Neurological Examination (Dubowitz & Dubowitz, 1981)	I. • Position prone and sidelying to promote flexion • Swaddle to encourage flexion • Huggel Bunting
II. State a. Irritable b. Poor self-regulation c. Disorganized d. Easily overstimulated e. Brief, alert periods, no quiet, alert state f. Distress cues • Color changes • Hiccoughs • Gaze aversion • Yawning • Sneezing • Frowning	II. Neonatal Individual Developmental Care and Assessment Program (NIDCAP) (Als, Duffy, & McAnulty, 1982) Assessment of Preterm Infant Behavior (APIB) (Als, Lester et al., 1982)	II. • Manipulate the environment (i.e., reduce noise levels, dim lights, etc.) • Provide auditory/tactile/visual stimulation, using one modality at a time (i.e., voice or face, rocking without visual or auditory input) • Swaddle to encourage organization • Vertical rocking • Respond to early distress cues by giving time out • Minimal handling, clustering care, containing limbs when changing positions
III. Feeding a. Immature, disorganized sucking/swallowing pattern b. Poor coordination between suckling, swallowing, and respiration c. Decreased/increased oral motor reflexes d. Frantic, disorganized sucking patterns e. Vomiting f. Regurgitation	III. Neonatal Oral Motor Assessment Scale (NOMAS) (Palmer, 1991)	III. • Place in prone after feeding if baby has been vomiting/regurgitating • Swaddle to encourage flexion and organization • Short, frequent feedings • Experiment with different nipples (e.g., preemie, Nuk, etc.) to regulate flow of formula • Provide oral stimulation during gavage feedings to increase frequency of

Table 11–1. *continued*

g. Require gavage feedings (i.e., nasogastric/orogastric feeding tubes) h. Oral tactile hypersensitivity i. Increased exposure to drugs if breastfeeding		swallowing, weight gain, association of fullness with oral motor sensation, and facilitate transition to oral feedings • Burp frequently, and allow frequent breaks during feeding • Provide chin and/or cheek support during feedings
IV. Mother-infant interaction a. Infant may exhibit distress cues (e.g., gaze aversion, hiccoughs, yawning)	The Mother's Assessment of the Behavior of Her Infant (Field, Dempsey, Mallock, & Shuman, 1978) Observation of Communicative Interaction (OCI) (Klein & Briggs, 1987)	IV. • Instruct mother on proper handling, positioning, and calming techniques • Instruct mother in reading infant's distress cues • Educate mother on dangers of breastfeeding while still using drugs
V. Hearing a. Neonate may be at risk for hearing loss due to low birthweight, prolonged mechanical ventilation, ototoxic drugs	Auditory Brain Stem Response (ABR)	V. • Prevent hearing loss by decreasing noise levels in NICU • If hearing loss found, immediate fitting of hearing aids to maximize hearing for language acquisition

Adapted from Vandenberg, 1991; Lesar, 1992; Lewis, Bennett, & Schmeder, 1989; Scheider & Chasnoff, 1987; Sparks, 1993; ASHA Joint Committee on Infant Hearing, 1993.

firm, gentle tactile stimulation around the face (Schneider et al., 1989). Drug-exposed newborns often sleep for extended periods of time, requiring awakening for feedings to ensure adequate nutritional intake (Sparks, 1993). Table 11–2 lists various assessment and intervention strategies for the drug-exposed newborn, focusing on motor, state, feeding, the caregiver-infant interaction, and hearing.

Infancy

During the infancy stage, the drug-exposed infant may exhibit increased extensor tone and delayed integration of primitive reflexes (Schneider & Chasnoff, 1987). The primary goal of intervention at this stage is enabling the infant to move appropriately in his or her environment (Lewis et al., 1989). Physical therapy may be a crucial aspect of the treatment plan. Parents should be provided with ideas for carrying and handling the infant in addition to positions appropriate for play (Schneider et al., 1989). Parents can encourage decreased extensor tone by carrying the infant in a flexed position with hands in midline (Schneider & Chasnoff, 1987) and by avoiding baby walkers (Lewis et al., 1989). Parents should be instructed on ways to handle and play with their infants. For example, although the drug-exposed infant may no longer require swaddling to organize or calm himself or herself, he or she may respond to gentle swinging rather than rough, rapid movements during play with the caregiver (Schneider et al., 1989). Table 11–3 provides behaviors, possible assessment tools, and intervention strategies that are pertinent to the infancy period.

Toddler Years

Assessment of the drug-exposed toddler should include age-appropriate, norm-referenced tests targeting the developmental areas in question. Central to realistic assessment is observation of play, behavior, language, and mother-child interactions in naturalistic settings (Sparks, 1993). Specific attention should be paid to self-regulatory behavior and coping abilities during typical social interactions and environmental transitions (Sparks, 1993).

Intervention should focus on the provision of the direct intervention services determined to be necessary within the context of the assessment process (i.e., speech-language therapy, occupational therapy, developmental monitoring, etc.). An early intervention program based on a multidisciplinary team model is strongly suggested for children identified to be at risk for developmental delays. Caregivers should be educated in how to manage behavior and provide developmentally appropriate activities. Service providers can later assist the child and family in making the transition from an early intervention program to a preschool or special education program. Table 11–4 shows specific assessment and intervention strategies for toddlers.

Preschool and School-Age Years

Although we cannot predict the exact long-term developmental outcome of the drug-exposed child (Lewis et al., 1989), we know that some of these children may have long-term cognitive, behavioral, and learning disabilities (Schneider & Chasnoff, 1987). A large number of these children may not be identified until they reach school age (Griffith, 1992), when subtle difficulties become more apparent.

To assist the drug-exposed preschool/school-age population, the service provider should use a caregiver-focused approach. Instruction in modifying the home and classroom environments to facilitate maximal learning and decrease the likelihood of behavioral outbursts is essential. Strategies for assisting children to develop self-regulation skills include providing predictable daily routines, establishing a small teacher-to-student ratio, and structuring transitions at home and in the classroom. Children and their parents should be taught to recognize warning signs that signal an approach to the threshold for loss of behavioral control and to develop adaptive self-regulatory strategies (Griffith, 1992). Table 11–5 shows specific assessment and intervention strategies for preschool and school-age children.

FAS/FAE Assessment and Intervention

Introduction

As described in previous sections, prenatal alcohol exposure can result in a variety of central nervous system abnormalities, including mental retardation, microcephaly, and developmental delay (Marcus, 1984). The FAS/FAE population manifests a high incidence of speech and language disorders (Church & Gerkin, 1988). However, in many children there is a discrepancy between seemingly high verbal skills and a limited ability to communicate effectively (Sparks, 1993).

Like the prenatally-drug exposed child, environmental factors can exacerbate the neurobehavioral manifestations of FAS/FAE. Due to the long-term effects of prenatal alcohol exposure, it is important to assess the family's coping strategies and stress levels (Olson, Burgess, & Streissguth, 1992). Educating caregivers about the effects of prenatal alcohol exposure is central to the development of intervention programs (Olson et al., 1992). Understanding the cause of the child's developmental delays and behavior difficulties may result in more realistic expectations on the part of the parent.

The teratogenic effects of prenatal alcohol exposure may result in lifelong disabilities (Olson et al., 1992). Early identification and intervention with the FAS/FAE population is essential. In addition to facilitating the development of appropriate intervention programs, early identification of FAS enables the referral of families for alcohol abuse treatment and can prevent the birth of future children with FAS (Olson et al., 1992).

Infancy

One of the most important steps involved in intervention with the FAS/FAE infant is provision of ongoing developmental monitoring with a family-centered focus (Olson et al., 1992). Caregivers need to be taught to read and understand the infant's behavioral cues and to respond appropriately. This type of instruction can help strengthen the parent-child relationship (Olson et al., 1992). Mothers should be prevented from breastfeeding because the infant may be a risk for continued exposure to alcohol (Sparks, 1993). Intervention ideas

Table 11–2. Newborn Stage (0–1 Month)

Goals:
1. Increase infant's alertness to enable appropriate parent-child interaction
2. Decrease irritability and poor self-regulation
3. Normalize tone
4. Improve oral feeding skills and decrease oral tactile hypersensitivity

Behaviors	Possible assessment tools	Intervention strategies
I. Motor a. Hyperextended postures b. Tremors c. Overshooting d. Stiffness or rigidity	I. The Neonatal Neurological Examination (Dubowitz & Dubowitz, 1981)	I. • Encourage flexion, using rolled-up blankets or by swaddling • Position in sidelying • Vertical rocking while swaddled • Hydrotherapy • Graded auditory and visual stimuli
II. State a. Rapid change from one extreme state to another b. Deep sleep state c. Agitated sleep state d. Vacillation between extremes of state e. Panicked awake state f. Poor transition from one state to another g. Prolonged and/or high-pitched cry h. Inability to sleep	II. Neonatal Behavior Assessment Scales (NBAS) (Brazelton, 1984)	II. • Appropriate positioning and handling (i.e., swaddling and slow vertical rocking) • Appropriate sensory stimulation (i.e., visual/tactile/auditory using multimodal stimulation as tolerated) • Soothe infant by holding snugly and close to body; swaddle if necessary • Aid sleep by reducing environmental stimuli and excessive handling
III. Feeding a. Persistence of immature suckling/swallowing pattern b. Poor oral motor control c. Oral tactile hypersensitivity d. Disorganized suckling/swallowing pattern e. Frantic sucking pattern	III. Prespeech Assessment Scale (Morris, 1982)	III. • Position to encourage flexion • Firm, strong touch to decrease oral/tactile hypersensitivity • Smaller amounts of formula fed more frequently • Allow more time for feeding, allowing frequent rest periods between suckling • Burp infant gently and frequently

Table 11–2. *continued*

f. Regurgitation g. Vomiting h. Tongue thrust i. Poor tongue stabilization in midline j. Tongue tremors k. Inadequate nutrition due to long periods of sleep l. Frantic sucking of fists		• Speak softly and calmly • Experiment with temperature and regulation of liquid flow, using various nipple shapes • Provide chin and/or cheek support to increase sucking ability • Place infant in prone or semi-upright position after feeding to avoid aspiration of formula and prevent gastroesophageal-like symptoms • Waken infant for feedings to ensure adequate nutritional intake • To decrease frantic sucking of fists, use infant shirts with sewn-in sleeves for mitts to prevent skin damage or use pacifier
IV. Parent-newborn interaction a. At risk due to • Gaze aversion • Poor state control • Abnormal motor behavior • Feeding difficulties	IV. Parent Behavior Progression (Bromwich et al., 1981)	IV. • Instruct parent on positioning/handling/feeding techniques, through demonstration and teaching • Teach parent calming, soothing techniques (i.e., swaddling, vertical rocking, pacifier, etc.) • Teach parent to read distress cues (e.g., yawning, frowning, gaze aversion)
V. Hearing Assess hearing if infant is at risk for hearing loss or demonstrates decreased response to sound	V. ABR	V. • Monitor and screen hearing if warranted (e.g., frequent middle ear infections, family history of hearing loss, etc.) • If hearing loss found, immediate fitting of hearing aids to maximize hearing for language acquisition

Adapted from Sparks, 1993; Lesar, 1992; Lewis, Bennett, & Schmeder, 1989; Schneider, Griffith, & Chasnoff, 1989; Finnegan & Macnew, 1979; MacDonald, 1992; Poulsen, 1989.

Table 11–3. Infancy (1–12 Months)

Goal:
Improve movement patterns to enhance interaction and exploration of environment

Behaviors	Possible assessment tools	Intervention strategies
I. Motor a. Weak pull-to-sit b. Tremors, trembling, extraneous movement c. Arms in W position d. Increased extensor tone e. Poor antigravity extensor strength	Movement Assessment of Infants (MAI) (Chandler, Skillen-Andrews, & Swanson, 1980) Bayley Scales of Infant Development (Bayley, 1969)	I. a. Weak pull-to-sit development: • Move infant from supine to sitting with head support. Hold infant semireclined, encourage to assist with pull-to-sit b. Decrease tremors: • Swaddle infant and hold close • Hold infant semireclined, keeping arms and shoulders forward. Hold infant's arms and legs close to body • Apply firm, calm touch to tremulous areas c. Arms in W position: • Swaddle infant with arms in midline • Carry infant in semireclined position with shoulders forward • Place infant in cloth, sling-style infant seat • Place infant in Tumbleform feeder chair, assisting in keeping arms midline d. Increased extensor tone: • Lift infant's pelvis up and flex legs toward chest to begin increased kicking movements with lower extremities • Rotate lower extremities side to side • Bring upper extremities down and forward at shoulder girdle, for reaching of objects

Table 11–3. *continued*

		e. Poor antigravity extensor strength: • Place infant in prone position • Discourage parents from leaving infant in supine or sitting position too long • Discourage supported standing in walkers and jumpers
II. State a. Poor sleeping patterns b. Hyperirritability c. Difficulty in consoling self d. Poor organization of behavior e. Decreased focused alertness f. Decreased use of adults for solace, play, and object attainment g. Poor self-regulation	II. Test of Sensory Function in Infants (TSFI) (DeGangi & Greenspan, 1989) Receptive-Expressive Emergent Language Scale (REEL) (Bzoch & League, 1971)	II. • Positioning, handling, and swaddling • Early maternal intervention to teach positioning, handling, and reading stress cues • Consistent, loving primary caregiver • Use of rituals, routines, mother-child interactive games • Structure an environment that prevents overstimulation • Use language to organize and explain experiences • Provide appropriate sensory and developmental stimulation using multimodal stimuli
III. Mother-infant interaction At risk for poor mother-infant interaction	III. See Newborn Section	III. • Teach parents appropriate carrying and handling techniques • Teach parents appropriate developmental and motor milestones, and developmentally appropriate activities • Teach parents ways of structuring and organizing environment to prevent overstimulation
IV. Hearing (see Newborn Section) Also may be at increased risk if history of frequent middle ear infections	IV. ABR or behavioral audiometry (audiogram/tympanogram)	IV. • Monitor speech sound development • Assess localization to sound and meaningful words

Adapted from Sparks, 1993; Lesar, 1992; Schneider, Griffith, & Chasnoff, 1989; Lewis, Bennett, & Schmeder, 1989; Finnegan & Macnew, 1974; Poulsen, 1989.

Table 11–4. Toddler Period (12–30 Months)

Goals:
1. Provide early intervention services to monitor and facilitate development skills
2. Teach caregivers, teachers, and service providers ways to structure environment to enhance child's ability for self-regulation and behavioral control
3. Provide direct intervention services (e.g., speech therapy) to identify areas of deficit

Behaviors	Possible assessment tools	Intervention strategies
I. State a. Hyperactivity b. Poor self-regulation c. Impulsivity d. Distractibility e. Prone to temper tantrums f. Poor organization of behavior	Bayley Scales of Infant Development (Bayley, 1969)	• Structure and organization of the environment • Predictable, consistent daily routines • Use of language to organize experiences • Consistent, loving primary caregiver and service providers • Providing environment that avoids over-stimulation • Use of rituals and mother-child games
II. Social attachment a. Bonding difficulties b. Difficulty in consoling self c. Difficulty in being comforted d. Decreased focused alertness e. Depressed interactive behaviors f. Decreased use of adults for solace, play, and attainment of objects g. Less secure attachment to parents		
III. Language a. Delayed language b. Slow language use c. Memory problems d. Limited play sequences e. Difficulty with processing information	Sequenced Inventory of Communication Development (Hedrick, Prather & Tobin, 1984) Rosetti Infant Toddler Language Scale (Rossetti, 1990)	• Direct speech/language therapy to address deficit areas • Provide caregivers with ideas for stimulating language development • Structured communication and play activities to stimulate language

Table 11–4. *continued*

IV. Mother-infant interaction At risk due to possible behaviors and developmental deficits		• Parent education in managing behavior and providing developmentally appropriate activities to facilitate play and stimulate language • Ongoing parent education
V. Hearing May be at risk if history of frequent middle ear infections	Behavioral audiometry (audiogram/tympanogram)	• Intervene as needed (i.e., pediatrician referral, hearing aid fitting, etc.)

Adapted from Lesar, 1992; Sparks, 1993; Poulsen, 1989; Griffith, 1992; Crites, Fischer, Stengel, & Siegal, 1992.

Table 11–5. Preschool/School Age

Goals:
1. Provide children with early intervention in hopes that they can be transitioned into a regular classroom
2. Find threshold for loss of behavioral control and teach adaptive self-regulation strategies to mother, teacher, and prenatally exposed child

Behaviors (possible)	Possible assessment tools	Intervention strategies
I. Language a. Delayed acquisition of words b. Difficulty in word-finding preschool level c. Decreased use of acquired words or gestures to communicate wants and needs d. Language delays e. Poor pragmatic skills f. Reduced mean length of utterance g. Syntactic disorganization, or syntax limited to simple sentences h. Receptive language impairment i. Poor/inappropriate pragmatic language abilities (e.g., poor turntaking skills) j. Multiple articulation errors k. Auditory processing difficulties l. Less spontaneous and developed imitative skills	Use norm-referenced tests to assess receptive/expressive/pragmatic language abilities Language: Examples Preschool Language Scale 3 (Zimmerman, Steiner, & Pond, 1992) Expressive One-Word Picture Vocabulary Test-Revised (Gardner, 1990) Receptive One-Word Picture Vocabulary Test (Gardner, 1985) Clinical Evaluation of Language Fundamentals-Preschool (CELF-Preschool) (Wing, Secord, & Semel, 1992)	• Direct speech/language therapy to enrich vocabulary skills and facilitate overall language abilities • Use whole language • Structured communication activities • Structured play activities • Use eye contact during interaction • Remediation of articulation errors • Provide good language model • Short, direct, clear verbal requests tailored to child's language level • Encourage child to use language and appropriate gesture to communicate • Tailor language input to child's level of understanding • Use cuing (visual, tactile) to assist child in understanding requests • Use short sentences, and use descriptive comments on activity you or child is engaged in • Acknowledge child's communication attempts
II. Motor and neurological a. Possible poor balance b. Tremulousness, increased startling c. Poor quality of visual following d. Fine motor dexterity difficulty e. Blanking out, bizarre eye movements	The Miller Assessment for Preschoolers (Miller, 1982)	• Direct occupational therapy to address visual-motor and sensory integrative deficits • Refer appropriately to occupational or physical therapy • Use developmentally appropriate activities

Table 11–5. *continued*

f. Problems with auditory/visual processing g. Poor motor planning		that promote motor planning strength and balance • Repetition of directions, command, provide cuing techniques
III. Social attachment a. Decreased/absent stranger and separation anxiety b. Aggressiveness with peers c. Decreased response to verbal praise d. Decreased use of adults for solace/comfort	Bruininks-Oseretsky Test of Motor Proficiency (School Age) (Bruininks, 1978)	• Structured play and communication activities to encourage social interactions among peers • Encourage attachment through consistency of teachers and service providers • Small student-to-teacher ratio to allow for individual attention
IV. Affective and behavioral a. Depressed affect, decreased laughter b. Irritable, explosive, and impulsive behaviors c. Inability to self-regulate d. Marked difficulty with transitioning		• Set firm, consistent limits on behavior • Anticipate and avoid stress • Use consistent, predictable, daily routines • Provide opportunity for physical affection during play • Structure/organize the environment • Structure transitions • Structure communication/play activity • Avoid thresholds of overstimulation • Teach child to recognize warning signs of overstimulation • Movement activities during play to encourage laughing, turn taking, eye contact
V. Problem-solving and attention strategies a. Poor on-task attention b. Increased distractibility to extraneous sounds and movements c. Inability to accommodate in problem-solving situations d. Impulsive responses before "reflecting" e. Continuous use of unsuccessful strategies		• Provide structured organized, predictable environment • Limit distractions • Teach adaptive, self-regulated strategies • Small student-to-teacher ratio • Help with focusing attention • Aid in decision making

Table 11–5. *continued*

VI. Mother-child/teacher-child interaction	• Service providers should work with caregivers and teachers on ways to structure environment, avoid overstimulation thresholds, and teach adaptive, self-regulation strategies
VII. Play a. Decreased amount of pretend play b. Does not exhibit the repertoire of play skills that normal peers do c. Difficulty selecting and organizing materials to play with d. Easily overstimulated by noise and other activities of other children and adults in the play environment	• Model appropriate play; participate in play with child • Use descriptive language to comment on what child is doing • Limit amount of toys available to decrease overstimulation

Adapted from Chapman, Worthington, Cooke, & Mayfield, 1992; Schneider & Chasnoff, 1987; Poulsen, 1989; MacDonald, 1992; Lewis, Bennett, & Schmeder, 1992; Griffith, 1992; Tyler, 1992; Sparks, 1993; Gregorchik, 1992.

described for the drug-exposed newborn/infant, such as swaddling and appropriate positioning and handling, may also benefit FAS infants displaying similar behaviors.

Preschool Years

Effects of FAS continue through the preschool years. Even though many of these children appear to be progressing normally, various problems often appear later in life (Olson et al., 1992). Affected children may be hyperactive, impulsive, show poor attention span and motor function, and exhibit fearlessness (Streissguth & LaDue, 1985). Many FAS/FAE children are small for their age and are often treated like younger children of a lower developmental level (Olson et al., 1992).

Intervention with the FAS/FAE preschool child should focus on assisting the primary caregivers and teachers to structure the home/school environment to facilitate cognitive and language development and to manage behavior (Sparks, 1993). Structuring may aid the FAS child who has difficulty making transitions (Olson et al., 1992) and reduce likelihood of temper tantrums and behavioral outbursts. Children may require specific interventions, such as occupational therapy, to address fine motor difficulties and oversensitivity to touch and other stimulation (Olson et al., 1992). FAS/FAE children may be prone to otitis media, dental problems, and possible feeding and/or gastrointestinal difficulties, and thus ongoing medical check-ups by a physician are essential.

School-Age Years

Learning disabilities, characterized by poor attention and memory and problem-solving difficulties, often appear at the school-age level. Hyperactivity, impulsivity, and distractibility may be exhibited (Olson et al., 1992) as well as emotional instability and clumsiness (Hill, Hegemier, & Tennyson, 1989). The FAS school-age child may have poor comprehension of social rules and expectations and not understand the consequences of his or her behavior. Stealing, lying, and potential for sexual exploitation are social problems that are of great concern for this population (Sparks, 1993).

School-age intervention should consist of appropriate school placement and the provision of necessary therapy and educational services. Direct speech therapy to address receptive, expressive, and pragmatic language abilities is often required. Therapy approaches that focus on functional language goals in school and social settings may be most appropriate (Sparks, 1993). Service providers should attempt to understand the child's communicative efforts, which may be exhibited through misbehavior, and provide language for feelings as a means of assisting the language-delayed FAS child (Olson et al., 1992). A service coordinator should be designated to serve as a liaison between the parents and school and medical and social service agencies (Sparks, 1993). Parents may benefit from counseling, respite care, and parent support groups (Olson et al., 1992).

Adolescence and Adulthood

After puberty, the dysmorphic facial features of FAS are not as distinctive (Streissguth et al., 1991), although affected individuals often remain short in stature and have small head size (Olson et al., 1992). Learning deficits persist into adolescence and adulthood. Low academic achievement and poor judgment can negatively affect the individual's ability to function appropriately in society (Sparks, 1993). (12) FAS adolescents and adults are often described as naive and immature (Olson et al., 1992) and need careful monitoring of home and school environment. Sexual behaviors need to be addressed through specific educational programs. Adolescence may be difficult for FAS children because they may begin to perceive themselves as different (Sparks, 1993). Behavioral problems may preclude placement in typical job training programs.

Conclusion

Substance abuse and its impact on child development is clearly an area that involves neurobiologic, environmental, linguistic, cognitive, socioemotional, and cultural issues. The effects of prenatal substance abuse pose a timely challenge for clinical professionals in the field of communication sciences and disorders. It has become apparent that nothing but an integrated team approach to intervention will be successful with these children. It must be an approach that views children and families as holistic units and unites professional disciplines within mutually supportive systems, which view children, families, humans, as active adaptive beings and whose individual professional members which have learned the skill of adaptation themselves.

References

Abel, E. L. (1980). Fetal alcohol syndrome: Behavioral teratology. *Psychological Bulletin, 87*(1), 29–50.

Abel, E., & Sokol, R. (1987). Incidence of fetal alcohol syndrome and economic impact of FAS related anomalies. *Drug Alcohol Depen., 19,* 51–70.

Abel, E., & Sokol, R. (1991). A revised conservative estimate of the incidence of FAS and its economic impact. *Alcohol. Clin. Exp. Res., 15,* 514–524.

Als, H., Lester, B. M., Tronick, E., & Brazelton, T. B. (1982). Toward a research instrument for the assessment of preterm infant behavior (APIB). In H. E. Fitzgerald, B. M. Lester, & M. W. Yogman (Eds.), *Theory and research in behavioral pediatrics* (pp. 35–132). New York: Plenum.

Als, H., Duffy, F. H., & McAnulty, G. (1992). *Neonatal individualized developmental care and assessment program.* N.I.D.C.A.P., Children's Hospital, 300 Longwood Ave., Boston, MA, 02115.

American Speech, Language, and Hearing Association. (1993). *Joint Committee on Infant Hearing 1993 position statement.* Rockville, MD: American Speech Language Hearing Association.

Aronson, M., Sandin, B. Sabel, K. G., Kyllerman, M., & Olegard, R. (1984). Children of alcoholic mothers: Outcome in relation to the social environment in which the children were brought up. *Rep. Depart. Appl. Psychol., 9*(2), 3–7.

Astley, S. J., & Little, R. E. (1990). Maternal marijuana use during lactation and infant development at one year. *Neurotoxicol. Teratol., 12,* 161–168.

Baily, D. N. (1989). Drug screening in an unconventional matrix: Hair analysis (Editorial). *J.A.M.A., 262,* 3331.

Baltaxe, C. A. M., D'Angiola, N., & Simmons, J. O. (1992). *Communication impairment and psychiatric disorders in children with prenatal drug exposure.* Paper presented at the annual convention fo the American Speech Language and Hearing Association, San Antonio, TX.

Bayley, N. (1969). *Bayley Scales of Infant Development.* San Antonio: The Psychological Corporation.

Braun, M., & Palmer, M. (1985). A pilot study for oral-motor dysfunction in at-risk infants. *Physical and Occupational Therapy in Pediatrics, 5,* 13–25.

Brazelton, T. B. (1984). *Neonatal Behavioral Assessment Scale.* London: Spastic International Medical Publications.

Bromwich, R. M., Khokha, E., Fust, L. S., Baxter, E., Burge, D., & Kass, E. W. (1978). Parent behavior progression. In R. Bromwich (Ed.), *Working with parents and infants: An interactional approach.* Baltimore: University Park Press.

Brown, R., Coles, C., Smith, I., Platzman, K., Silverstein, J., Erickson, S., & Falck, A. (1991). Effects of prenatal alcohol exposure at school age. II. Attention and behavior. *Neurotoxicol. Teratol., 13,* 369–367.

Bruininks, R. H. (1978). *Bruinicks-Oseretsky test of motor proficiency.* Circle Pines, MN: American Guidance Services.

Burns, K., Chetnik, L., Burns, W. J., & Clark, R. (1991). Dyadic disturbances in cocaine abusing mothers and their infants. *Journal of Clinical Psychology, 47,* 316–319.

Carzoli, R. P., Murphy, S. P., Hammer-Knisely, J., & Houy, J. (1991). Evaluation of auditory brainstem response in full-term infants of cocaine abusing mothers. *A.J.D.C., 145,* 1013–1016.

Chandler, L., Skillen-Andrews, M., & Swanson, M. (1980). *Movement assessment of infants.* Rolling Bay, WA.

Chapman, J. K., Worthington, L. Cook, M., & Mayfield, P. (1992). Cocaine exposed infants: A potential generation of at-risk and vulnerable children. *Infant Toddler Intervention, 2,* 223–237.

Chasnoff, I. J., Burns, W. J., Schnoll, S. H., & Burns, K. A. (1985). Cocaine use in pregnancy. *New Engl. Journal of Med., 313*(11), 666–669.

Chasnoff, I. J. (1987). Perinatal effects of cocaine. *Contemporary OB/GYN, 29*(5), 163–179.

Chasnoff, I. J., Lewis, D. E., & Squires, L. (1987). Cocaine Intoxication in a breast-fed infant. *Pediatr., 80*(6), 836–838.

Chasnoff, I. (1988). Drug use in pregnancy: Parameters of risk. *The Pediatric Clinics of North America, 35,* 1403–1411.

Chasnoff, I. J. (1989). Drug use and women: Establishing a standard of care. *Annals of the New York Academy of Science 562,* 208–210.

Chasnoff, I. J., Lewis, D. E., Griffith, D. R., & Wiley, S. (1989). Cocaine and pregnancy: Clinical toxicological implications for the neonate. *Clinical Chemistry, 35,* 1276–1278.

Chasnoff, I. J. (1990). The prevalence of illicit drug and alcohol use during pregnancy and discrepancies in mandatory reporting in Pinellas County Florida. *New Engl. J. of Med., 322*(7), 1202–1206.

Chasnoff, I. J., Griffith, D. R., Freir, C., & Murray, J. (1992). Cocaine/polydrug use in pregnancy: Two year follow-up. *Pediatr., 89*(2), 284–289.

Church, M. W., & Gerkin, K. P. (1988). Hearing disorders in children with fetal alcohol syndrome: Findings from case reports. *Pediatrics, 82*(2), 147–154.

Clapp, J., Wesley, M., Cooke, R., Pekals, R., & Holstein, C. (1986). The effects of marijuana smoke on gas exchange in ovine pregnancy. *Alcohol Drug Res., 7,* 85–92.

Clarren, S. K., & Smith, D. W. (1978). The fetal alcohol syndrome. *N. Engl. J. Med., 298,* 1063–1067.

Cnattingus, S., Haglund, B., & Meirik, O. (1988). Cigarette smoking as risk factor for late fetal and early neonatal death. *Br. Med. J., 297,* 258–261.

Coles, C. D., Smith, I. E., Lancaster, J. S., & Falek, A. (1987). Persistence over the first month of neurobehavioral differences in infants exposed to alcohol prenatally. *Inf. Behav. Dev., 10,* 23–37.

Crites, L., Fischer, K., Stengel, M., & Siegel, C. (1992). Working with families of drug-exposed children: Three model programs. *Infant Toddler Intervention, 2,* 13–23.

Day, N. L., & Richardson, G. A. (1991). Prenatal marijuana use: Epidemiology, methodologic issues, and infant outcome. *Clin. Perinatal., 18,* 77.

Day, N. L., Robles, N., Richardson, G. A., Sambamoorthi, U., Taylor, P., Scher, M., Stoffer, D., & Cornelius, M. (1991). The effects of prenatal alcohol use on the growth of children at three years of age. *Alcohol. Clin. Exp. Res., 15,* 67–71.

DeGangi, G., & Greenspan, S. (1989). *Test of sensory function in infants.* Los Angeles: Western Psychological Services.

Department of the Treasury, U.S. Customs Service. (1988). Crack: A non-traditional form of freebasing. *Narcotic Identification Manual,* 44–47.

Dixon, S. D., & Bejar, R. (1989). Echoencephalographic findings in neonates associated with maternal cocaine and methoamphetamine use: Incidence and clinical correlates. *J. Pediatr., 115,* 7709.

Dominguez, R., Vila-Coro, A. A., Slopes, J. M., & Bohan, T. P. (1991). Brain and ocular abnormalities in infants with in utero exposure to cocaine and other street drugs. *A.J.D.C, 145,* 688–695.

Dubowitz, L., & Dubowitz, V. (1981). *The neurological assessment of the pre-term and full-term infants.* Philadelphia: J. B. Lippincott.

Eckerman, C. O., Lynne, A. S., & Gross, S. J. (1985). Different developmental courses for very-low birthweight infants differing in early head growth. *Dev. Psych., 21,* 813–827.

Ernhart, C. B., Wolf, A. W., Linn, P. L., Sokol, R., Kennard, M., & Filopvich, H. (1985). Alcohol related birth defects: Syndromal anomalies, intrauterine growth retardation and neonatal behavioral assessment. *Alcohol. Clin. Res., 9,* 447–453.

Finnegan, L. P., & Macnew, B. A. (1979). Care of the addicted infant. *American Journal of Nursing, 74*(4), 685–693.

Frank, D. A., Zuckerman, B., Amaro, H., Aboagye, K., Bauchman, H., Cabral, H., Fried, L., & Hingson, R. (1988). Cocaine use during pregnancy: Prevalence and correlates. *Pediatrics, 8*(6), 888–895.

Freeman, S., & Mayo, R. (1992). *Managing drug-exposed children: Survey of rehabilitation and clinical models*. The University of North Carolina at Chapel Hill, unpublished report.

Fried, P. A., & Makin, J. E. (1987). Neonatal behavioral correlates of prenatal exposure to marijuana, cigarettes, and alcohol in a low-risk population. *Neurobehav. Toxicol. Teratol., 9,* 1–7.

Fried, P. A., & O'Connell, C. M. (1987). A comparison of the effects of prenatal exposure to tobacco, alchohol, cannabis, and caffeine on birth size and subsequent growth. *Neurotoxicol. Teratol., 9,* 79–85.

Fried, P. A., & Watkinson, B. (1988). 12- and 24-month neurobehavioral follow-up of children prenatally exposed to marijuana, cigarettes, and alcohol. *J. Dev. Behav. Pediatr., 10,* 305–313.

Fried, P. A., & Watkinson, B. (1990). 36- and 48-month neurobehavioral follow-up of children prenatally exposed to marijuana, cigarettes, and alcohol. *Developmental and Behavioral Pediatrics, 11*(2), 49–58.

Fried, P. A. (1992). Clinical implications of smoking: Determining long term teratogenicity. In I. S. Zagon and T. A. Slotkin (Eds.), *Maternal substance abuse and the developing nervous system* (pp. 77–96). San Diego: Academic Press.

Fulroth, R., Phillips, B., & Durand, D. J. (1989). Perinatal outcome of infants exposed to cocaine and/or heroin in utero. *Am. J. Obstet. Gynecol., 150,* 23–27.

Gardner, M. F. (1985). *Receptive one-word picture vocabulary test.* Novato, CH: Academic Therapy Publications.

Gardner, M. F. (1990). *Expressive one-word picture vocabulary test–revised.* Novato, CH: Academic Therapy Publications.

Gawin, F. H. (1991). Cocaine addiction: Psychology and neurophysiology. *Science, 251,* 1580–1585.

Gittler, J., & McPherson, M. (1990). Prenatal substance abuse: An overview of the problem. *Children Today,* July–August, 3–7.

Goodlett, C. R., & West, J. R. (1992). Fetal alcohol effects: Rat model of alcohol exposure during the brain growth spurt. In I. S. Zagon & T. A. Slotkin (Eds.), *Maternal substance abuse and the developing nervous system* (pp. 45–75). San Diego: Academic Press.

Gregorchik, L. (1992). The cocaine exposed children are here. *Phi Delta Kappan,* 709–711.

Griffith, D. (1992). Prenatal exposure to cocaine and other drugs: Developmental and educational progress. *Phi Delta Kappan,* September, *74,* 30–34.

Gusella, J., & Fried, P. (1984). Effects of maternal social drinking and smoking on offspring at 13 months. *Neurobehav. Toxicol. Teratol., 6,* 13–17.

Hadeed, A. J., & Siegal, S. R. (1989). Maternal cocaine use during pregnancy: Effect on the newborn infant. *Pediatrics, 84,* 205–210.

Haglund, B., & Cnattingus, S. (1990). Cigarette smoking as a risk factor for sudden infant death syndrome: A population based study. *Am. J. Pub. Health, 80,* 29–32.

Hamilton, H. E., Wallace, J. E., Shimek, E. L., Land, P., Harris, S. C., & Christenson, J. G. (1977). Cocaine and benzoylecgonine excretion in humans. *J. Forensic Toxicol., 22,* 697–702.

Handler, A., Kistin, N., Davis, F., & Ferre, C. (1991). Cocaine use during pregnancy: Perinatal outcomes. *Am. J. Epidemiol., 133,* 818–825.

Hannig, V. L., & Phillips, J. A. (1991). Maternal cocaine abuse and fetal anomalies: Evidence for teratogenic effects of cocaine. *Southern Medical Journal, 84*(4), 498–499.

Harrison, H. (1983). *The premature baby book.* New York: St. Martin's.

Hedrick, D. L., Prather, E. M., & Tobin, A. R. (1984). *Sequenced inventory of communication development–revised.* Seattle, WA: University of Washington Press.

Herd, D. (1988). Drinking by black and white women: Results from a national survey. *Soc. Prob., 35,* 493–505.

Hill, R., Hegemier, S., & Tennyson, L. (1989). Fetal alcohol syndrome: A multihandicapped child. Presented at the Sixth International Neurotoxicology Conference. *Neurotoxicology, 10,* 585–596.

Hilton, M. E. (1988). The demographic distribution of drinking patterns in 1984. *Drug Alcohol Depend., 22,* 37–47.

Howard, I., Beckwith, L., Rodnig, C., & Kropenske, V. (1989). The development of young children of substance-abusing parents: Insights from seven years of intervention and research. *Zero to Three, National Center for Clinical Infant Programs, 9,* 8–12.

Hoyme, H. E., Jones, K. L., Dixon, S. D., Jewet, T., Hanson, J. W., Robinson, L. K., Msall, M. E., & Allanson, J. E. (1990). Prenatal cocaine exposure and fetal vascular disruption. *Pediatrics, 85,* 743–747.

Jacobson, S. W., Fein, G. G., Jacobson, J. L., Schwartz, P., & Dowler, J. (1984). Neonatal correlates of prenatal exposure to smoking, caffeine, and alcohol. *Inf. Behav. Dev., 7,* 253–265.

Johnson, J. M., Foose, S., Seikel, J. A., & Madison, C. L. (1992). *Language abilities of 21 preschool children exhibiting cocaine intoxication at birth.* Paper presented at the annual convention of the American Speech Language and Hearing Association in San Antonio, TX.

Jones, K. L., & Smith, D. W. (1973). Recognition of fetal alcohol syndrome in early infancy. *Lancet, 2,* 991–1001.

Kaplan-Sanoff & Rice, K. (1992). Working with addicted women in recovery and their children: Lessons learned in Boston City's Women and Infant's Clinic. *Zero to Three, National Center for Clinical Infant Programs, 9,* 17–22.

Karakostav, P. (1985). *Passive smoking among pregnant women and its effect on the weight and height of the newborn.* Abstract in Smoking Bulletin Abstr. No. 31644, Office of Smoking and Health, Rockville, MD.

Kharasch, S. J., Glotzer, D., Vinci, R., Weitzman, M., & Sargent, J. (1991). Unsuspected cocaine exposure in young children. *A.J.D.C., 145,* 204–206.

Klein, M. D., & Briggs, M. H. (1987). Observation of communicative interaction. In M. D. Klein & M. H. Briggs, Facilitating mother–infant communicative interactions in mothers of high-risk infants. *Journal of Communication Disorders, 10*(2), 95–106.

Kristjansson, B., Fried, P. A., & Watkinson, B. (1989). Maternal smoking during pregnancy affects children's vigilance performance. *Drug Alcohol Depen., 24,* 11–19.

Krug, S. E. (1989). Cocaine abuse: Historical, epidmiological, and clinical perspectives for pediatricians. *Current Problems in Pediatrics, 74,* 451–487.

Lemoine, P., Harrousseau, H., Borteyru, J. P., & Menuet, J. C. (1968). Les enfants de parents alcooliques: Anomalies observèes: à propos de 127 cas. *Ouest Med., 8,* 476–482.

Lesar, S. (1992). Prenatal cocaine exposure: The challenge to education. *Infant Toddler Intervention, 2,* 37–52.

Lester, B. M., Corwin, M. J., Sepkoski, C., Seifer, R., Peucker, M., McLaughlin, S., & Golub, H. L. (1991). Neurobehavioral syndromes in cocaine exposed newborn infants. *Child Dev., 62,* 694–705.

Lewis, K., Bennett, B., & Schmeder, N. (1989). The care of infants menaced by cocaine abuse. *MCN, 14,* 324–329.

Lipschultz, S. E., Frassica, J. J., & Orav, E. J. (1991). Cardiovascular abnormalities in infants prenatally exposed to cocaine. *J. Pediatr., 118,* 44–51.

Little, B. B., Snell, L. M., Rosenfeld, C. R., Gilstrap, L. C., & Gant, N. F. (1990). Failure to recognize fetal alcohol syndrome in newborn infants. *Am. J. Dis. Child, 144,* 1142–1146.

Little, B. B., & Snell, L. M. (1991). Brain growth among fetuses exposed to cocaine in utero asymmetrical growth retardation. *Obstetrics and Gynecology, 77*(3), 361–364.

MacDonald, C. C. (1992). Perinatal cocaine exposure: Predictor of an endangered generation. *Infant and Toddler Intervention, 2,* 1–11.

MacGregor, S. N., Keith, L. G., Chasnoff, I. J., Rosner, M. A., Chisum, G. M., Shaw, P. D., & Minogue, J. P. (1987). Cocaine use during pregnancy: Adverse perinatal outcome. *Am. J. Perinatal Outcome, 157,* 686–690.

Majewski, F., & Majewski, B. (1988). Alcohol embryopathy: Symptoms, auxological data, frequency, among the offspring and pathogenesis. *Excerpta Medica. International Conference Series, 805,* 837–844.

Makin, J., Fried, P. A., & Watkinson, B. (1991). A comparison of active and passive smoking during pregnancy: Long-term effects. *Neurotoxicol. Teratol., 13,* 5–12.

Marcus, J. C. (1984). *Neurological findings in the fetal alcohol syndrome.* Paper presented at the 36th meeting of the American Academy of Neurology, Boston, MA.

Martin, T. R., & Bracken, M. B. (1986). Association of low birth weight with passive smoke exposure in pregnancy. *Am. J. Epidemiol., 124,* 663–642.

McCarthy, P. (1972). *McCarthy Scales of Children's Abilities.* San Antonio: The Psychological Corporation.

Meyer, M. B., Jonas, B. S., & Tonascia, J. A. (1976). Perinatal events associated with maternal smoking during pregnancy. *Am J. Epidemiol., 103,* 464–476.

Miller, L. J. (1982). *The Miller assessment for preschoolers.* Littleton, CO: The Foundation for Knowledge in Development.

Morris, S. E. (1982). *The Pre-Speech Assessment Scale.* Clifton, NJ: J. A. Preston.

Morris, S. E. (1987). *Pre-feeding skills.* Tucson, AZ: Therapy Skill Builders.

Myer, B., Olson, H. C., & Kallenback, K. (1992). Cocaine exposed infants: Myths and misunderstandings. *Zero to Three: Bulletin of the National Center for Clinical Infant Programs, 13*(1), 1–5.

Nahas, G. (1976). *Marijuana: Chemistry, biochemistry, and cellular effect.* New York: Springer-Verlag.

National Institute on Drug Abuse. (1991). *National Household Survey on Drug Abuse: Main findings, 1990* (DHHS Publication No. ADM 91-1788). Rockville, MD: U.S. Department of Health and Human Services.

Crack's toll among babies: A joyless view of even toys. *New York Times,* Sept. 17, 1989.

Olson, H., Burgess, D., & Streissguth, A. P. (1992). Fetal alcohol syndrome and fetal alcohol effects: A lifespan view, with implications for early intervention. *Zero to Three, National Center for Clinical Infant Programs, 9,* 24–29.

Osofsky, J. (1976). Neonatal characteristics and mother-infant interaction in two observational situations. *Child Development, 47,* 1138–1147.

Ostrea, E. M., Brady, M., Gause, S., Raymundo, A., & Steven, M. (1992). Drug screening of newborns by meconium analysis: A large scale prospective epidemiologic study. *Pediatrics, 89,* 107–113.

Palmer, M. (1991). *The Neonatal Oral Motor Assessment Scale.* Presented at the Developmental Interventions in Neonatal Care Conference, Boston, MA.

Peabody Picture Vocabulary Test

Petitti, D. B., & Coleman, C. (1990). Cocaine and the risk of low birth weight. *A.J.P.H., 80*(1), 25–28.

Phibbs, C., Bateman, D., & Schwartz, R. (1991). The neonatal costs of maternal cocaine use. *J.A.M.A., 266,* 1521–1526.

Picone, T. A., Allen, L. H., Olsen, P. N., & Ferris, M. E. (1982). Pregnancy outcome in North American women. II. Effects of diet, cigarette smoking, stress, and weight gain on placentas, and on neonatal physical and behavioral characteristics. *Am. J. Clin. Nutr., 36,* 1214–1224.

Poulsen, M. K. (1989). *Perinatal substance abuse: Risk factors seen in children at risk due to prenatal drug exposure and intervention strategies for infant preschool programs.* Early Intervention Technical Assistance Network Group, Los Angeles, CA.

Reynell, J., & Huntley, M. (1989). *Reynell developmental language scales.* Windsor, Berkshire, England: Nser-Nelson Publishing Company Ltd.

Risch, H. A., Weiss, N. S., Clarke, E. A., & Miller, A. B. (1988). Risk factors for spontaneous abortion and its reoccurrence. *Am. J. Epidemiol., 128,* 420–430.

Rivers, K. O., & Hedrick, D. L. (1992). Language and behavioral concerns for drug-exposed infants and toddlers. *Infant and Toddler Intervention, 2*(1), 63–73.

Rodnig, C., Beckwith, L., & Howard, J. (1990). *Characteristics of attachment organization and play organization in prenatally drug exposed toddlers.* Paper presented at the Workshop on Children and Parental Illicit Drug Use: Research, Clinical, and Policy Issues, Washington, DC, National Research Council, Institute of Medicine.

Rossetti, L. (1990). *The Rossetti Infant-Toddler Scale.* East Moline, IL: Linguisystems Inc.

Rush, D., & Callahan, K. (1989). Exposure to passive cigarette smoking and child development. A critical review. Prenatal abuse of licit and illicit drugs. *Ann. N. Y. Acad. Sci., 562,* 74–100.

Ryan, L., Ehrlich, S., & Finnegan, L. (1987). Cocaine abuse in pregnancy: Effects on the fetus and newborn. *Neurotoxicol. Teratol., 9,* 295–299.

Salamy, A., Eldredge, L., Anderson, J., & Bull, D. (1990). Brain stem transmission time in infants exposed to cocaine in utero. *J. Pediatr., 17,* 627–629.

Schneider, J., & Chasnoff, I. (1987). Cocaine abuse during pregnancy: Its effects on infant motor development—a clinical perspective. *Top Acute Care Trauma Rehabilitation, 2,* 59–69.

Schneider, J. W., Griffith, D. R., & Chasnoff, I. J. (1989). Infants exposed to cocaine in utero: Implications for developmental assessment and intervention. *Infants and Young Children, 2,* 25–36.

Shaywitz, S., Cohen, D., & Shaywitz, B. (1980). Behavior and learning difficulties in children of normal intelligence born to alcoholic mothers. *J. Pediatr., 96,* 978–982.

Shih, L., Cone-Wesson, B., & Reddix, B. (1988). Effects of maternal cocaine abuse on the neonatal auditory system. *Int. J. Pediatr. Otorhinolaryngol., 15,* 245–251.

Shutzman, D. L., Frankenfield-Chernicoff, M., Clatterbaugh, H. E., & Singer, J. (1991). Incident of intrauterine cocaine exposure in a suburban setting. *Pediatrics, 88*(4), 825–827.

Slotkin, T. A. (1992). Prenatal exposure to nicotine: What can we learn from animal models? In I. S. Zagon & T. A. Slotkin (Eds.), *Maternal substance abuse and the developing nervous system* (pp. 97–124). San Diego: Academic Press Inc.

Smith, D. W. (1982). *Recognizable patterns of human malformation: Genetic, embryologic and clinical aspects* (3rd ed.). Philadelphia: W. B. Saunders.

Smith, N., Austen, J., & Rolles, C. J. (1982). Tertiary smoking by the fetus. *Lancet, 1,* 8283.

Sparks, S. N. (1993). *Children of prenatal substance abuse.* San Diego: Singular Publishing Group.

Spohr, H. L., & Steinhausen, H. C. (1987). Follow-up studies of children with fetal alcohol syndrome. *Neuropediatrics, 18,* 13–17.

Streissguth, A. P., Herman, C. S., & Smith, D. W., (1978). Intelligence, behavior, and dysmorphogenesis in fetal alcohol syndrome: A report on 20 patients. *J. Pediatr., 92*(3), 363–367.

Streissguth, A. P., Barr, H., Martin, D. C., & Herman, C. S. (1980). Effects of maternal alcohol, nicotine, and caffeine use during pregnancy on infant mental and motor development at eight months. *Alcohol. Clin. Exp. Res., 4,* 152–164.

Streissguth, A., Barr, H., & Martin, D. (1983). Maternal alcohol use and neonatal habituation assessed with the Brazelton Scale. *Child Dev., 545,* 1109–1118.

Streissguth, A. P., Martin, D. C., Barr, H. M., Sandman, B. M., Kirchner, G. L., & Darby, B. L. (1984). Intrauterine alcohol and nicotine exposure: Attention and reaction time in 4-year-old children. *Dev. Psychol., 20,* 533–541.

Streissguth, A. P., & LaDue, R. (1985). Psychological and behavioral effects in children prenatally exposed to alcohol. *Alcohol Health and Research World, 10,* 6–12.

Streissguth, A. P., Clarren, S. K., & Jones, K. L. (1985). Natural history of the fetal alcohol syndrome: A ten year follow-up ot eleven patients. *Lancet, 2,* 85–92.

Streissguth, A. P., Barr, H. M., Sampson, P. D., Parrish-Johnson, J. C., Kirchner, G. L., & Martin, D. C.

(1989). IQ at age 4 in relation to maternal alcohol use and smoking during pregnancy. *Dev. Pharmacol., 25,* 3.

Streissguth, A. P., Randels, S. P., & Smith, D. (1991). A test-retest study of intelligence in patients with fetal alcohol syndrome: Implications for care. *J. Am. Acad. Child. Adolesc. Psychiatry, 30*(4), 584–587.

Streissguth, A. P., Aase, I. M., Clarren, S. K., Randels, S. P., LaDue, R. A., & Smith, D. F. (1991). Fetal alcohol syndrom in adolescents and adults. *J.A.M.A., 265,* 1961–1967.

Streissguth, A. P. (1992). Fetal alcohol syndrome and fetal alcohol effects: A clinical perspective of later developmental consequences. In I. S. Zagon & T. A. Slotkin (Eds.), *Maternal substance abuse and the developing nervous system* (pp. 5–25). San Diego: Academic Press.

Tyler, R. (1992). Prenatal drug exposure: An overview of associated problems and intervention strategies. *Phi Delta Kappan,* September, *74,* 705–708.

Vandenberg, K. (1990). Nippling management of the sick neonate in the NICU: The disorganized feeder. *Neonatal Network,* 9, 9–16.

Vandenberg, K. (1991). *Assessment and intervention for the high risk infant in the NICU and after discharge.* Presented at the Developmental Interventions in Neonatal Care Conference, Boston, MA.

Wang, L. H., Rudolph, A. M., & Benet, L. Z. (1980). Pharmacokinetics of drugs and metabolites in the maternal placental fetal unit: General principles. In C. N. Chiang & C. Lee (Eds.), *Prenatal drug exposure: Kinetics and dynamics* (pp. 25–38). Washington, DC: U.S. Department of Health and Human Services, NIDA Research Monograph Series 60.

Washington Post, September 17, 1989.

Wiig, E. H., Secord, W., & Semel, E. (1992). *Clinical evaluations of language fundamentals—preschool.* San Antonio, TX: The Psychological Corporation.

Williamson, D. F., Serdula, M. K., Kendrick, J. S., & Binkin, N. J. (1989). Comparing the prevalence of smoking in pregnant and non-pregnant women, 1985–1986. *J.A.M.A., 261,* 70–74.

Zimmerman, I. L., Steiner, V. G., & Pond, R. E. (1992). *Preschool Language Scale–3.* San Antonio, TX: The Psychological Corporation.

Zuckerman, B. (1988). Marijuana and cigarette smoking during pregnancy: Neonatal effects. In I. Chasnoff (Ed.), *Drugs, alcohol, pregnancy, and parenting* (pp. 73–89). Dordrecht, Holland: Kluwer Academic.

Zuckerman, B., Frank, D., Hingson, R., Amaro, H., Levenson, S. M., Kayne, H., Parker, S., Vinci, R., Aboagye, K., Fried, L. E., Cabral, H., Timperi, R., & Bauchner, H. (1989). Effects of maternal marijuana and cocaine use on fetal growth. *New Engl. J. Med., 320,* 762.

Zuckerman, B. (1991). Selected methodological issues in investigations of prenatal effects of cocaine; lessons from the past. *National Institute of Drug Abuse Research Monograph, 114,* 45–54.

Zuckerman, B., & Frank, D. A. (1992). Prenatal cocaine and marijuana exposure: Research and clinical implications. In I. S. Zagon & T. A. Slotkin (Eds.), *Maternal substance abuse and the developing nervous system* (pp. 125–153). San Diego: Academic Press.

12

Multicultural Populations and Language Disorders

JACK S. DAMICO, PH.D.,
MICHAEL SMITH, PH.D., AND
LLOYD E. AUGUSTINE, PH.D.

Introduction

The treatment of childhood language disorders presents a number of challenges to the practicing speech-language pathologist. There are issues involving the etiology of such disorders; the impact that language disorders have on the various cognitive, linguistic, and social abilities exhibited by these students; and the vast array of clinical issues that must be addressed every day when clinicians sit down and face their caseloads. Based on the concept of the adaptive nature of immature systems, many of these issues are addressed in this volume.

One issue of particular and growing concern will be the focus of this chapter: How can speech-language pathologists best serve students from multicultural backgrounds who are suspected of exhibiting childhood language disorders? This is not a trivial issue. There are growing numbers of students from multicultural backgrounds entering the public education system in the United States. One need only review recent demographic data to recognize this fact. According to statistics from the Bureau of the Census, in 1990 nearly 25% of the population in the United States was listed in a "traditional minority" category (e.g., African American, Hispanic, Asian or Pacific Islander, Native American) and the percentages of individuals from culturally/linguistically diverse (CLD) backgrounds has increased dramatically over the past decade. For example, in the United States there was a 107.8% increase in Asian and Pacific Islanders from the 1980 census to the 1990 census and a 53% increase in Hispanics in that same period. Such rapid increases in CLD individuals require more attention to these populations and their specific problems when entering an educational system that is not particularly oriented to cultural and/or linguistic diversity.

Due to their training and their perceived roles as language experts in the public schools, speech-language pathologists are frequently called on to assess the language/learning abilities of students from multicultural backgrounds, determine the presence or absence of a language disorder, and recommend appropriate educational placements for these students. The speech-language pathologist may also be required to provide intervention services to these students if a language or learning disorder is identified. When attempting to fulfill this role as the language expert with multicultural populations, however, the speech-language pathologist must resolve a number of complex issues if appropriate service delivery is to be provided.

The honest clinician recognizes that students from culturally and linguistically diverse backgrounds present complexities that go beyond the issues of service delivery to mainstream and monolingual English speakers who exhibit potential language disorders. Most obviously, speech-language pathologists do not generally speak the student's home language and/or are not familiar with the student's home culture. Additionally, the clinicians must consider the potential impact of second-language acquisition, cultural assimilation, prejudice, disempowerment, and a host of other factors that create many difficulties when trying to differentiate between true language disorders and cultural/language differences. These complexities cause many clinicians to believe that they cannot provide sufficient service delivery to students from multicultural populations.

As perplexing as these complexities are, however, it is possible for the typical (and monolingual) speech-language pathologist to provide appropriate and effective service delivery to students from multicultural populations. This chapter will discuss this issue and offer models for practical assessment techniques and intervention strategies.

To appreciate the complexities of working with this population and to recognize the advantages of the strategies that will be presented, it is necessary to discuss some of the differences between children from the multicultural population and those from the mainstream and monolingual English population.

The Scope of Linguistic and Cultural Diversity

When considering the differences between children from the mainstream and from multicultural populations, two major areas of diversity are important for the practicing speech-language pathologist: linguistic/communicative differences and other cultural differences.

Linguistic/Communicative Differences

Many of the CLD children in the schools come from homes in which mainstream English is not the first or preferred language or dialect. Rather, the children and their families may speak other languages or different dialects of English. Indeed, these students may come to school with little or no English language proficiency. In these situations, the children may exhibit language and/or communicative difficulties when they enter the schools even though they exhibit normal language-learning proficiency. The problem, of course, is that they do not speak mainstream English, which is the language of interaction and instruction in the schools.

When CLD students (who are normal language learners) are placed in mainstream situations and forced to use mainstream English, they may manifest language and/or communicative difficulties that are similar to the problems exhibited by mainstream children with language disorders. For example, both groups may exhibit low verbal output, a reluctance to interact in the classroom, superficial difficulties with the English grammar system, and comprehension difficulties (Damico & Hamayan, 1992). Further, both groups may experience academic problems that are reflected in their test scores and classroom performances. When evaluating the abilities of these students, the practicing speech-language pathologist must be able to differentiate between communicative and academic difficulties due to differences versus those due to deficits. To make these distinctions, speech-language pathologists must be aware of the linguistic and communicative differences exhibited by CLD children.

LINGUISTIC CODES AND STYLES

The most obvious linguistic differences between mainstream children and CLD children arise from differences in the selection and usage of specific language codes and styles. Of the code and stylistic differences, the most significant ones involve intelligibility issues. Even though CLD students may be proficient users of their home languages, they are in English-only environments and are required to use the language of the mainstream. Proficiency in their home languages does not help them negotiate meaning in the typical mainstream classroom and often stigmatizes them. To avoid this situation, the CLD students attempt to use English—usually their weaker language—in the academic environment. If their English intelligibility is restricted, these CLD students simply cannot interact well enough with members of the mainstream or with the academic curriculum to benefit from exposure to the English context. Consequently, the CLD students experience difficulty with communication and learning and may "turn off" to the mainstream opportunities. In many of these cases, socialization and academic achievement are greatly reduced.

Less obvious code differences may also interfere with learning and socialization. Although many CLD students can speak English, they may employ English in conjunction with communicative styles or interactional patterns that might be misinterpreted by individuals uninformed about language diversity. For example, the students may engage in conversational style shifting that is different from the mainstream. This is not an unusual occurrence. Different cultures frequently exhibit different types of speech styles or different rules for selecting one speech style over another (Irvine, 1985). Although this is normal and culturally based communicative behavior, it may be inappropriately interpreted as evidence of a language disorder (Damico & Damico, 1993a).

Other examples of less obvious code differences that might alter communicative effectiveness and that might be misperceived involve code switching and the presence of language transfer phenomena. In code switching, CLD speakers typically switch back and forth between their first and second linguistic systems for social and/or psychological reasons (Auer, 1984; Lipski, 1985). So, for example, a Spanish-English bilingual might begin an utterance in English and end in Spanish (e.g., "I put the forks en las mesas"). This common second-language phenomenon is typically not reflective of any linguistic deficit; research shows code switching to be systematic and rule governed. Many uninformed listeners, however, may inappropriately interpret code switching as evidence of some sort of language-learning or language usage deficit.

Language transfer phenomena may also cause difficulties. Language transfer refers to a frequent phenomenon that occurs when an individual is learning a second language. In the process of acquiring the second language, there may be a transfer of some of the grammatical, phonological, semantic, or pragmatic patterns or rules from the first language into the second. For example, Navajo speakers may exhibit a transfer of nasalized patterns from their first language into English. Although this is a normal acquisitional phenomenon (Hakuta, 1986; Schumann, 1978; Vigil & Oller, 1976), it may appear to be faulty language learning from the monolingual English perspective, and these behaviors may be seized on (inappropriately) as an indication of a language-learning deficit (Garcia & Ortiz, 1988).

CONVERSATIONAL DIFFERENCES

Another type of communicative diversity between mainstream children and CLD children involves the use of conversational discourse. Because conversation is mutually constructed, there are many opportunities for discontinuities to occur and to affect the CLD student's interactions with others in the mainstream context. One frequent result of these discontinuities is a reduction of incidental learning. Further, various affective variables may be negatively influenced because the individuals misperceive one another and miscommunicate. Although there are a number of potential conversational difficulties, a few examples are provided here.

Contextualization cues are verbal and nonverbal cues used by the speaker to highlight or emphasize certain aspects of the conversation (Gumperz, 1983). These cues enable the listener to read between the lines and grasp the intended meaning from what is said. Because CLD students may use different contextualization cues or may not use the mainstream English cues appropriately, their intended meanings may be missed or misunderstood. In every culture, numerous features—such as prosody, lexical choices, the rate of speech, facial expressions, pauses, silences, and proxemics—act as contextualization cues, and significant diversity has been demonstrated. Goodwin (1981, 1990) and Heath (1983) have discussed such expressive differences between African American children and white children in various informal conversational activities, whereas Duranti (1985), Hakuta (1986), and Schieffelin and Ochs (1986) have documented differences in a number of other languages and cultures.

Many other conversational strategies vary widely across cultures, and these may also lead to confusion and to possible misinterpretation. In many cultures, there are differences regarding who an individual may speak to and when these interactions may occur (Borofsky, 1987; Philips, 1983). Frequently, these speaker rights are due to social status differences. Ochs (1986), for example, found that Samoan children were expected to listen and not ask questions of adults. Because they were low status, Samoan children could not pose questions to adults (who were higher status) without violating cultural norms.

The diversity within conversational discourse can be noted in many other interactional patterns and strategies that determine how well CLD students may communicate in the mainstream context. For example, the way that different cultures employ discourse to tease individuals and even the reasons for teasing have been studied and found to be different from the patterns and reasons expected in mainstream English settings (Clancy, 1986; Crago, 1988; Eisenberg, 1986). Similarly, the employment of various interactional routines (Crago, 1988; Peters & Boggs, 1986; Tannen, 1984), the transmission of affective status (Irvine, 1982), and the negotiation of disputes (Young, 1982) are subtle but important conversational strategies that may result in difficulties if the CLD students use nonmainstream strategies rather than those expected in the mainstream context.

DIFFERENCES BETWEEN FIRST- AND SECOND-LANGUAGE ACQUISITION

Finally, although research does not substantiate the belief that there are great qualitative differences between the process of first-language acquisition and acquisition of a second language—particularly in the case of simultaneous bilingualism (Genesee, 1992)—there are some important differences between the two processes that emerge when the second language is learned after the first. Differences appear in the impact that age has on the acquisition of a second language, in the types of motivations for learning a second language, in the kinds of language models and opportunities for learning that are provided to second-language learners, and in the kinds of expectations and reinforcements directed toward second-language learners.

Given the concept of the adaptive nature of developmental immaturity (Bjorklund & Schwartz, this volume), it should not be surprising that age does play a role in the readiness and ease of second-language acquisition. Although the first language is acquired when the developmentally immature cognitive and semiotic systems can act as supports and mediational filters for this process, this may not be the case when the second language is learned at a later time. If an individual attempts to learn a second language after the cognitive/semiotic systems have matured, this acquisition may not be as easily attained. Although second-language acquisition is still possible, more effort and different strategies may have to be applied by older language learners. These differences may result in problems. For example, some of these different strategies may not fit into the mainstream classroom practices or the time frames expected for learning new material. Consequently, it may appear that the student is simply a poor learner rather than an individual engaged in different types of acquisitional and learning strategies (e.g., Cummins, 1984; Trueba, 1983).

There are also motivational differences. Unlike acquisition of a first language when individuals are highly motivated to acquire the language for communication and for constructing comprehensible maps of the world (Oller, 1989; Vygotsky, 1978), second-language learners already employ their first languages for these purposes. Consequently, their primary motivations for acquiring the second language are different. Rather than acquiring the second language for sense making, second-language acquisition is generally guided by social motivations and the desire for assimilation. If the second-language learner is highly motivated to assimilate into that cultural/linguistic community (i.e., the perceived social distance between the second-language learner and the second-language community is small), then acquisition will be more successful. If this social motivation is not strong, acquisition will not be as successful (Schumann, 1976, 1978). Consequently, social motivations rather than epistemological motivations most often characterize second-language acquisition, and this difference can affect the rate and extent of acquisition.

Another difference between first- and second-language acquisition involves the opportunities and models available for learning the second language. In first-language acquisition, the child is constantly exposed to native speakers of this language, and nearly all acquisition occurs in naturalistic settings. The child spends all of his or her waking hours acquiring the first language in contextually embedded and meaningful situations with strong language models. In contrast, the second-language learner often has limited exposure to the second language in terms of location, time, and language models. Typically, the school-age child acquiring the second language receives second-language instruction in an English as a Second Language (ESL) classroom or a bilingual setting for only a portion of the day. Further, the language-learning tasks may be more artificial and the models that the student is exposed to may not be presented by native users of the language. Consequently, limited exposure to the second language in terms of the models available, the time spent on acquisition, and the authenticity of the language-learning contexts may be less than for the first-language learner.

The role and impact of both the expectations of individuals for second-language learners and the types of reinforcement given to them also tend to differ from first-language acquisition. When an infant is acquiring a first language, there are no expectations that the child is required to produce perfect language or communication. This acquisitional process is recognized as developmental in nature, and the focus is on meaning transmission and on the attempts to communicate. During second-language acquisition—especially when it occurs after the preschool years—the expectations are different. The attention is often on correct production of superficial aspects of language structure, such as accent and grammar. Although the importance of meaning and the tenacity to attempt communication may be recognized and supported, these variables play a less significant role. Consequently, the types of feedback and the types of reinforcement given to first-language learners and those acquiring the second language may differ significantly (Beebe, 1988; Vigil & Oller, 1976).

Each of these acquisitional differences can have a strong impact on the social, conversational, and academic performances of CLD students. Even though they might possess normal language and learning proficiency, these CLD students may exhibit some temporary difficulties as a function of the acquisition process that they must work through (Damico & Hamayan, 1992). They may require additional support in the form of tutoring or other non–special education practices, but usually these students are not language or learning disordered. To the uninformed teacher or specialist, however, these behaviors may appear to indicate language and/or learning disabilities.

Other Cultural Differences

It should be expected that if there are linguistic and communicative differences between CLD students and students from the mainstream, other cultural aspects will also differ and play a role in the CLD student's academic and social performances. Research supports this contention (Chamberlain & Medeiros-Landurand, 1991; Deyhle, 1987; Heath, 1983; Philips, 1983; Schieffelin & Ochs, 1986; Tannen, 1984; van Kleeck, 1994; Westby, 1994). There are a number of cultural differences that may result in difficulties both for CLD students in the mainstream setting and for speech-language pathologists who must provide service to them.

One important cultural difference that can affect academic and social performance is the way in which individuals establish and maintain their "face." As discussed by Goffman (1972), "face" is a descriptor that has been used to refer to one's socially generated self-image. Based on past experiences and interactions with others, each individual has developed an internalized psychological construct of who he or she is and how he or she should react and interact in various contexts.

This construct is highly embedded in one's initial cultural context. That is, the values, norms, and traditions that help structure one's face come directly from primary experiences obtained in the home culture. Because of this local influence, the values and behavioral norms that define one's face may vary significantly from one culture to another. For example, in some cultures, the concept of cooperation in learning is highly prized and is an important value to maintain when constructing one's face. In other cultures, competition appears to be more important (Goldman & McDermott, 1987; Philips, 1983). Consequently, for some CLD students the competitive learning activities characteristic of our mainstream schools may be a violation of their face. In such cases, the students are presented with a dilemma: They can violate their internalized construct or they can perform poorly (or not at all) in the competitive tasks and maintain their face. Such a dilemma places these students at a serious disadvantage in the mainstream schools (Seymour, 1981).

When CLD students experience conflicts between the maintenance of face versus other behavioral objectives, they will typically choose the maintenance of face over other goals or purposes (Brandt, 1981; Eriks-Brophy & Crago, 1993; Philips, 1983; Scollon & Scollon, 1981). The result may be poor performance in the academic or social setting that may be interpreted by the uninformed as evidence of a language or learning disorder rather than a cultural discontinuity.

Many other cultural differences may also exist between the CLD student and the mainstream student. Chamberlain and Medeiros-Landurand (1991) have identified a number of cultural variables that may differ and may result in communicative and/or learning difficulties when the diversity is not addressed. For example, in testing situations or in social settings, one's use of touch to establish comfort and acceptance, one's definition of personal space, one's respect for and adherence to time constraints, one's use of eye-gaze strategies, and the conceptions of taboos and offensive behavior are all culturally determined variables that may be in conflict across cultures and may affect performance.

Westby (1994) has discussed the impact of cultural diversity on the ways that CLD students handle oral and written texts. Based on local cultural practices, many students are more oriented to some literary genres and oral styles than to others. These findings are consistent with the work of Heath (1983) and Michaels

(1981, 1985). Without question, these differences—if not recognized and addressed during literacy development—will result in poor literacy skills and possible misdiagnosis of CLD students as learning disabled.

These potential cultural differences may be even more subtle. For example, cultural background often influences one's perceptual style, one's cognitive style, and even one's learning preferences with respect to different modes and channels of information transmission and practice (Deyhle, 1987; Philips, 1983). Even the importance of education to the individual and one's perceptions of punishment and reward are highly culturally based. Finally, a student's belief in individual responsibility and the role such a belief plays in academic motivation, completion of homework, and test preparation vary from one cultural context to another. Simply put, if an individual is raised in a culture that believes in fate more than in individual responsibility, less specific effort may be applied to academic preparation.

If teachers or specialists do not account for these cultural differences and, consequently, hold inappropriate expectations for CLD students, these students may not perform as well as possible. In such circumstances, observed difficulties, rather than being due to problems internal to the student, may reside in the lack of individualized and culturally sensitive instruction.

An excellent example of how the failure to account for diversity can directly affect service delivery has been provided by van Kleeck (1994). In an excellent review, she discussed how numerous child-rearing practices vary across cultures. The value of talk during child rearing, the amount of acceptable talk, how displays of knowledge are handled, how status is handled during interactions, and the actual language-teaching beliefs and how they influence child rearing may vary considerably. If the speech-language pathologist does not take these differences into consideration, many of the parent-training programs and the child-rearing suggestions directed to parents and children from diverse cultures may be biased and ineffective.

Given these examples of diversity and recognizing that many more are possible, speech-language pathologists may be tempted to throw up their hands in despair. They may believe that the complexities of working with CLD students overwhelm their levels of expertise and ability. As language experts in professional settings, however, it is the responsibility of speech-language pathologists to address the needs of CLD students as well as the needs of students from the mainstream. Fortunately, there are a number of service delivery strategies that can be applied to accomplish these professional obligations. The remainder of this chapter will discuss these strategies.

Addressing Diversity in Service Delivery

Regardless of their own cultural and linguistic backgrounds, speech-language pathologists can provide effective services to students from CLD backgrounds. To do so, however, clinicians must recognize that there are differences between these CLD students and mainstream students, and they should apply a number of assessment and intervention strategies that are designed to account for these differences in practical and clinically relevant ways.

Assessment of CLD Students

To evaluate CLD students adequately, assessment practices must recognize that an individual's linguistic proficiency and communicative competence are not easily described. Many variables must be considered from a realistic perspective. Further, there must be a set of practical strategies in place during assessment to overcome the clinician's potentially limited expertise with diversity issues and the inherent biases built into the traditional assessment process when CLD students are involved (Taylor, 1977; Taylor & Payne, 1983).

THE ADVANTAGE OF A DESCRIPTIVE APPROACH TO ASSESSMENT

To provide effective service delivery and to understand the extent of a CLD child's linguistic/communicative difficulties, a descriptive approach to language assessment that accounts for the complexity of communication and its diversity should be employed. A descriptive approach can accomplish two primary assessment objectives.

First, when CLD students are suspected of exhibiting potential language disorders, it is the task of the speech-language pathologist to determine whether difficulties actually exist. To accomplish this task, the speech-language pathologist should ask whether the individual is a successful or unsuccessful communicator in the contexts of interest. That is, does the child adequately use his or her language proficiency and communicative competence to accomplish the goals and objectives of communication when interacting with other individuals or with the academic curriculum? Additionally, the speech-language pathologist must be able to describe the child's communicative strengths, weaknesses, and any problematic behaviors that serve as potential indexes of underlying language or communicative deficits. Once this is accomplished, the clinician must attempt to complete the second assessment objective: to determine the underlying causal factors for the identified difficulties (if any exist). That is, are the documented communicative or academic difficulties due to cultural and/or linguistic differences, a language disorder, or a combination of these two factors?

To accomplish these two objectives, it is not sufficient to rely solely on norm-referenced tests that only provide scores, percentiles, or age ranges. Rather, the clinician should be able to create a detailed description of what the children say, how they behave, and what types of materials they effectively use in communicative, social, and academic contexts (Damico, Secord, & Wiig, 1992). This information is then interpreted to make defensible inferences about the child's linguistic and learning capabilities. Basically, the descriptive approach provides both quantitative and qualitative data that can be used for interpretive purposes (Damico, 1991b; Silliman & Wilkinson, 1994; Westby, Stevens-Dominguez, & Oetter, in press).

COLLECTION OF AUTHENTIC DATA

In addition to the descriptive approach, it is important that the data collected and analyzed for assessment be as authentic as possible. That is, assessment must be structured to observe language during actual communicative activities within real contexts (Damico, 1991b; Oller, 1979). For our purposes, authenticity means that the methods used in assessment focus on data that possess linguistic realism, ecological validity, and representativeness.

Linguistic realism requires that assessment procedures treat linguistic behavior as a complex and synergistic phenomenon that exists primarily for the transmission and interpretation of meaning (Crystal, 1987; Oller, 1983a, 1989; Shuy, 1981; Smith, 1983). Consequently, the data of interest in assessment should be actual utterances and other meaningful chunks of linguistic behavior that serve to transmit an idea or intention from a speaker or writer to a listener or reader.

Ecological validity is another aspect of authenticity that must be accommodated during assessment. Rather than trying to isolate the assessment process from contextual influence, assessment should be accomplished in naturalistic settings in which true communicative performance is occurring and is influenced by contextual factors. Such practices will enable the evaluator to discern the effects of contextual variables on the student's communicative performance and will enable assessment to remain consistent with the emphasis on relativism in behavior analysis (Oller, 1979).

Representativeness is a third aspect of authenticity. When focussing on observed behaviors and using these behaviors to comment on a child's underlying linguistic, communicative, or academic ability, it is important to ensure that the behaviors are truly representative of the child's actual performance. Without this assurance, the speech-language pathologist runs the risk of determining potential difficulties and deficits on the basis of behaviors that may not be a true indication of the child's underlying proficiency.

If possible, data collection should be oriented toward collecting examples of the child's best performances, worse performances, and most typical performances. Gathering data across this behavioral range will greatly increase the descriptiveness and interpretive ability of the speech-language pathologist (Nelson, 1993; Silliman & Wilkinson, 1991, 1994).

ADOPTION OF A PRACTICAL ASSESSMENT STRATEGY

Finally, to assess effectively the linguistic proficiency and communicative competence of CLD students, speech-language pathologists should engage in a four-component assessment strategy. They should (1) engage in a collaborative approach to assessment, (2) implement a prereferral intervention structure, (3) build a diversity framework into the assessment process, and (4) ensure that assessment is conducted from a functional focus. If these four components are implemented and linked to the two previous assessment suggestions, the assessment of language proficiency in CLD children can be greatly enhanced (Damico & Hamayan, 1992). A discussion of each of the four components follows.

Component 1: Collaboration. When assessing children from multicultural backgrounds, many variables must be considered. As discussed previously, these variables include knowledge of the home language and culture, a clear understanding of the processes of second-language acquisition and cultural assimilation, knowledge of the potential effects of disempowerment on CLD students, and a host of other variables (Damico & Hamayan, 1992; Langdon & Cheng, 1992). Additionally, the speech language pathologist may not have the time or opportunity to conduct an assessment that would be sufficient to address all the issues of the CLD child. For this reason, it is important for the speech-language pathologist to engage in a process of collaboration when providing services to CLD students.

Over the past several years, collaboration as a process has been repeatedly proposed and discussed in speech-language pathology (Nelson, 1993; Secord, 1990; Secord & Wiig, 1991; Simon, 1987). From a service delivery perspective, collaboration is both an approach to group interaction and a problem-solving approach that enables a collection of people who share common objectives but diverse backgrounds and expertise to work efficiently and effectively for those common objectives. In the case of assessment of CLD students, the collaborative approach means that several people may be involved in the assessment process.

As discussed by Secord and Wiig (1991), the major advantage of collaboration is that it produces leverage. That is, by combining the knowledge, experiences, expertise, and opportunities of each member of the collaborative team, there is a significant enhancement of each of these factors. Using appropriate collaboration generates a synergistic interaction which produces a much greater capacity for assessment than can be accomplished by the speech-language pathologist alone. For example, the speech-language pathologist can bring knowledge of appropriate functional assessment measures and information regarding the academic curriculum to the assessment process, whereas a linguistic informant can apply these assessment measures in the student's first language. Additionally, a cultural informant can interact with the parents in the home and provide information on home/school cultural discontinuities, the teacher can provide observations of actual classroom strengths and weaknesses, the bilingual educator can assess the role of language transfer and subtractive bilingualism in the student's current level of functioning, and the student and parents can provide their perspective on what aspects of the school experience they consider most important. In such a collaboration, multiple input best serves the needs of both the service delivery agents and the CLD students. Our experience with the CLD population for 2 decades indicates that the best assessment with these students is collaborative assessment.

Component 2: Prereferral Intervention. One of the real difficulties in working with CLD students is that they may be inappropriately referred for special education assessment. The classroom teachers note communicative and/or learning difficulties in the classroom, and they refer these students on the basis of these difficulties. As previously discussed, however, many of these difficulties may be caused by linguistic and cultural differences rather than by true childhood language or learning disorders. Due to the numbers of these inappropriate referrals, the collaborative assessment team has less opportunity to assess the students referred. Additionally, when a special education referral is made, there is a tendency for evaluators to find an identifiable impairment within the student. This is especially true when dealing with CLD students (Cummins, 1984; Damico, 1991b; Garcia & Ortiz, 1988).

To overcome this tendency for inappropriate referral (and diagnosis), a regular education initiative that attempts to deal with the CLD students' problems before they are referred for special education assessment is needed. This type of initiative will empower teachers to work with CLD students in their classrooms rather than routinely and prematurely referring them for special education evaluations. Because most CLD children with normal language/learning proficiency will eventually work through the barriers presented by their diversity—especially if they receive support from non-special education programs—the regular education initiative will be beneficial to all involved parties. The CLD students will have the time and regular support to assimilate into the mainstream, regular education teachers will become more empowered to handle their students, and special educators will have fewer referrals and more time for students with true disabilities, with the result that there will be less potential for inappropriate diagnoses.

A prereferral intervention process that initially accounts for diversity in the classroom is the preferred type of regular education initiative. Several prereferral processes that can be easily adapted for service delivery to CLD students have been discussed in the literature. Chalfant, Pysh, and Moultrie (1979), for example, have described a particular approach to the design and functioning of teacher assistance teams that works well. When the prereferral process utilizes trained regular educators selected by their peers and supported by the school-based administration, many students with difficulties can have their problems addressed without the input of special education. Through a problem-solving approach that provides the regular educator with a set of specific interventions designed for individual students, the special education realm can be avoided.

Similarly, Garcia and Ortiz (1988) have provided a variation on the teacher assistance team concept that is specifically oriented to the CLD student. Using a set of prereferral flowchart recommendations and some practical suggestions for dealing with bilingual collaboration, an effective and efficient prereferral intervention framework is discussed and demonstrated. Experience with this approach indicates significant improvement in the ways that both regular educators and special educators address the problems of CLD students (Damico & Hamayan, 1992).

The aforementioned references regarding the prereferral intervention process are specific and should be scrutinized carefully. In our experience, most school districts around the United States and Canada use some version of a prereferral framework. The vast majority of these frameworks, however, are not regular education initiatives or are not designed or implemented correctly. Consequently, most of the frameworks in use provide little benefit to the students or the service providers. To ensure some benefit from this second component of the recommended assessment strategy, a true and effective regular education initiative based on prereferral interventions should be implemented. The work of Chalfont, Pysh, and Moultrie (1979), and Garcia and Ortiz (1988) can guide this implementation.

Component 3: A Diversity Framework. Because the primary concern when conducting assessments of CLD students involves the issue of diversity, there must be a framework built into the assessment process that allows the speech-language pathologist to account for this diversity. It is not enough to recognize that poor performance may be due to differences as well as deficits; the speech-language pathologist must be able to account systematically for this possibility in a way that is institutionalized. That is, an expected phase of each evaluation should involve an attempt to determine how many of the specific difficulties can be explained as a result of the student's cultural and/or linguistic diversity.

This diversity framework can be accomplished through the use of a bilevel analysis paradigm that incorporates an initial descriptive analysis of communicative performance with a detailed explanatory analysis of language proficiency (Damico, 1991b). The first level of analysis in this paradigm is descriptive analysis. At this descriptive level, the speech-language pathologist (or a collaborator) typically uses functional assessment procedures to observe the student's communicative and academic performances in the contexts and modalities of interest and to determine whether the student is communicatively successful. By using functional and authentic assessment procedures, data are provided to document the student's strengths and weaknesses, the student's overall success as an English language user, and the student's progress over time (when pre- and postanalyses are conducted). At this level of analysis, the evaluator functions primarily as an agent of the mainstream culture to determine what types of difficulties the CLD student exhibits. If there are no difficulties noted after a descriptive analysis is performed, then the assessment is concluded. If there are difficulties indicated at this level of analysis and if there are concerns regarding the student's language-learning proficiency, then the second level of analysis is necessary.

The second level of the analysis paradigm involves explanatory analysis, which seeks to determine the causal factors for the communicative difficulties noted in the descriptive analysis. At this analytic level, the examiner notes the CLD student's strengths and weaknesses and seeks to determine why these behaviors occurred. At this time, the evaluator addresses the diversity issues and functions more as an advocate for the CLD student than an agent of the mainstream culture.

The explanatory level of analysis typically does not involve additional data collection or assessment procedures. Rather, this level involves a deeper interpretation of the data collected at the descriptive level. The evaluator attempts to explain how variables such as aspects of the context, the student's social/cultural experience, or the individual's cognitive abilities or linguistic proficiency can account for the described difficulties. The evaluator attempts to determine the adequacy of the student's underlying language proficiency or comment on the effectiveness of the student's deeper semiotic capacities (see Oller & Damico, 1991).

To conduct an explanatory analysis, a number of strategies employing sets of guiding questions or focus items have been developed and may be systematically applied. These question sets have the advantage of focussing the evaluator(s) on the potential variables that may influence the CLD student's communicative and/or academic performances. Several types of questions have been developed. For example, Wolfram (1985) has applied his sociolinguistic expertise to discuss a detailed and systematic approach to reviewing phonological differences versus deficits. Kovarsky (1992) has adapted work from the ethnography of communication to create a set of questions for comparing language use across contexts. Silliman and Wilkinson (1991) have structured an analysis of performance based on observational assessment procedures that focus on different levels of behavioral analysis. Addressing CLD students directly, Damico (1991b) has structured a set of six general questions that focus on issues such as bias, acquisitional phenomena, cultural interference, inadequate assessment practices, dialectal issues, and disempowerment. Additionally, Damico discusses procedures for identifying underlying deficits due to language and/or learning disabilities.

It is at this explanatory level of analysis that the speech-language pathologist, in collaboration with others, must make a decision regarding the origin of the communicative/academic difficulties. That is, are these difficulties due to differences, disorders, or a combination of the two? The work of Damico (1991b) and others (Kovarsky, 1992; Wolfram, 1985) can assist in this task.

Component 4: A Focus on Functionality. As discussed in the previous section, during descriptive analysis the focus should be on functional assessment. This is because there is a bias inherent in the assessment of language structure with CLD groups (Damico, Oller, & Storey, 1983; Nelson, 1993; Oller, 1979). To create a functional focus, the evaluator should conduct authentic observation with one primary question in mind: "How successful is this student as a communicator in the contexts and modalities of interest?" This question is based on how well the student functions on three criteria: the effectiveness of meaning transmission, the fluency of meaning transmission, and the appropriateness of meaning transmission (Damico, 1991b).

These three criteria enable the descriptive assessment process to focus on the functional dimension of communicative ability in a manner that transcends the need to divide language proficiency into a variety of skills, modules, or components at the time of assessment. Consequently, the synergistic quality of language, which is so important within communicative settings, is preserved. Additionally, this initial focus on functionality enables the evaluator to answer real and pragmatic questions about the CLD student's ability to function in the mainstream contexts.

To remain consistent with the descriptive assessment approach, the assessment tools and procedures utilized must be able to analyze language use in authentic situations from a functional perspective. Over the past 15 years, a number of procedures and tools have been developed that fit these requirements. In general, these procedures can be conveniently organized according to their different data collection formats and the primary behavioral manifestations that these procedures target. In keeping with Damico et al. (1992), these tools and procedures will be organized into four major data collection formats (structured probes, behavioral sampling, rating scales and protocols, and direct and on-line observation) and two general language usage manifestations (conversational and academic). Although these divisions are too general to provide a rigorous classification system, they will permit sufficient organization for this discussion.

The first classification of potential assessment tools and procedures to incorporate a functional perspective involves structured probe activities. The probe format is the most widely used of the four data collection strategies. It has been used in the design of norm-referenced tests and many integrative and descriptive procedures. There are numerous variations within this category, including picture elicitation probes, question and answer probes, elicited imitation probes, interactive computer probes, direct translation probes, and role-playing activities. Probes are structured tasks or activities that elicit a specific language behavior from the individual being assessed. With probes, the evaluator may anticipate the type of response that will be elicited from the student. This is because the task performed is carefully designed to elicit a specific behavior.

For conversational purposes, a number of probe activities are available. Brinton and Fujiki (1992), for example, have structured an assessment activity used to probe a student's ability to revise utterances, maintain topics, and ask relevant questions during conversation. Olshtain and Blum-Kulka (1985) have suggested several elicitation techniques that focus on language usage, whereas Oller (1979) and Jonz (1987) have adapted cloze procedures for discourse or conversational assessment. In working with adolescents, Brown, Anderson, Shillicock and Yule (1983) have suggested a number of task-based activities that tap the student's ability to use transactional language during interactions.

Academically, probe activities are widely used. The current trend toward criterion-referenced assessment in second-language testing (Cloud, 1991) and some applications of curriculum-based assessment (Marston & Magnusson, 1987) are dependent on probe activities. Wade (1990) has provided a method to use "think-alouds" to describe students' reading comprehension, and Creaghead (1992) recommended a probe-oriented approach to determine what kinds of classroom scripts or routines children possess. Simon (1989) has developed a comprehensive analysis of classroom communicative abilities needed in the transition from elementary to secondary school that employs several probe strategies in addition to other formats. Her work has been found to be successful in allowing CLD students to function in the mainstream classroom environment. Especially for academic purposes, the probe format is effective (Cloud, 1991; O'Malley, 1989).

The second assessment format involves behavioral sampling procedures. Within this format, the student being assessed completes some required (but less structured) task, and this performance is audiorecorded (or videorecorded) and transcribed or documented in some other way. Following data collection, the behavioral sample is analyzed. This format has been extensively applied over the past 25 years, and there are numerous procedures available for both conversational assessment and for evaluation of many academic activities.

Conversationally, a number of functional language-sampling procedures are available. Loban (1976) emphasizes dimensions of clarity of expression, fluency, command of lexical expression, and comprehension. Adams and Bishop (1990) focus on exchange structures, clarity, and cohesion; and Damico (1991a) employs a set of 17 problematic behaviors that focus specifically on the functional criteria previously mentioned (i.e., effectiveness, fluency, appropriateness).

A number of effective, academically related behavior-sampling procedures are available for performance assessment. For example, many excellent narrative analyses can be used for assessment purposes. Westby (1992) and Hedberg and Stoel-Gammon (1986) have demonstrated the effectiveness of several complex story grammar and narrative analyses for evaluative purposes. Although narrative development and organization are culturally dependent (Heath, 1986; Westby, 1994), these behavioral analyses provide important data regarding English language task expectations.

Curriculum-based assessment from a subject-based perspective (Deno, 1985; Marston & Magnusson, 1987) and reading miscue analysis (Goodman, Watson, & Burke, 1987) frequently involve behavioral sampling to accomplish the actual goals of the assessment. Two other promising approaches along these lines are Nelson's "curriculum-based language assessment" (1992, 1993) and dynamic assessment techniques (Lidz, 1987; Palincsar, Brown, & Campione, 1994; Palincsar & Klenk, 1992). Nelson uses think-alouds and behavioral analysis from an ethnographic perspective to determine whether the student possesses the communicative strategies essential for effective functioning in a classroom setting. The dynamic assessment techniques are designed to determine a child's zone of instructional sensitivity and comment on his or her actual learning potential.

Finally, when targeting academically related assessment, portfolio assessment must be considered. This behavioral sampling procedure is currently receiving much attention in education. Arising from the literacy and language arts fields (Flood & Lapp, 1989; Jongsma, 1989; Mathews, 1990; Valencia, 1990; Wolf, 1989), this procedure is somewhat different from many behavioral sampling procedures in that a primary evaluation of the artifacts placed in the student's portfolio involves generalized comparisons rather than detailed analyses. However, this procedure is effective in documenting the student's current performance level and his or her progress over time.

The third data collection format involves rating scales and protocols. This format enables the examiner to observe the student as a communicator in the context of interest and then rate or describe that student according to a set of reliable and valid indices of communication. Following the observation, the examiner completes a rating scale or protocol when the student being assessed is no longer present. Two frequent variations of this format are checklists and interview questions. Typically, procedures within this format comprise measurable indicators (e.g., numerical scale, age range, semantic differential, forced judgment of appropriate/inappropriate) for each behavior on the scale or protocol.

For conversational purposes, a number of rating scales have been developed. Damico and Oller (1985) created a functional language-screening instrument, *Spotting Language Problems,* that effectively screens school-age individuals for communication difficulties; whereas Mattes (1985; Mattes & Omark, 1984) and Cheng (1987) have designed several protocols involving both verbal and nonverbal behaviors which are helpful in the descriptive assessment of Spanish and Asian CLD students. A widely known descriptive protocol, the *Pragmatic Protocol* (Prutting & Kirchner, 1987), focuses on a large number of language usage behaviors and requires that the evaluator rate the student's ability to use these behaviors appropriately or inappropriately.

Academically, many rating scales, protocols, checklists, and interview questionnaires focus on the functional needs of the student in the classroom. For example, Cloud (1991) has provided several questionnaires to describe home background from an academic perspective, classroom environment, and previous educational experience. O'Malley (1989) provides an Interpersonal and Academic Skills Checklist that focuses on 30 skills important for cognitive academic language proficiency and a Literacy Development Checklist to guide the evaluator in functional assessment of language minority students. Specific to speech-language pathology, Larson and McKinley (1987) have also provided checklists that may be beneficial in describing academic success or difficulty.

The final division of assessment procedures employs direct and on-line observation. This format involves the direct observation of a student's communicative interaction and real-time/immediate coding of the communicative and academic behaviors observed. Consequently, these procedures are able to provide detailed and objective data on the student's performance.

There are a number of procedures and recommendations currently available. In terms of an overall framework, Silliman and Wilkinson (1991, 1994) have discussed direct observation through the use of a photographic metaphor which describes different lenses that relate to different levels of analyses. Westby et al. (in press) have proposed an on-line narrative recording procedure during direct observation that can focus on a wide range of behaviors. These authors also describe the actual process of team collaboration when using this "performance-competence model."

A number of authors have suggested direct observations that avoid predetermination what might be observed and recorded. Some of these suggestions are based on anecdotal assessment (Goodman, 1985; Goodman, Goodman, & Hood, 1989; Kemp, 1990; Pils, 1991), which enables many individuals to observe and record information during daily classroom and home activities. Others suggest a much more detailed and elaborate process based on modifications of participant observation methods employed in ethnographic research (Cheng, 1990; Kovarsky, 1992; Nelson, 1993; Spradley, 1980). Each of these recommendations may be applied to the description of both conversational skills and classroom performance.

Finally, there are a few observational procedures that are more structured than those previously mentioned. For example, the Social Interactive Coding System was designed by Rice, Sell, and Hadley (1990) to describe the speaker's verbal interactive status in conjunction with the setting, the conversational partner, and the activities in which the speaker is engaged. Similarly, Systematic Observation of Communicative Interaction (Damico, 1992a) was designed to employ a balanced set of low-inference and high-inference items to achieve a reliable coding of illocutionary acts, verbal and nonverbal problematic behaviors, and the appropriateness of the student's communicative interaction. Along with the previously mentioned suggestions, these more structured procedures provide the speech-language pathologist with a wide selection of direct observational techniques.

Regardless of which assessment procedures are utilized, the speech-language pathologist can greatly enhance the assessment of CLD students by employing this practical four-component assessment strategy. Applied as recommended, this strategy will enable appropriate and effective assessment of these students regardless of the cultural and linguistic background of the speech-language pathologist.

Intervention with CLD Students

Once the initial assessment phase is completed, issues of intervention must be addressed. Again, the speech-language pathologist must recognize the complexities of providing supportive services and/or direct intervention to the CLD students. The same kinds of diversity issues must be addressed, and care must be taken to avoid the biases when treatment and intervention are considered and implemented.

As with assessment, specific processes and strategies can be applied with good success. The speech-language pathologist should remember that the key to effective intervention is that the techniques employed must involve authentic skills, tasks, and activities. As discussed by Oller (1983b) and others (Damico & Damico, 1993b; Nelson, 1993; Norris & Hoffman, 1993), any activities that follow the logic and flow of experience, that fulfill expectancies about the way the world operates, and that are meaningful, relevant, well structured, and motivating will result in positive effects.

ADOPTION OF A PRACTICAL INTERVENTION STRATEGY

In parallel with the practical considerations for the assessment of CLD students, speech-language pathologists should implement a five-component intervention strategy. They should (1) engage in a collaborative approach to intervention, (2) determine the most appropriate placement for the CLD student, (3) create an individualized language usage plan, (4) structure an additive language/learning environment, and (5) utilize a holistic/pragmatic intervention paradigm. Each of these components is discussed next.

Component 1: Collaboration. If it is possible, a collaborative intervention system is even more necessary than collaboration in assessment. This is primarily because the speech-language pathologist cannot hope to spend enough time or provide enough support by himself or herself to meet the needs of the CLD student.

When a student is identified as needing language, communicative, or academic support or direct intervention, a plan to provide continuous support in all environments is necessary. Anything less is likely to be insufficient. Consequently, the speech-language pathologist should never be the sole intervention agent. Rather, a collaborative team should determine how best to provide support to the student at all times and in all settings. In this situation, the speech-language pathologist can help design the collaborative intervention plan and participate as appropriate in the implementation of this plan. The clinician may provide direct intervention, consultative support to others, and follow-up in varying degrees to ensure that the collaborative plan is appropriately implemented (Damico & Nye, 1990).

In designing a collaborative intervention plan, the teacher and/or classroom aides, parents or siblings, the bilingual educator and/or the ESL teacher, cultural/linguistic informants, and peers will likely be involved in service delivery. When addressing the needs of the CLD student, therefore, speech-language pathologists should not consider themselves the primary intervention agents. Rather than an individual, the primary intervention agent is a synergistic professional entity that consists of a number of individuals with roles to play in helping students overcome their difficulties.

Component 2: Determination of Appropriate Placement. When addressing the needs of CLD students, it is important that the most appropriate placements are provided to these students. Placement of students into programs or intervention structures that do not meet their needs will typically produce negative results (Cummins, 1989; Damico & Hamayan, 1992).

In general, six potential placement decisions can be made: (1) placement in regular education with no support or intervention needed, (2) placement in regular education with in-class support, (3) placement in regular education with ESL support, (4) placement in bilingual education, (5) placement in special education, and (6) placement in special education with bilingual or ESL support. As discussed by Willig and Ortiz (1991), appropriate placement is dependent on the assessment conducted and the willingness of the professionals to meet the student's needs rather than to provide a placement that merely meets administrative or legal requirements. If the four-pronged assessment strategy is followed, a valid assessment and useful information should be obtained. If the professionals take ethical responsibility for their actions and decisions (Damico & Hamayan, 1991), this information will be used appropriately.

Component 3: Creation of a Language Usage Plan. When working with linguistically diverse students, professionals should strive to provide as much support as possible in the students' strongest language (Cummins, 1989). This is primarily because students should have an opportunity to use their strongest language-learning proficiency in remedial or intervention activities. Additionally, these students should never be isolated from their language of socialization and comfort; because these languages are usually the first or home languages, they should neither be sacrificed nor discouraged—such discouragement may result in negative and disruptive affective factors (Hamayan & Damico, 1991).

When working with these students, there is usually no need to decide between the students' two languages. Both languages can be used for the benefit of the student if a collaborative service delivery plan is implemented. The collaborative intervention team can create a language usage plan to determine who works with the student, in what language, and at what times (Willig & Ortiz, 1991). The language usage plan should be incorporated as a document into the student's individualized education plan. The creation of a language usage plan will help ensure that instruction is consistent with the student's language status, that appropriate support is provided, and that needs are recognized.

Component 4: An Additive Language-Learning Environment. To provide the most effective interventions to CLD students, the interventionist(s) must create an environment that will encourage active learning and risk taking on the part of the CLD students (Bashir, 1989; Cummins, 1989; Edelsky, Draper, & Smith, 1983; Fradd & Weismantel, 1989). When the additive language-learning environment is structured to allow students to believe in themselves as learners and communicators, when the environment avoids projection of negative judgments on the students' home cultures or first languages, and when the environment is structured so that these students have the encouragement and opportunity to use their home cultures and first languages to support additional language learning and academics, then CLD students are empowered as learners and will exhibit greater and more rapid growth (Cummins, 1989; Damico & Armstrong, 1991; Lambert, 1975; Ortiz, 1988; Wong-Fillmore, 1986). To assist in determining an effective additive environment for CLD students, Ortiz (1988) has provided a checklist consisting of 25 items that can indicate how well the needs of the students are being met. Additionally, several general principles can be applied to promote an additive learning environment. Fradd and Weismantel (1989) have discussed the following principles for establishing an additive language-learning environment for students learning English as a second language:

1. Expect and respect a silent period in which students listen actively, take in language, and express themselves nonverbally or in their first language.
2. Expect errors in speech and celebrate approximations to correct form, but not at the expense of meaning.
3. As students talk, remember that their oral language proficiency in their second language does not necessarily reflect a level of cognitive functioning (thinking ability).
4. As students talk, pay attention to what they are saying (meaning) rather than how they say it (accent, grammar, vocabulary).
5. Use instructional methodologies which focus on learning by doing and which require higher level thinking processes.
6. Develop nonverbal ways in which students can demonstrate their knowledge.
7. Celebrate the different languages and cultures represented by the students throughout the school year.
8. Arrange the environment so that all students can actively participate in and contribute to the success of the class regardless of language or culture.
9. Encourage high levels of interaction among students, and utilize experiences familiar to the students as part of the curriculum.

Additionally, by planning a general intervention program that addresses the following elements, an additive environment is typically established:

1. Plan goals and objectives tailored to naturalistic principles and relevancy.
2. Give the students as many opportunities as possible to read, write, talk, and listen in various group structures.
3. Allow the students to think and discuss options, make decisions, and establish accountability for what they do when working with you.
4. Immerse the students with print to build a literacy-rich environment.
5. Treat the students with respect and work to empower them as learners.
6. Utilize interesting and meaningful materials and activities.

Once the additive intervention environment is in place, it is essential to sustain positive learning opportunities through the use of meaningful, relevant, and effective intervention strategies and approaches.

Component 5: The Holistic/Pragmatic Intervention Paradigm. Over many years, the disciplines of applied linguistics and language arts have progressively embraced a holistic/pragmatic intervention paradigm (Norris & Damico, 1990). This has occurred for one simple reason: This paradigm works (Carrasquillo & Hedley, 1993; Damico & Damico, 1993b; Edelsky, 1986; Norris & Hoffman, 1993; Oller, 1983b, 1993 Smith, 1988). There are several reasons why this paradigm appears to be so effective.

First, this paradigm is based on a philosophy of teaching/intervention as opposed to an approach to teaching/intervention (Edelsky, Altwerger, & Flores, 1990; Goodman, 1986). Consequently, the paradigm does not merely exist in the activities or materials used for teaching and intervention. Rather, the strength of the paradigm lies in the dynamic interaction between the activities, the interventionist, the materials, and the students (Damico, 1992b). This philosophy addresses the entire learning/teaching context.

Second, this holistic/pragmatic paradigm is built on data obtained from normal developmental research, which states that language acquisition (in all skill areas) is a constructive process that is best accomplished when both the language and the intervention are meaningful, relevant, authentic, and contextually embedded. Just as children acquire their native language in a home environment, all other forms of language and the intervention process itself must be natural and directed toward "meaning-making" (Wells, 1986).

Further, to benefit maximally from the power of language to create meaning and to understand that this meaning-making is the general purpose of all forms of language, it is important to provide students with opportunities to work in all language skill areas. Consequently, when working with CLD students, speech-language pathologists (and other interventionists) should engage the students in plenty of reading, writing, and listening activities as well as speaking tasks. Better yet, these four skills should be interwoven in all teaching activities.

Finally, once the language-teaching activities focus on these three previous points, the students will become empowered to be active language learners and meaning-makers (Beed, Hawkins, & Roller, 1991; Damico & Armstrong, 1991). Through the assistance provided to them, these students will begin to assist themselves as language users and as learners in general, with the result that they will enhance their own learning processes.

Numerous authentic language activities may be used within the holistic/pragmatic paradigm (Goodman & Goodman, 1983; Oller & Richard-Amato, 1983; Willig & Ortiz, 1991). Damico (1992b) discusses no less than 35 different activities that can be incorporated into this intervention framework. For example, dialogue journals (Staton, 1983) and response journals (Wollman-Bonilla, 1989) meet the criteria for promoting authenticity in language-teaching activities because they encompass interactive written and spoken dialogues between a student and another individual. In these activities, the focus centers on attention to meaning and function rather than grammatical form. Consequently, the students are more willing to communicate and take risks with language forms when attempting to communicate. Because these activities result in the interactants getting to know one another as unique individuals, motivation and interest are increased on the part of both parties.

Theme building (Norris & Damico, 1990; Stabb, 1991) is another excellent authentic instructional activity. This generalized strategy utilizes repeatable context and experience. In theme building, recurring activities and events are designed around a particular theme that is chosen by the students themselves as an area of investigation. Multiple formats, various language functions, and numerous activities can be incorporated into a theme-building unit.

To engage in theme building, the language teacher develops activities surrounding a theme and incorporates relationships among people, objects, and events. The following steps may be used when designing theme-building activities: (1) Determine the theme (content) that will be the initial focus; (2) determine the modalities to be employed during the activities; (3) determine the language functions to be focused on during the activities; (4) determine the various language texts, formats, and strategies that will be used; and (5) determine the actual sequence and organization of activities that will be incorporated into the theme-building instructional unit.

Another authentic language activity that can incorporate all forms of text in a meaningful and relevant manner is the establishment of a writing workshop in the classroom or during the intervention period. As advocated by Atwell (1987), writing workshops fit easily into the holistic/pragmatic paradigm. Writing activities are meshed with discussions and reading assignments. The primary focus of the activities, however, is the writing process itself, during which the student receives encouragement and instruction within this text manifestation. The focus of writing, therefore, is not skill building but writing for well-motivated meaning transmission through a process-oriented approach.

Although the typical speech-language pathologist may not have much experience implementing such academically related tasks (especially writing workshops), these kinds of activities are appropriate as speech-language intervention strategies. For too long, clinicians have limited themselves to oral language activities, like categorization drills and discussions of topics, that are tangential to the interests of their students and to the classroom curricula. Reading, writing, and discussions of what we read and write are the true communicative activities of the classroom; speech-language pathologists must embrace these activities—especially with their CLD students.

Many other instructional techniques, activities, and strategies can be effectively incorporated within this intervention paradigm. For example, mediation of learning techniques (Damico, 1992b; Nelson, 1993), script building (Creaghead, 1990), communicative reading strategies (Norris, 1989), story telling (Peck, 1989), and literature study circles (Samway et al., 1991) are all reflective of the goals of intervention with CLD students and can be implemented by speech-language pathologists as well as other interventionists.

Several other types of language intervention techniques that fit within the holistic/pragmatic paradigm should be mentioned. First, speech-language pathologists can use peer teaching and cooperative learning groups (Damico, 1992b; De Avila, Cohen, & Intili, 1981; Slavin, 1986; Willig & Ortiz, 1991). These two strategies are designed to enable CLD students to receive academic support from their classroom peers through interactive group learning activities and incidental learning. In peer tutoring, specific peers of the CLD student are selected and used to provide one-on-one support to the CLD student in areas of greatest difficulty. These students work together to complete academic tasks.

Cooperative learning groups are adaptations of traditional classroom structures and activities that allow students to work in small groups that encourage mutual cooperation during learning activities. These groups are organized so that there is a heterogeneous mixture of students from various backgrounds and levels of learning proficiency, and these individuals work together to accomplish group learning goals. Due to the way that the groups are structured, each student in these small groups (four to five students) becomes an active and contributing member of the group. This is the case even for students who are experiencing language and/or learning difficulties.

Finally, there are a number of techniques and strategies that can be used to assist the classroom teacher in more effectively teaching CLD students. Hamayan and Perlman (1990) have made suggestions for adapting materials for content-based language instruction, preparing the student for content-based lessons, and making the classroom language more comprehensible. In terms of adapting materials for content-based instruction, a six-step process is suggested. The teacher and/or other interventionist should (1) modify the content to fit the students' proficiency level, (2) build on students' prior knowledge, (3) highlight specific text in the material, (4) control new vocabulary and simplify contextual vocabulary, (5) simplify the grammar of the material, and (6) structure paragraphs carefully. If appropriately implemented, these suggestions will give the teacher control over the content and its complexity, reduce cultural bias, and improve the learning potential of the CLD students.

In preparing the student for content-based lessons, Hamayan and Perlman (1990) offer suggestions regarding teaching the core vocabulary in advance and contextualizing the lesson. To assist the teacher in making language more comprehensible, Hamayan and Perlman discuss sheltered instruction activities and a host of other strategies that enable teachers to communicate better with students in the classroom.

As with the assessment strategy, implementing the five-component intervention strategy will help ensure that the CLD student—whether in need of regular education support or special education—can better negotiate communicative and academic contexts. Further, this collaborative approach enables the speech-language pathologist to provide the support necessary for effective and efficient service delivery.

Conclusion

CLD students demand the best efforts of speech-language pathologists. Due to the way that mainstream schools typically handle diversity, this group of students can least afford poor service delivery from the "language experts" in the schools. Regardless of our ability to speak their languages or recognize their cultural differences, we, as speech-language pathologists, often are these students' last and best chance for the assessments and interventions most appropriate to their situations.

Given the types of assessment and intervention strategies discussed in this chapter, even the most monolingual and culturally restricted professional can create an effective service delivery process through collaboration and a genuine interest in CLD students. We must use our expertise in a proactive manner to implement assessment processes that allow us to meet the needs of our CLD students at the same time that we meet the needs of our school systems and programs. To do so, there must be a focus on procedures that generate authentic and pragmatic results. By adopting a descriptive approach to assessment, this can be accomplished. In terms of intervention, we must determine the most appropriate placements and then structure the most effective teaching/intervention programs possible. We must remember that our students must be motivated, interested, and given the opportunity to become meaning-makers for real and relevant purposes.

As professionals, we are committed to providing effective service delivery to meet the needs of our students. Further, we want to help them become independent users of language and communication in all of their various forms and manifestations. If we demand this of ourselves, our CLD students will be well served.

References

Adams, C., & Bishop, D. V. M. (1990). Conversational characteristics of children with semantic-pragmatic disorder. I: Exchange structure, turntaking, repairs, and cohesion. *British Journal of Disorders of Communication, 24,* 211–239.

Atwell, N. (1987). *In the middle: Writing, reading, and learning with adolescents.* Portsmouth, NH: Heinemann.

Auer, J. (1984). *Bilingual conversation.* Amsterdam: John Benjamins.

Bashir, A. (1989). Language intervention and the curriculum. *Seminars in Speech and Language, 10,* 181–191.

Beebe, L. (1988). *Issues in second language acquisition.* New York: Newbury House.

Beed, P., Hawkins, E., & Roller, C. (1991). Moving learners toward independence: The power of scaffold instruction. *The Reading Teacher, 44,* 648–655.

Borofsky, R. (1987). *Making history: Pukapukan and anthropological constructions of knowledge.* Cambridge, UK: Cambridge University Press.

Brandt, E. A. (1981). Native American attitudes toward literacy recording in the Southwest. *Journal of the Linguistic Association of the Southwest, 4,* 185–195.

Brinton, B., & Fujiki, M. (1992). Setting the context for conversational language sampling. *Best Practices in School Speech-Language Pathology, 2,* 9–19.

Brown, G., Anderson, A., Shillicock, R. & Yule, G. (1983). *Teaching talk.* Cambridge, UK: Cambridge University Press.

Carrasquillo, A., & Hedley, C. (Eds.). (1993). *Whole language and the bilingual learner.* Norwood, NJ: Ablex.

Chalfant, J., Pysh, M., & Moultrie, R. (1979). Teacher assistance teams: A model for within-building problem solving. *Learning Disability Quarterly, 2,* 81–96.

Chamberlain, P., & Medeiros-Landurand, P. (1991). Practical considerations in the assessment of bilingual students. In E. V. Hamayan & J. S. Damico (Eds.), *Limiting bias in the assessment of bilingual students* (pp. 111–156). Austin, TX: Pro-ed.

Cheng, L. (1987). *Assessing Asian language performance.* Rockville, MD: Aspen.

Cheng, L. (1990). The identification of communicative disorders in Asian-Pacific students. *Journal of Childhood Communicative Disorders, 13,* 113–119.

Clancy, P. (1986). The acquisition of communicative style in Japanese. In B. B. Schieffelin & E. Ochs (Eds.), *Language socialization across cultures* (pp. 213–250). New York: Cambridge University Press.

Cloud, N. (1991). Educational assessment. In E. V. Hamayan & J. S. Damico (Eds.), *Limiting bias in the assessment of bilingual students* (pp. 220–245). Austin, TX: Pro-ed.

Crago, M. B. (1988). *Cultural context in communicative interaction of young Inuit children.* Unpublished doctoral dissertation, McGill University, Montreal.

Creaghead, N. A. (1990). Mutual empowerment through collaboration: A new script for an old problem. *Best Practices in School Speech-Language Pathology, 1,* 109–116.

Creaghead, N. (1992). What does this student know about school? Analysis of classroom scripts for interaction. *Best Practices in School Speech-Language Pathology, 2,* 65–72.

Crystal, D. (1987). Towards a "bucket" theory of language disability: Taking account of interaction between linguistic levels. *Clinical Linguistics and Phonetics, 1,* 7–22.

Cummins, J. P. (1984). *Bilingualism and special education: Issues in assessment and pedagogy.* San Diego: College-Hill Press.

Cummins, J. (1989). *Empowering minority students.* Sacramento, CA: California Association of Bilingual Educators.

Damico, J. S. (1991a). Clinical Discourse Analysis: A functional language assessment technique. In C. S. Simon (Ed.), *Communication skills and classroom success: Assessment and therapy methodologies for language and learning disabled students* (pp. 125–150). Eau Claire, WI: Thinking Publications.

Damico, J. S. (1991b). Descriptive assessment of communicative ability in limited English proficient students. In E. V. Hamayan & J. S. Damico (Eds.), *Limiting bias in the assessment of bilingual students* (pp. 157–217). Austin, TX: Pro-ed.

Damico, J. S. (1992a). Systematic observation of communicative interaction: A valid and practical descriptive assessment technique. *Best Practices in School Speech-Language Pathology, 2,* 133–144.

Damico, J. S. (1992b). *Whole language for special needs children.* Chicago, IL: Riverside Publishers.

Damico, J. S., & Armstrong, M. B. (1991). Empowerment in the clinical context: The speech-language pathologist as advocate. *NSSLHA Journal, 18,* 34–43.

Damico, J. S., & Damico, S. K. (1993a). Language and social skills from a diversity perspective: Considerations for the speech-language pathologist. *Language, Speech, and Hearing Services in Schools, 24,* 236–243.

Damico, J. S., & Damico, S. K. (1993b). Mapping a course over different roads: Language teaching with special populations. In J. W. Oller, Jr. (Ed.), *Methods that work: A smorgasbord of language teaching ideas* (2nd ed., pp. 320–331). New York: Newbury House.

Damico, J. S., & Hamayan, E. V. (1991). Implementing assessment in the real world. In E. V. Hamayan & J. S. Damico (Eds.), *Limiting bias in the assessment of bilingual students* (pp. 303–316). Austin, TX: Pro-ed.

Damico, J. S., & Hamayan, E. V. (1992). *Multicultural language intervention: Addressing cultural and linguistic diversity.* Chicago: Riverside Publishers.

Damico, J. S., & Nye, C. (1990). Collaborative issues in multicultural populations. *Best Practices in School Speech-Language Pathology, 1,* 127–140.

Damico, J. S., & Oller, J. W., Jr. (1985). *Spotting language problems.* San Diego: Los Amigos Research Associates.

Damico, J. S., Oller, J. W., Jr., & Storey, M. E. (1983). The diagnosis of language disorders in bilingual children: Pragmatic and Surface-oriented criteria. *Journal of Speech and Hearing Disorders, 48,* 385–394.

Damico, J. S., Secord, W. A., & Wiig, E. H. (1992). Descriptive language assessment at school: Characteristics and design. *Best Practices in School Speech-Language Pathology, 2,* 1–9.

De Avila, E., Cohen, E., & Intili, J. (1981). *Multicultural improvement of cognitive abilities.* Final report to the California State Department of Education.

Deno, S. L. (1985). Curriculum-based measurement: The emerging alternative. *Exceptional Children, 52,* 219–232.

Deyhle, D. (1987). Learning failure: Tests as gatekeepers and the culturally different child. In H. E. Trueba (Ed.), *Success or failure?* (pp. 85–108). Cambridge, MA: Newbury House.

Duranti, A. (1985). Socio-cultural dimensions of discourse. In T. Van Dijk (Ed.), *Handbook of discourse analysis* (pp. 193–230). New York: Academic Press.

Edelsky, C. (1986). *Writing in a bilingual program: Habia Una Vez.* Norwood, NJ: Ablex.

Edelsky, C., Altwerger, B., & Flores, B. (1990). *Whole language: What's the difference?* Portsmouth, NH: Heinemann.

Edelsky, C., Draper, K., & Smith, K. (1983). Hookin' em in at the start of school in a "Whole language classroom". *Anthropology and Education Quarterly, 14,* 257–281.

Eisenberg, A. (1986). Teasing: Verbal play in two Mexican homes. In B. Schieffelin & E. Ochs (Eds.) *Language socialization across cultures* (pp. 182–198). New York: Cambridge University Press.

Eriks-Brophy, A., & Crago, M. (1993). Maintaining face: Elements of classroom discourse with Inuit children. In D. Kovarsky, M. Maxwell, & J. Damico (Eds.), *Language interaction in clinical and educational settings* (pp. 10–17). Rockville, MD: American Speech-Language-Hearing Association.

Flood, J., & Lapp, D. (1989). Reporting reading progress: A comparison portfolio for parents. *The Reading Teacher, 42,* 508–514.

Fradd, S. H., & Weismantel, M. J. (1989). *Meeting the needs of culturally and linguistically different students: A handbook for educators.* Boston: College-Hill Press.

Garcia, S. B., & Ortiz, A. A. (1988). Preventing inappropriate referrals of language minority students to special education. *New Focus: Occasional Papers in Bilingual Education, 5,* 1–12.

Genesee, F. (1992). *Learning through two languages: Studies of immersion and bilingual education.* Boston: Heinle and Heinle.

Goffman, E. (1972). On face-work: An analysis of ritual elements in social interaction. In J. Laver & S. Hutcheson (Eds.), *Communication in face to face interaction* (pp. 35–68). Middlesex, UK: Penguin Books.

Goldman, S., & McDermott, R. (1987). The culture of competition in American schools. In G. Spindler (Ed.), *Education and cultural process* (2nd ed., pp. 282–299). Prospect Heights, IL: Waveland Press.

Goodman, K. (1986). *What's whole in whole language?* Portsmouth, NH: Heinemann.

Goodman, K., & Goodman, Y. (1983). Reading and writing relationships: Pragmatic functions. *Language Arts, 60,* 590–599.

Goodman, K., Goodman, Y., & Hood, W. (Eds.). (1989). *The whole language evaluation book.* Portsmouth, NH: Heinemann.

Goodman, Y. (1985). Kid watching: An alternative to testing. *National Elementary Principal, 57*(4), 41–45.

Goodman, Y. M., Watson, D. J., & Burke, C. L. (1987). *Reading miscue analysis: Alternative procedures.* New York: Robert C. Owens.

Goodwin, C. (1981). *Conversational organization: Interaction between speakers and hearers.* New York: Academic Press.

Goodwin, M. (1990). *He-said-she-said: Talk as social organization among black children.* Bloomington: Indiana University Press.
Gumperz, J. (1983). *Discourse strategies.* Cambridge, UK: Cambridge University Press.
Hakuta, K. (1986). *Mirror of language: The debate on bilingualism.* New York: Basic Books.
Hamayan, E. V., & Damico, J. S. (1991). Developing and using a second language. In E. V. Hamayan & J. S. Damico (Eds.), *Limiting bias in the assessment of bilingual students* (pp. 40–76). Austin, TX: Pro-ed.
Hamayan, E. V., & Perlman, R. (1990). *Helping language minority students after they exit from bilingual/ESL programs.* Washington, DC: NCBE.
Heath, S. B. (1983). *Ways with words.* Cambridge, UK: Cambridge University Press.
Heath, S. B. (1986). Taking a cross-cultural look at narratives. *Topics in Language Disorders, 7,* 84–94.
Hedberg, N. L., & Stoel-Gammon, C. (1986). Narrative analysis: Clinical procedures. *Topics in Language Disorders. 7,* 58–69.
Irvine, J. (1982). Language and affect: Some cross-cultural issues. In H. Byrnes (Ed.), *Georgetown University Roundtable on Languages and Linguistics 1982* (pp. 31–47). Washington, DC: Georgetown University Press.
Irvine, J. T. (1985). Status and style in language. *Annual Review of Anthropology, 14,* 557–581.
Jongsma, K. S. (1989). Portfolio assessment. *The Reading Teacher, 43,* 264–265.
Jonz, J. (1987). Textual cohesion and second-language comprehension. *Language Learning, 37,* 409–438.
Kemp. M. (1990). *Watching children read and write.* Portsmouth, NH: Heinemann.
Kovarsky, D. (1992). Ethnography and language assessment: Toward the contextualized description and interpretation of communicative behavior. *Best Practices in School Speech-Language Pathology, 2,* 115–122.
Lambert, W. E. (1975). Culture and language as factors in learning and education. In A. Wolfgang (Ed.), *Education of immigrant students* (pp. 15–27). Toronto: OISE.
Langdon, H. W., & Cheng, L-R.L. (1992). *Hispanic children and adults with communicative disorders: Assessment and prevention.* Gaithersburg, MD: Aspen.
Larson, V. L., & McKinley, N. L. (1987). *Communication assessment and intervention strategies for adolescents.* Eau Claire, WI: Thinking Publications.
Lidz, C. S. (Ed.). (1987). *Dynamic assessment: Foundations and fundamentals.* New York: Guilford.
Lipski, J. (1985). *Linguistic aspects of Spanish-English language switching.* Tempe, AZ: Center for Latin American Studies.
Loban, W. (1976). *Language development: K–12.* Urbana, IL: NCTE.
Marston, D., & Magnusson, D. (1987). *Curriculum-based measurement: An introduction.* Minneapolis, MN: Minneapolis Public Schools.
Mathews, J. K. (1990). From computer management to portfolio assessments. *The Reading Teacher, 43,* 420–421.
Mattes, L. J. (1985). *Spanish language assessment procedures: A communication skills inventory.* San Diego: Los Amigos.
Mattes, L. J., & Omark, D. R. (1984). *Speech and language assessment for the bilingual handicapped.* San Diego: College-Hill Press.
Michaels, S. (1981). Sharing time: Children's narrative styles and differential access to literacy. *Language in Society, 10,* 423–442.
Michaels, S. (1985). Hearing the connections in children's oral and written discourse. *Journal of Education, 167,* 36–56.
Nelson, N. W. (1992). Targets of curriculum-based language assessment. *Best Practices in School Speech-Language Pathology, 2,* 73–86.
Nelson, N. W. (1993). *Childhood language disorders in context: Infancy through adolescents.* New York: Merrill/Macmillian.
Norris, J. A. (1989). Providing language remediation in the classroom: An integrated language-to-reading intervention model. *Language, Speech, and Hearing Services in Schools, 20,* 205–218.
Norris, J. A., & Damico, J. S. (1990). Whole language in theory and practice: Implications for language intervention. *Language, Speech, and Hearing Services in Schools, 21,* 212–220.
Norris, J. A. & Hoffman, P. R. (1993). *Whole language intervention with school-age children.* San Diego: Singular Press.
Ochs, E. (1986). *Culture and language acquisition: Acquiring communicative competence in a Western Samoan village.* New York: Cambridge University Press.
Oller, J. W., Jr. (1979). *Language tests at school: A pragmatic approach.* London: Longman.
Oller, J. W., Jr. (1983a). A consensus for the 80's? In J. W. Oller, Jr. (Ed.), *Issues in second language testing research* (pp. 351–356). Rowley, MA: Newbury House.
Oller, J. W., Jr. (1983b). Some working ideas for language teaching. In J. W. Oller, Jr. & P. Richard-Amato (Eds.), *Methods that work* (pp. 3–19). Rowley, MA: Newbury House.
Oller, J. W., Jr. (1989). Conclusions toward a rational pragmatism. In J. W. Oller, Jr. (Ed.), *Language and experience* (pp. 223–250). Lanham, MD: University Press of America.

Oller, J. W., Jr. (Ed.). (1993). *Methods that work* (2nd ed.). Boston: Heinle & Heinle.
Oller, J. W., Jr., & Damico, J. S. (1991). Theoretical considerations in the assessment of LEP students. In E. V. Hamayan & J. S. Damico (Eds.), *Limiting bias in the assessment of bilingual students* (pp. 77–110). Austin, TX: Pro-ed.
Oller, J. W., Jr., & Richard-Amato, P. (Eds.). (1983). *Methods that work.* Rowley, MA: Newbury House.
Olshtain, E., & Blum-Kulka, S. (1985). Cross cultural pragmatics and the testing of communicative competence. *Language Testing, 2,* 16–30.
O'Malley, J. M. (1989). Language proficiency testing with limited English-proficient students. In D. Tannen (Ed.), *Georgetown University Round Table on Languages and Linguistics* (pp. 235–244). Washington, DC: Georgetown University Press.
Ortiz, A. A. (1988). Evaluating educational contexts in which language minority students are served. *Bilingual Special Education Newsletter, 7,* 1–4, 7.
Palincsar, A. S., Brown, A. L., & Campione, J. C. (1994). Models and practices of dynamic assessment. In G. P. Wallach & K. G. Butler (Eds.), *Language learning disabilities in school-age children and adolescents: Some principles and applications* (pp. 132–144). New York: Macmillan.
Palincsar, A. S., & Klenk, L. (1992). Fostering literacy learning in supportive contexts. *Journal of Learning Disabilities, 25,* 211–225, 229.
Peck, J. (1989). Using storytelling to promote language and literacy development. *The Reading Teacher, 42,* 138–141.
Peters, A., & Boggs, S. (1986). Interactional routines as cultural influences upon language acquisition. In B. B. Schieffelin & E. Ochs (Eds.), *Language socialization across cultures* (pp. 80–96). New York: Cambridge University Press.
Philips, S. (1983). *The invisible culture.* New York: Longman.
Pils, L. (1991). Soon anofe you tout me: Evaluation in a first-grade whole language classroom. *The Reading Teacher, 45,* 46–50.
Prutting, C. A., & Kirchner, D. M. (1987). A clinical appraisal of the pragmatic aspects of language. *Journal of Speech and Hearing Disorders, 52,* 105–119.
Rice, M. L., Sell, M. A., & Hadley, P. A. (1990). The Social Interactive Coding System (SICS): An online, clinically relevant descriptive tool. *Language, Speech, and Hearing Services in Schools, 21,* 2–14.
Samway, K., Whang, G., Cade, C., & Gamil, M., Lubandina, M. A., & Phommachanh, K. (1991). Reading the skeleton, the heart, and the brain of a book: Students' perspectives on literature study circles. *The Reading Teacher, 45,* 196–206.
Schieffelin, B. B., & Ochs, E. (Eds.). (1986). *Language socialization across cultures.* New York: Cambridge University Press.
Schumann, J. (1976). Social distance as a factor in second language acquisition. *Language Learning, 26,* 135–143.
Schumann, J. (1978). *The pidginization process: A model for second language acquisition.* Rowley, MA: Newbury House.
Scollon R., & Scollon, S. K. (1981). *Narrative, literacy and face in interethnic communication.* Norwood, NJ: Ablex.
Secord, W. A. (1990) (Ed.). *Best Practices in School Speech-Language Pathology, 1,* 1–141.
Secord, W. A., & Wiig, E. H. (1991). *Developing a collaborative language intervention program.* Chicago: Riverside Publishers.
Seymour, S. (1981). Cooperation and Competition: Some issues and problems in cross cultural analysis. In R. Monroe & B. Whiting (Eds.), *Handbook of cross cultural human development* (pp. 192–219). New York: Garland.
Shuy, R. (1981). A holistic view of language. *Research in the Teaching of English, 15,* 101–111.
Silliman, E. R., & Wilkinson, L. C. (1991). *Communicating for learning: Classroom observation and collaboration.* Gaithersburg, MD: Aspen.
Silliman, E. R., & Wilkinson, L. C. (1994). Observation is more than looking. In G. P. Wallach & K. G. Butler (Eds.) *Language learning disabilities in school-age children and adolescents: Some principles and applications* (pp. 145–173). New York: Macmillian.
Simon, C. S. (Ed.). (1987). *Journal of Childhood Communication Disorders, 11.* Topical issue on making the collaborative consultation model work.
Simon, C. S. (1989). *Classroom communication screening procedure for early adolescents: A handbook for assessment and intervention.* Tempe, AZ: Communi-Cog Publications.
Slavin, R. (1986). *Using student team learning.* Baltimore: Johns Hopkins University.
Smith, F. (1988). *Joining the literacy club.* Portsmouth, NH: Heinemann.
Smith, M. (1983). Fragile first attempts at articulation and meaning. In J. L. Locke (Ed.), *Assessing and treating phonological disorders.* New York: Thieme Medical Publishers.
Spradley, J. P. (1980). *Participant observation.* New York: Holt, Rinehart & Winston.
Stabb, C. (1991). Classroom organization: Thematic centers revisited. *Language Arts, 68,* 108–113.

Staton, J. (1983). Dialogue journals: A new tool for teaching communication. *ERIC/CLL News Bulletin*, March.

Tannen, D. (1984). The pragmatics of cross-cultural communication. *Applied Linguistics, 5,* 189–195.

Taylor, O. L. (1977). The sociolinguistic dimension of standardized testing. In M. Saville-Troike (Ed.), *Linguistics and anthropology* (pp. 84–97). Washington, DC: Georgetown University Press.

Taylor, O. L., & Payne, K. T. (1983). Culturally valid testing: A proactive approach. *Topics in Language Disorders. 3,* 8–20.

Trueba, H. T. (1983). Adjustment problems of Mexican-American children: An anthropological study. *Learning Disabilities Quarterly, 5,* 395–415.

Valencia, S. (1990). A portfolio approach to classroom reading assessment: The whys, whats, and hows. *The Reading Teacher, 43,* 338–340.

van Kleeck, A. (1994). Potential cultural bias in training parents as conversational partners with their children who have delays in language development. *American Journal of Speech-Language Pathology, 3,* 67–78.

Vigil, N., & Oller, J. W., Jr. (1976). Rule fossilization: A tentative model. *Language Learning, 26,* 281–295.

Vygotsky, L. S. (1978). *Mind in society.* Cambridge, MA: Harvard University Press.

Wade, S. (1990). Using think alouds to assess comprehension. *The Reading Teacher, 43,* 442–451.

Wells, G. (1986). *The meaning makers: Children learning language and using language to learn.* Portsmouth, NH: Heinemann.

Westby, C. E. (1992). Narrative assessment. *Best Practices in School Speech-Language Pathology, 2,* 53–64.

Westby, C. E. (1994). The effects of culture on genre, structure, and style of oral and written texts. In G. P. Wallach & K. G. Butler (Eds.), *Language learning disabilities in school-age children and adolescents: Some principles and applications* (pp. 180–218). New York: Macmillian.

Westby, C. E., Stevens-Dominguez, M., & Oetter, P. (in press). A performance/competence model of observational assessment. *Language, Speech, and Hearing Services in Schools.*

Willig, A. C., & Ortiz, A. A. (1991). The non-biased Individualized Educational Program: Linking assessment to instruction. In E. V. Hamayan & J. S. Damico (Eds.), *Limiting bias in the assessment of bilingual students* (pp. 241–302). Austin, TX: Pro-ed.

Wolf, D. P. (1989). Portfolio assessment: Sampling student work. *Educational Leadership, 46*(7), 35–39.

Wolfram, W. (1985). The phonologic system: Problems of second language acquisition. In J. M. Costello (Ed.), *Speech disorders in adults* (pp. 59–76), San Diego: College-Hill Press.

Wollman-Bonilla, J. (1989). Reading journals: Invitations to participate in literature. *The Reading Teacher, 42,* 112–119.

Wong-Fillmore, L. (1986). Teaching bilingual learners. In M. C. Wittrock (Ed.), *Handbook of research on teaching* (3rd ed., pp. 648–685). New York: Macmillian.

Young, L. W. L. (1982). Inscrutability revisited. In J. J. Gumperz (Ed.), *Language and social identity* (pp. 72–84). Cambridge, UK: Cambridge University Press.

13

Early Intervention in Communication Development

A Collaborative Model for Professionals Consulting with Families

YVONNE GILLETTE, PH.D.

Introduction

Families now have unprecedented opportunities for promoting the adaptive abilities and, in turn, the social inclusion of the youngest of developmentally at-risk children (infants and toddlers, birth to 36 months of age). These opportunities are due largely to legislation and entitlements implemented by states in response to congressional actions that led to the passage of Public Law (P.L.) 99-457, commonly referred to as the Individuals with Disabilities Education Act (IDEA). Two closely linked mandates characterize local and national IDEA initiatives: (1) that intervention programs must be designed, first and foremost, to enhance the family's capacity to meet the developmental needs of fragile children; and (2) that family-centered teams conduct the work of early intervention, with highest priority assigned to the promotion of social, emotional, cognitive, and linguistic growth among fragile children. Successful efforts will increasingly reduce the demand for later—and more costly—educational or institutional services (Early Intervention, 1989).

This legislation has significant implications for speech-language pathologists who choose to practice in early intervention (EI) programs. First, in response to the IDEA mandates, the role of EI clinicians is to provide family-centered communication interventions, thus accentuating the family's capacity to energize their child's development. Second, the communication interventions implemented by clinicians must reflect directly the contents of an individualized family service plan (IFSP). As an instrument of advocacy, the IFSP is designed to document the child's present behavioral status and, concurrently, promote the child's developmental progression within the family context. The result is that the IFSP is the defining force behind early intervention programming, and its contents determine the options that may be taken along the evaluation-intervention continuum. By acknowledging the advantages of shared responsibility, human service professionals and family members can now work together, as equals, in efforts to identify specific strengths and needs and implement appropriate services (Crais, 1991; Dunst, 1989; Gillette, 1992).

In the early intervention melieu, we may initially assume the role of family consultant as the IFSP takes shape and moves through the negotiation process. In this role, we serve families who differ significantly from one another and who must adjust to communities that vary in the availability of program resources and ready access to practicing professionals representing a variety of backgrounds and disciplines. In light of these realities and to function as responsive consultants, EI clinicians require a flexible system of concrete guidelines for evaluating communicative competence and designing effective intervention programs. Consistent with the practical implications of Bjorklund and Schwartz's adaptability hypothesis (this volume), what we have come to call the Ecological Communicative Program, or ECO, provides a system by which we can accommodate the strengths and respond to the needs of individual families and, in the process, take into account a community's capacity to work hand in hand with family members (Gillette, 1989; MacDonald, 1989).

The Ecological Communication Program

Throughout the 1980s, James MacDonald and I conducted a series of research and development projects, known collectively as the ECO Program (The Nisonger Center for Mental Retardation and Developmental Disabilities at Ohio State University). These projects were motivated by the realization that our far-reaching, traditional reliance on one-to-one, behaviorally oriented therapies has often rendered us ineffective when working with young children in need of resolving communication breakdowns with family members and other significant talkers. The ECO Program takes a contextual perspective, pairing emergent communicators with familiar communicating partners—namely, those native speakers with a vested interest in transforming instances of ineffective language use into acts of communication. The close and frequently exclusive ties between young children and their families prompted a need for early intervention models capable of setting developmental priorities and, in turn, giving concrete direction to families engaged in establishing rapport with their socially and communicatively fragile offspring.

The ECO Program (MacDonald & Gillette, 1984–1988) evolved from our extensive fieldwork with families and early childhood educators. We acted as their consultants no less than they acted as our consultants. Our method focused on the building and maintenance of communicative partnerships rather than communicative modifications of singular individuals. As part of the ECO system, the evaluation process addresses two primary questions: (1) How do children interact and communicate with familiar partners across daily routines? and (2) How do communication partners enhance and meaningfully extend children's communication experiences?

The first evaluation question addresses an individual child's range of interactive experience and, in particular, the study of the child's preferred social routines. It may be unfair to judge children's ability or performance without representative knowledge of their significant or preferred life experiences. Far too many children have alarmingly few opportunities to exercise their communicative skills, let alone realize developmental growth. For example, consider the plight of children with severe physical impairments for whom daily care routines occupy large amounts of time and energy, or children in high-risk groups for whom experience is restricted due to adverse family circumstances. Obviously, the impact of such differences in daily experience must be factored into the diagnostic equation.

The second question addresses issues related to the course of intervention. Recently, various researchers (Bjorklund & Schwartz, this volume; Goodman, 1992) have challenged the appropriateness of using behavioral techniques to impose more mature and sophisticated forms of behavior on an immature child. They argue that instruction keyed to and literally resonating with the child's current level of functioning is developmentally appropriate and is more apt to produce enduring developmental growth.

Evaluations and interventions conducted under ECO systems address four communication outcomes. Each specific outcome is associated with the formation and maintenance of partnerships between children and their trusted companions:

- Active and consistent participation in a suitable variety of social and functional routines
- Balanced interaction of communication partners within an increasing variety of social and functional routines
- Match of intent and content between the actions and messages that partners contribute to engaging routines
- Successful communication and shared enjoyment (conversation and persuasion) between partners.

The first outcome addresses the content and variety of the child's common (expected) experiences. The subsequent outcomes address functional communication development, with the child's communication partners taking on the role of primary agents of change and, with it, targeting what we call balance, match, and emotionality (what ECO takes to be the central features of developmentally appropriate intervention plans).

The effective use of ecologically grounded approaches to evaluation and intervention may require major shifts in orientation for clinicians who have become allied with traditional clinician-to-client therapy models. Our own collaborative work with clinicians suggests that an ecological approach—both as process and product—is more attuned to clinicians' intuitions and sense for what constitutes responsive intervention: therapy models that are compellingly interactive and contextually sound. Increasingly more, clinicians report that a programmatic emphasis on child-and-partner behaviors yields functional clinical outcomes; the ECO Program simply organizes these intuitions in a clinically useful manner.

This chapter is designed to guide EI clinicians in the practice of early intervention through the use of developmentally appropriate activities with families and young children. First we will discuss the multiple factors that influence a family's decision to feature communication intervention in the IFSP text. Next we consider the specifics of conducting evaluations in which the child—as emergent communicator—is the focus of communicating partnerships. Following this, we consider the design and day-to-day conduct of interventions that activate communication partnerships. We conclude with a brief review of case studies selected to illustrate both the stability and flexibility of ECO principles as used in three common early intervention settings (home, day care, and center/classroom settings).

Nature and Differentiating Features

Early developmental vulnerabilities and at-risk conditions frequently remain undetected in spite of legislation designed to enable families to obtain the assistance and services they need for their young children. For example, Meisels and Wasik (1990) reported on data from the state of Michigan, but not unique to it, indicating that in the recent past no more than 0.7% of infants and toddlers (birth to 36 months) were identified as being at risk for or having significant developmental disabilities. Compare this figure to the much higher percentage of children identified at the age of 9 years—no less than 12.6%. An identification rate of this order merits our undivided attention, and it clearly indicates that early intervention programs face formidable challenges. Simply put, there is much work to be done by EI practitioners if we are to reverse the costly direction of such identification growth patterns.

Early intervention or IDEA standards define disability along the lines first proposed by Tjosemm (1976), who classified developmental risk conditions under three categories: established diagnosis, biological vulnerability, and environmental risk. Established diagnosis includes children who will experience a range of known developmental disabilities associated, for example, with Down syndrome, spina bifida, or cleft palate. Biological vulnerability includes children at risk for experiencing the consequences of a fragile biological history associated, for example, with prematurity, maternal substance abuse, or anoxia. Environmental risk acknowledges those children at risk due to intrusive domestic forces and unstable family dynamics, including social isolation and inadequate day care, substandard housing, inadequate health care, or poor nutrition. These factors impose stressful demands on families and the youngest of children.

The potential for overlap among the diverse categories of established diagnosis, biological vulnerability, and environmental risk is inherent to the problems of determining eligibility for participation in early intervention programs. Clinicians practicing as members of the early intervention team must be aware that child performance data alone are rarely sufficient for adequate identification in early intervention. Multiple factor approaches vary considerably in their composition, with the most successful including biological and environmental histories along with child diagnostic and performance data. Data from Bee, Barnard, and Eyres (1982) illustrate the complexity of identification by indicating that different information is more predictive at different time points. For example, family functioning and family perception of the child appears most predictive at birth. However, at age 2, child performance on standardized tests paired with systematic observation of the home environment appears most useful and predictive.

Clinicians face an additional problem beyond identification for early intervention services. They must determine which families qualify for specific services in speech-language intervention. Because IFSPs are individualized, the pattern of family strengths and needs will influence which services the plan includes and their priority within the plan. Although the professionals on the team provide input to the family, it is the family who ultimately decides the priority for each service in the plan.

Evaluation

Clinicians working in an ecological model conduct evaluations that assist families as they make decisions regarding their overall intervention plan and the priority of communication intervention within the plan. Because the ECO Program components and related clinical tools (Gillette, 1989; MacDonald, 1989; Gillette & MacDonald, 1989; MacDonald, Gillette, & Hutchinson, 1989) are so comprehensive, three new tools adapted from the ECO Program but directed toward infants and toddlers in particular will be featured here: the ECO Daily Life Chart, the Ecological Communication Guidelines, and the ECO Intervention Planning Guide. The ECO Program promotes a contextual perspective, evaluating the child within daily life routines and in relationship to communicating partners. When designing an evaluation in response to an IFSP, it is essential to take this contextual perspective. To do this systematically, a three-step procedure should be followed:

1. Conduct an ecological evaluation, viewing the child in the context of daily life. Note where and with whom the child spends time and determine the frequency and variety of social and functional routines in which the child participates.
2. Conduct a partnership evaluation, viewing the child in the context of communication partners. Evaluate this partner-child relationship within routines by noting the following: (1) balance in child and partner contributions to routines, (2) similarities between child and partner behavior/communication within routines (progressive match), and (3) mutual enjoyment during the routines.
3. Conduct a dynamic evaluation (Feuerstein, Rand, & Hoffman, 1979; Olswang, Bain, & Johnson, 1992) to determine how the child's behavior changes in relationship to changes in routines and partner strategies. Interact with the child by varying routines and partner strategies until positive change in the child's behavior occurs.

Ecological Evaluation

An ecological evaluation should be conducted to determine the intensity of the child's participation in daily life. Children develop in diverse circumstances, and few assumptions can be made about the life of any child. Conducting an ecological communication evaluation requires that clinicians become aware of the actual circumstances in which each child develops. This will enable clinicians to avoid making incorrect assumptions. The measures relevant to ecological evaluation include (1) where the child spends time (situations), (2) how much time is spent in each situation (3) with whom the child spends time (partners), (4) the frequency and variety of social and functional routines in which the child participates, and (5) typical amounts of time spent in specific routines with partners.

This information may be gathered from interviews, observations, or a combination of available sources. When carrying out an ecological evaluation, clinicians should sample behavior across the range of settings in which the child often spends time. These can include the family home, day care, the home of a relative or neighbor, the grocery store, or a familiar park. Finally, a representative evaluation must include reference to commonly occurring routines and relevant participants.

To assist in organizing the data collected, the ECO Daily Life Chart (Fig. 13–1) provides a helpful format. As a display, it allows intervention teams, in company with families, to review the child's present life circumstances in a realistic manner. With a visual display of the essential variables (situation, partners, and routine) it is possible for all team members to contribute ideas to a communication intervention plan designed to enrich the child's participation in daily life. Often, teams will create opportunities for communication in naturally occurring events once they understand that more participation in life leads to improved communication skills.

Partnership Evaluation

A partnership evaluation acknowledges that no individual operates in isolation. Partners influence the child's interaction and communication across situations within interactive routines. To conduct a partnership evaluation, the clinician needs to observe the child's communicative behavior in functional and social routines. Examples of such routines might include mealtime interactions with a day care teacher, playing with a parent at home, and discussing a television program with a grandparent.

What at first appear to be obstacles (e.g., issues of organization and direction of interactions) to the efficient planning and execution of dynamic partnership evaluations can be overcome through the use of the Ecological Communication (ECO) Guidelines (Fig. 13–2). These guidelines feature child skills and partner strategies that lead to desirable communication experiences framed within familiar routines. The ECO Guidelines provide a vantage point from which clinicians can plan for communication outcomes in terms of specific child skills and partner strategies. The theoretical and empirical bases for the outcomes that comprise the ECO Guidelines are described next.

OUTCOME 1: PARTICIPATE IN VARIED SOCIAL AND FUNCTIONAL ROUTINES

These routines include social interactions (Stern, 1977), formats (Bruner, 1983), and joint activities (Bronfenbrenner, 1979) to which both partners contribute turns (Kaye & Charney, 1980) in the form of actions and messages. Routines may be socially motivated, such as in games of peek-a-boo or pat-a-cake and play with preferred toys or dolls. Routines may also be functionally motivated, such as those occurring during mealtime, bath time, shopping trips, or riding together in a car or on public transportation. Social and functional routines provide opportunities for partners to engage in appropriate actions and exchange messages that

Partners Situations/Routines											

Rate each in square as O = Often, S = Sometimes
(Do not include infrequent routines)

Figure 13–1. ECO daily life chart.

gradually increase the child's understanding of the world and how to use acts of communication to become an active part of the world.

Bruner (1983) maintains that the routines allow the child to witness first hand how language works. He draws parallels between the basic formats of social games and the underlying structures of language. Games, like language, have underlying structures that are realized in a variety of surface structures through the application of realization rules. Bruner illustrates this point by citing the early appearance of the peek-a-boo routine. At the surface, peek-a-boo appears to be a simple activity. However, it can vary considerably in regard to who initiates the

OUTCOME 1: Participate in varied social and functional routines

Child Skills
- Stay with others in play/daily living routines
- Contact others to initiate a variety of routines
- Interact/converse for a variety of reasons

Partner Strategies:
- Contact the child frequently
- Follow the child's lead

Measures of Participation:
- Where the child spends time (situations)
- How much time spent in each situation
- With whom the child spends time (partners)
- The frequency and variety of social and functional routines in which the child participates
- Typical amounts of time spent in routines with partners

OUTCOME 2: Balance participation in routines

Child Skills:
- Show a turntaking play style
- Imitate others

Partner Strategies:
- Maintain and balance turntaking in play
- Maintain and balance turntaking in conversations
- Wait, signal, and expect
- Respond with actions and messages
- Imitate the child at times

Measures of Balance:
- Ratio of actions each partner contributes to the routine
- Ratio of messages each partner contributes to the routine

OUTCOME 3: Act and communicate in progressively matched ways

Child Skills:
- Imitate actions and messages partners use
- Use actions and messages in functional and meaningful ways
- Use varied messages (gestures, sounds, signs, words, phrases)
- Make self understood

Partner Strategies:
- Model actions and messages the child can imitate
- Match child behavior, play in childlike ways
- Communicate in ways close to the child
- Comment more than question or command
- Develop verbal topics with the child

Measures of Match:
- Number, range, and functionality of actions each partner contributes to a routine
- Number, range, complexity, and appropriateness of messages each partner contributes to a routine
- Similarity between these measures for each partner

OUTCOME 4: Share enjoyment

Child Skills:
- Show enjoyment through face and voice
- Contact others for fun

Partner Strategies:
- Be animated
- Use positive comments
- Have social, friendly conversations with the child

Measures of Enjoyment:
- A rating of the pleasure each partner derives from being together in routines

Figure 13–2. Ecological communication guidelines.

activity (child or partner), how the activity is initiated (gesture, touch, vocalization, or word), the length of pauses between turns, how one's face is covered (hands or scarf), the intensity or number of turns taken, the amount and type of accompanying verbal behavior, and who terminates the activity and in what fashion. Clearly, peek-a-boo has many variations and may never unfold in exactly the same way from one time to another. Much the same can be said for any routine dissected in this manner.

Variation within and across routines expands the child's dynamic experiences and adds meaning to participation in joint activities. Unfortunately, young children who are at risk or disabled often participate in daily life in limited ways (Mahoney, 1988; Massie, 1980; Merighi, Edison, & Zigler, 1990). At the least, this limited participation may contribute to an overall delay in communication development. In contrast, regular and repeated experience with motivating routines enables the young child to build and extend interaction skills and, thus, engage in increasingly sophisticated acts of communication (Bjorklund & Schwartz, this volume; Goodman, 1992).

Outcome 1, or the participation in varied social and functional routines, of the ECO Guidelines (Fig. 13–2) lends organization to our descriptions of the child's preferred routines and the nature of the interactions that typically occur. We are presented with practical information related to specific child skills, partner strategies for maintaining and extending activities, and concrete measures of participation (MacDonald, 1989; MacDonald & Carroll, 1992).

OUTCOME 2: BALANCED PARTICIPATION IN ROUTINES

A key concept in Bronfenbrenner's (1979) views on the ecology of human development is the balance of power. His work suggests that development best occurs within relationships in which the balance of power gradually shifts toward the developing person. With these shifts, the youngest of children are primed to become active learners and the major participants in joint activity routines.

Bruner (1983) also notes the importance of balanced participation in the framework of the handover principle and the descriptive motto "Where before there was a spectator, let there now be a participant." Along similar lines, Stern (1977) referred to "attunement," Kaye and Charney (1980) to "turnarounds," and Als, Tronick, and Brazelton (1979) to "mutual feedback systems." Whatever the descriptor used, there is a growing consensus among researchers that children begin to learn language by making repetitive contributions—along with their partners—to the interactive routines of daily life.

As Stern (1977) pointed out, the critical ingredients to managing gradual power shifts and, next, maintaining balanced participation are timing and structure. A variety of factors affect the interplay of timing and structure, with a prominent one being the physical stability (in degrees) of individuals and the extent to which they can explore and regularly participate in the environment. Clearly, because children with disabilities experience less stability in their daily lives than their peers do, child and partner dyads must work harder at negotiating delicate balances and maintaining productive interactions. If this work is not done, the risk is that children with disabilities will effectively default, become dominated by partners, and grow into less than fulfilled adults (Buckhalt,

Rutherford, & Goldberg, 1978; Cunningham, Blackwell, Reuler, & Deck, 1981; Jones, 1980; Mahoney, Finger, & Powell, 1985; Merighi et al., 1990; Records, Tomblin, & Freese, 1992).

It will likely take patient adjustments on the part of native-speaking partners to achieve balance with a child who experiences instability and is slower to respond due to sensory or motor impairments. The literal pacing of interaction will be critical, with the child given the necessary freedom and the time to formulate spontaneous contributions to communicative routines.

To determine whether participation in routines is balanced, clinicians may use the ECO Guidelines to observe a variety of social and functional interactions across partners noting the following child skills and partner strategies:

Child Skills

- Show a turn-taking play style.
- Imitate others.

Partner Strategies

- Maintain and balance turn-taking in play (take one turn, then wait for the child to take a turn).
- Wait, signal, and expect the child to take a turn.

If the child is verbal

- Maintain and balance conversations with the child (comment once, then wait for the child to do the same).

Strategies that shift the balance of power toward the child

- Respond to the child with action and/or messages.
- Imitate the child at times.

OUTCOME 3: ACT AND COMMUNICATE IN PROGRESSIVELY MATCHED WAYS

Interactions structured to increase a child's contributions to routines include a factor known as a progressive match (MacDonald & Gillette, 1985, 1986, 1988). Progressive match is achieved when the partners behave in ways that the child can and occasionally a challenging step above. Many scholars have acknowledged the importance of this notion in development. Piaget (1951) notes that children form schemas based on experiences that are moderately incongruent with their existing mental structures and cannot incorporate those that are highly novel. Hunt (1965) calls the notion a "minimal discrepancy," Vygotsky (1962) calls it "the zone of optimal development," and Bruner (1983) calls it "fine tuning." The notion is also central to Van Dijk's sequence of interpersonal methods (Stillman & Battle, 1984).

Children learn through observation and practice when partners provide models of behavior that are similar to the child's. Bandura's social learning theory (1977) is grounded in the notion that learning occurs through observation and practice. Social learning theory postulates that children learn much of what they know by observing adult models and repeating their behavior. Once learned, the behavior becomes part of the child's repertoire without the necessity of the model's presence.

Bandura cites a study by Valentine (1930) that shows that infants imitate their mothers more than others and that although they often fail to respond to initial demonstrations, they will do so when an action is repeated a number of times. He concludes from Valentine's study that infants appear to vary in their performance based on who the models are, what they select to model, and how they do model. Bandura also notes the importance of affective responding to infant behavior. He cites the work of Lovaas (1967), which indicates that "young children imitate accurately when they have incentives to do so, but their imitations deteriorate rapidly if others do not care how they behave" (p. 32).

The notion of progressively matched modeling strongly suggests that effective partners do things the child can do as well as model novel actions and messages that are only slightly discrepant with the child's performance. This indicates that it is essential for the child's partners to understand the child's current performances, in terms of both action and vocalization/verbalization, to provide the appropriate match (Goodman, 1992). Imitating the child fosters a sensorimotor understanding of the child's current performance. However, imitating the child is rarely a sufficient intervention. The child also needs models of progressively matched behaviors and messages to practice and incorporate into his behavioral and verbal repertoire.

An experiment by Kaye (1976) indicated that mothers were likely to model a learning task for a child if the child came close to performing it on a pretest. However, mothers were directive if the child did not exhibit a close performance. This experiment indicates that partners may need intervention before they consider a teaching strategy which consists of adjusting their models to match more closely the children's performances. Without intervention, many partners may continue to rely on the strategy of directing children to perform outside of their capabilities. A study by Cheseldine and McConkey (1979) also indicates that modeling may not be the strategy of natural choice for all partners. They instructed parents to teach 20 target words to their children with Down's syndrome. The results showed that parents who were the most effective language teachers provided the child with models of target words. Some parents used questions and commands, but they were the least successful.

These studies have strong implications for communication interventions with partners. Not all partners will intuitively use modeling as a teaching strategy. Partners who rely on questions do not provide models of the communicative behavior they expect. Partners who direct a child's behavior verbally by telling them what to do do not provide action and verbal models for the child to follow (Goodman, 1992).

Clinicians may now use the ECO Guidelines to organize an evaluation of the child skills and partner strategies which contribute to the outcome and communicate in progressively matched ways.

Child Skills

- Imitate actions partners use.
- Use actions in functional and meaningful ways.

As the child increases verbal skills

- Imitate messages partner's use.
- Use varied messages (gestures, sounds, signs, words, phrases).
- Make self understood.

Partner Strategies

- Model actions and messages the child may be able to imitate.
- Match the child's behavior.
- Play in childlike ways.
- Communicate in ways close to the child.
- Communicate about immediate experiences.
- Comment more than question or command.

If the child is verbal

- Develop verbal topics with the child.

OUTCOME 4: SHARE ENJOYMENT

Bronfenbrenner (1979) hypothesized that developmental impact will be enhanced if the context of a primary dyad is characterized by mutuality of positive feeling (one learns more from a teacher with whom one has a close relationship). Greenspan (1985), Bruner (1983), and Stern (1986), among others, also note the importance of emotional attachment to development and to effective communication.

Positive emotion is an essential ingredient in the process of learning and living together. It may be the most difficult component to prescribe and measure in a communication intervention program because clinicians may fear that by prescribing enjoyment they are implying a judgment about how a partner feels about a child. However, it is easier to perform this portion of the evaluation by remembering that it is never clear which partner runs the show in terms of the emotionality of the partnership (Bell, 1968, 1971, 1977).

Murray and Trevarthen (1986) devised an ingenious experiment to determine whether infants affect maternal behaviors. Eight dyads including 2- to 3-month-old infants interacted over video monitors. In one condition, both members of the dyads were shown to each other live. In the other condition, the infant behavior from the live interaction was replayed to the mother, who thought the infant's video was live. In the live condition, mothers worked off infant behavior, commented positively about the infant, and responded to what the infant did. In the replay, mothers directed the child, called the child's attention, corrected the child, and made negative comments. From this experiment, it is clear that infant behavior influences mother behavior.

Tronick, Als, and Adamson (1979) studied infant influences in another way. They had mothers interrupt a happy play routine by showing the infant a passive face. The infants reacted by vocalizing, turning their heads, and waving their hands to regain the partner's attention. When they finally gave up, they became notably distressed. This observation indicates that infants do appear to be aware that they influence partner behavior.

With these studies in mind, it is apparent that emotion-based child outcomes and partner strategies are essential to a successful communication intervention plan. This fourth guideline may be used to observe systematically the affective nature of partnerships in terms of child skills and partner strategies:

Child Skills

- Show enjoyment in face and voice.
- Contact others for fun.

Partner Strategies

- Be animated (show enjoyment through facial and vocal expression).
- Use positive comments.

If the child is verbal

- Have social, friendly conversations with the child.

Dynamic Evaluation

Describing the child's present communicating partnerships is not sufficient for contributing potential communication outcomes to an IFSP. Next, determine the child's ability for greater participation in daily life routines by conducting a dynamic evaluation. To conduct a dynamic evaluation, engage the child in a variety of routines and alter partner strategies to determine if greater participation results from these changes. Use strategies from the ECO Guidelines while interacting with the child. In particular, use the strategies the partners used which led to the most successful interactions. In addition, use strategies which observation suggested could have contributed to more successful interaction. These commonly include waiting, commenting, behaving in ways similar to the child's, and simply having fun. Note changes that occur in the child's behavior when altering routines and partner strategies. The results of the dynamic evaluation will become the fuel for planning effective intervention programs.

ECO Evaluation: Summary

Evaluations that reflect children in the context of their daily routines and partners lead to effective communication intervention programs. An evaluation for intervention includes three components: ecological evaluation, partnership evaluation, and dynamic evaluation. The ECO Daily Life Chart organizes the information needed for the ecological evaluation. It provides a visual display of the child's opportunities for communication skills to develop in terms of situations, partners, and routines. The ECO Guidelines provide a flexible structure for conducting the partnership evaluation and dynamic evaluation. The next section provides explicit guidance for developing intervention plans from information gathered in the evaluations.

Intervention

The ECO Program promotes interventions designed on the basis of evaluation of children in the context of their daily lives and partners. To facilitate this process, information gathered during the ecological, partnership, and dynamic evaluations with the ECO Daily Life Chart and the Ecological Communication Guidelines translates directly to the ECO Intervention Planning Guide (Fig. 13–3). This tool provides an outline which clinicians can use to focus the group discussion involved in planning communication interventions with families and teams. The ECO Intervention Planning Guide addresses the requirements of an IFSP by including the following plan components:

SITUATIONS: Home School Other __________ __________

ROUTINES: (Social) __________ __________ __________
(Functional) __________ __________ __________

PARTNERS: __________ __________ __________

OUTCOMES: (participate, balance, match, enjoy)

1. __________

Measure: __________

2. __________

Measure: __________

CHILD SKILLS: __________

PARTNER STRATEGIES:

PRACTICE SCHEDULE:

Routine: __________ Time of Day: __________ Length of Time: __________

Routine: __________ Time of Day: __________ Length of Time: __________

Routine: __________ Time of Day: __________ Length of Time: __________

Figure 13–3. ECO communication intervention planning guide.

1. Situations, partners, and routines in which intervention will occur
2. Communication outcomes
3. Child skills and partner strategies which facilitate achieving outcomes
4. Measures of progress
5. A practice schedule.

Models of Intervention

Although many options to service delivery exist, communities vary in terms of the range of models in which they deliver services. Service providers typically locate within schools, hospitals, or other community centers. Some speech-language services for infants and toddlers may be provided directly by the clinician in one-to-one sessions, small groups, or as part of a classroom program. However, the mandates of family-centered intervention prompt clinicians to provide services as consultants to families or to interdisciplinary programs. In any case, families and intervention teams work together to design the program that best meets the needs of the child within the family. If families do not feel that the plan developed meets their child's needs, they can take advantage of the due process required by law if the situation is not resolved with their team (Biklen, 1992).

The ECO Consultant Model

Developing the skills necessary to function as an effective consultant is a never-ending process (Weinberg, 1985). However, clinicians who provide intervention within the framework of the ECO Program have a distinct advantage because the ECO principles and the ECO clinical tools greatly facilitate their role as a consultant. The principles promote the central role of the child's daily life routines and partners in successful communication intervention. The three ECO clinical tools described in this chapter require input from the family and intervention team for successful completion. Once intervention begins, the ECO consultant model (Gillette, 1989) recommends that intervention sessions be conducted with the child and partners to complete four clinical processes within each intervention session: assess, plan/educate, practice, and integrate into daily life. These clinical processes are described next.

ASSESS

We assess to begin new programs, monitor progress in existing programs, and plan continued intervention. Assessment for and of intervention is guided by a review of the ECO Guidelines in conjunction with a review of any previously developed ECO Intervention Planning Guides. Assessment involves sampling the child's current life situations, the routines and partners within each situation, and the child skills and partner strategies that contribute to the four ECO communication outcomes: participation, balance, match, and enjoyment.

PLAN/EDUCATE

At the outset, clinicians should plan a preliminary intervention using the ECO Intervention Planning Guide to select the targets of the plan in terms of situations, routines, partners, outcomes, measures, child skills, and partner strategies and to determine a practice schedule. Note that the plan developed here is preliminary and will change depending on how well the plan endures during the discussions of the education process and actual rehearsal of some aspects of the plan during the practice process. This preliminary plan will be finalized during the last process, in which the team decides how to integrate the plan into daily life.

The child's partners will function best if they understand the reasons behind the plan's components. Because the plan contains a variety of components, it may be necessary to target one or two for open discussion. The educational needs of the partners may change as they participate in the intervention process. Often, initial sessions must focus on the role that daily life routines and partners play in conducting intervention. This is because so many partners assume that communication intervention occurs between the child and the clinician in a one-to-one session. Later, the significance of the ECO communication outcomes to the success of the program becomes essential. Partner strategies or child skills also make valuable contributions to the continuing education of the partner.

Educating the partners can occur through a variety of methods. Discussion during the planning portion of the intervention session is one important method. However, partners will learn during the practice portion of the session as well. Some partners find it useful to view videotaped samples of their interactions with the child and to use the samples as the basis of their discussion. Video models of routines between other partners and children can also be useful (Gillette, 1993; MacDonald & Gillette, 1989; McConkey, 1988). Once they leave the session, some partners may find it helpful to read further information. Descriptions of some outcomes, child skills, and partner strategies can be found in the ECO Resources (Gillette & MacDonald, 1989).

Clinicians familiar with the ECO model have found these guidelines to be essential in planning and educating partners (adapted from Gillette, 1989, p. 13):

1. *Start small and build.* Rather than constructing an elaborate plan that the partner may find cumbersome and difficult to follow, work for a small but noticeable change. Partners will often be eager to build on these small but successful plans, whereas they may get discouraged with too much planning and not enough action early on.
2. *Use strengths as well as concerns in the plan.* Plans rarely succeed when built on concerns. Consider the child is entire profile to construct the intervention plan logically. For example, a partner may not be balanced or matched in interactions with the child. However, this same partner is conscientious and so can be counted on to practice according to the schedule determined in the plan. Conscientiousness can provide the fuel for change.
3. *Trust your working partner.* Professionals often assume the attitude that "we know best." However, in the ECO model, partner contributions to the plan and its execution are essential to success. Let the partner's input guide your plan. Through negotiation, you will create a realistic plan as well as one which the partner feels invested in and committed to.

PRACTICE

It is rarely sufficient to tell a partner what to do. Modeling is often a more effective tool for behavior change. Just as clinicians expect the partners to model for the child, clinicians will be most successful with partners when they model routines with the child which partners observe and practice.

This three-step approach often produces effective results (Gillette, 1989):

- Model a routine with the child as the partner observes.
- Observe the partner in a similar routine with the child.
- Provide feedback on the performance, relating it to child outcomes and partner strategies. Typical forms of feedback include another model or verbal comments.

Ideally, the consultant and a partner take turns practicing brief (less than 1 minute) routines with the child. Feedback should also be brief, focusing on one or two points. It often works best if the consultant provides a positive comment before suggesting directions for change.

Practice provides the partner with a model to observe as well as a sensorimotor experience of how the plan works with the child. Alternatives include providing video examples of other similar pairs which the partners view or providing video examples of the clinician performing with the child. These alternatives may be helpful when the program design does not allow much direct contact with the child's partners.

INTEGRATE INTO DAILY LIFE

The purpose of this step is to bridge the gap between a practice session and the child's daily life with partners. Ideally, intervention motivates the child's total life experience toward promoting his or her communication skills. The child and partners who accomplish this integration successfully will establish a habit of participating together in regularly occurring balanced, enjoyable routines. The child learns new actions and messages when the partners provide progressively matched models within these routines.

Clinicians should recommend that partners establish regular practice times for themselves and the child and incorporate the strategies into their spontaneous contacts with the child. Scheduled practice will allow the partner to focus on practicing the strategies that are part of the plan. Spontaneous practice will assist in achieving the goal of integration into daily life.

Clinicians should advise partners to monitor their practice in some way. Some partners may feel comfortable monitoring the outcomes and their own use of strategies in a systematic chart. Others may prefer some sort of diary. Partners who keep some record of their program provide more systematic input to the shape of the plan as the program continues to develop (Gillette & MacDonald, 1989). Common measures of participation in ecological programs include the number and range of routines and the length of time in the routine. For example, measure balance by comparing the number of partner turns compared to child turns. Use number and complexity of actions and messages used in the routine (by both partners) to measure match. Enhance the measures with examples of typical actions and messages. Finally, measure enjoyment by rating your perceptions of the amount of pleasure each partner derived from being together.

ECO Intervention: Summary

Ecologically based intervention programs include these components:

Assess

- Compare the partnership observed to the ideal described by the ECO Communication Guidelines.

Plan/Educate

- Plan child outcomes, partner strategies, and routines for practice. Educate partners so they understand the reasons that motivate the plan.

Practice

- Use a three-step approach to provide partners with experiences in interacting and communicating effectively with the child: (1) model routines, (2) observe the partner, and (3) provide feedback. Practice several routines using this design.

Integrate into daily life

- Recommend that partners practice in scheduled and spontaneous contacts. Decide on a practice schedule and a method partners use to monitor the program.

The following section uses case examples to illustrate how the ECO Program can be implemented, with the clinician acting as a consultant in three three distinct service delivery models.

Models of ECO Intervention

Models of treatment vary in intensity and will be influenced by the decisions the intervention team makes when it designs the IFSP (Gillette, 1992). Three typical models of ECO interventions are presented here: (1) a clinician consulting with a parent-child partnership as a primary component of an IFSP; (2) a clinician consulting to a caregiver in a day care setting attended by one child with a disability; and (3) a clinician consulting to a teacher providing a multidisciplinary program to a group of 10 children with disabilities.

Model 1: Parent-Child Intervention

This mother and child pair became involved in communication intervention due to an interdisciplinary developmental assessment and a consensus between the mother and her team members during an IFSP update. The professionals had sufficient knowledge of communication development to make an appropriate referral and fostered the mother's decision to incorporate communication intervention in her IFSP. The referral shows the importance of interdisciplinary collaboration.

DEVELOPMENTAL ASSESSMENT

The child, Christie, had been born prematurely and was routinely evaluated every 3 months through the neonatal follow-up clinic at a hospital. The clinic's assessment team had developed an IFSP with the mother which primarily included attendance at this clinic for medical and developmental follow-up. This single mother came to the clinic as she was scheduled even though transportation was a major problem.

At this 12-month assessment, the team had completed the Hawaii Early Learning Profile (HELP; Furono et al., 1985) with the mother; it indicated that Christie functioned at a 9-month level in motor, cognition, and self-help skills. However, social and communication measures of 6 months indicated that Christie had not changed much in these skills since her last assessment.

IFSP UPDATE

At the conclusion of the clinic visit, the mother and her team updated the IFSP. In light of the information the mother had obtained from the HELP regarding Christie's communication skills, she decided to take part in the communication intervention program the team recommended. They suggested that the service could be offered as a home-based or center-based program. Due to her transportation problems, the mother decided that home-based programming was her choice and signed a form requesting once-a-week contact with a speech-language pathologist in her home.

COMMUNICATION INTERVENTION

At this first visit, the clinician wanted to motivate the mother to participate in the intervention. She knew that if the mother were involved in the assessment, had some success in practicing the intervention, and felt she knew what to do on her own, she would likely be more motivated. Conducting an ECO assessment for intervention would lead immediately to the active intervention plan she needed. She used the four clinical processes—assess, plan/educate, practice, and integrate into daily life—during her first visit.

Assess. The Clinician used the ECO Guidelines to guide to guide her assessment. The first outcome, "Participate in a variety of social and functional routines," could be measured through an interview using the ECO Daily Life Chart. Because the clinician and the mother would need to complete the chart together, the clinician knew it could also help her begin to build a relationship with the mother.

To complete the analysis, the mother and the clinician discussed a typical day with Christie, determining where and with whom Christie spent time and what she did with others. Once completed, it was apparent that Christie spent most of her day in the house with her mother and in functionally based routines like feeding, diapering, bathing, and bedtime.

When the clinician asked the mother to play with Christie, it was apparent that play was something the mother expected Christie to do on her own. The mother surrounded her child with dolls and other toys, but Christie did not do much with them yet. The mother primarily observed or suggested things for Christie to do, such as "Make the dolly walk" or "Give mommy the ball."

Plan/Educate. The pair's isolated life concerned the clinician but would probably require another revision to the IFSP to address completely. So, for today, she would develop an intervention plan that helped the two of them play together, establish balance, act and communicate in progressively matched ways, and enjoy one another. Although this was a lot to expect to accomplish, the clinician felt that once the mother could observe some successful routines, she would learn quickly. At the same time, the clinician would be educating the mother about the importance of these kinds of interactions for herself and her child.

Practice. To start things off, the clinician took the dolly and hugged it, saying "ooo ooo." Then she extended it to Christie and waited with a smile. The routine took off as follows (C stands for Christie, CL for clinician):

C: (Took the doll and held it close.)
CL: (Tickled Christie's cheek to get her attention, and held out her hand to signal "my turn." Then she waited with anticipation.)
C: (Extended the doll.)
CL: (Hugged the doll again.) "baby, baby." (Extended it to C.)
C: (Laughed and took the doll, patting the doll's back.)

CL: (Reached over and imitated, patting the doll, adding) "ooo ooo."
C: (Extended the doll sounding "ah" to call attention.)

At this point, the clinician decided to involve the mother, so she took the doll, patted the doll's head, said "baby," and extended the doll to the mother, lending support through a smile. This led to a three-way practice session (M stands for mother):

M: (Held the doll.) "nice baby, nice baby." (Looked up and wondered what to do.)
CL: (Pointed to C to signal M to give C the doll.)
C: (Took the doll, smiled at her mother.)
M: (Smiled back.)
C: (Held the doll close, made soft sounds.)
CL: (Leaned over and imitated the soft sounds near C, then signaled to the mother to do the same.)
M: (Imitated the sounds, then leaned back and waited.)
C: (Made more soft sounds, then extended the doll to her mother.)

The clinician gave the mother this feedback: "Christie responded so well when you used the kinds of actions and messages she uses herself. Imitating her sounds got her to make more sounds, just what we want. I was so glad you waited to see if she'd give you the doll; now we know what she can do." The mother responded, "I'd never really played that way with Christie before. I guess I didn't realize that what I did could make such a difference in what she did."

The feedback and response became an outline of the child skills and partner strategies the clinician would recommend in the ECO Intervention Planning Guide she would develop with the mother. The clinician suggested that they practice a few more routines. The three of them practiced rolling a ball and pushing a car back and forth and simply had fun imitating each other's sounds and movements.

Integrate into Daily Life. The mother and the clinician developed a plan which included the four play routines they had practiced, outcomes, child skills for Christie, and strategies for the mother based on the ECO Guidelines. The clinician also gave the mother some suggestions of messages to use in the routines. After discussing various ways to monitor the program, the mother decided to complete a diary on their kitchen calendar, including how many times they practiced each routine and a particularly interesting point about their best routine each day.

They agreed to meet again in a week. The mother had something to do that would help her and Christie communicate together more effectively. The clinician had an idea of where to go with this program, expanding this pair's routines to include more play. Once this mother-child pair played together regularly, the clinician could incorporate the ecological components of the plan into functional routines as well. The clinician would also need to involve the team to consider the merits of expanding the limits of the world in which Christie and her mother lived. But, for today, mother and child were already smiling more at each other—possibly the most important goal of all.

Model 2: The Integrated Day Care Setting

The clinician had an hour to make an impact on Sam's day care program. The teacher had wanted to work with Sam but was worried that a special program might be better because Sam mostly stayed by himself and did not seem to know how to play.

ASSESS

The reason for referral and a brief observation indicated that Sam spent most of his time on his own. Although he was 2 years old, his cerebral palsy did not allow him to walk and he scooted with difficulty from place to place. He could say many single words but used a soft volume and was difficult to understand. A brief interview with the day care teacher indicated that she and her staff did try to go to Sam and talk for a while every day. However, the other kids commanded much of their attention, pulling and tugging at them all day long.

PLAN/EDUCATE

The clinician suggested that they try two approaches to working with Sam. First, contact him for brief interactions lasting less than a minute. Do this off and on throughout the day—that is, salt and pepper the day with brief interactions (MacDonald & Gillette, 1985). Second, bring a child to Sam every now and then; those who pulled and tugged for attention might be best. This would develop a buddy approach to communication intervention (Gillette, 1989). They did not think these brief encounters would be a problem, but would that be enough? The clinician thought that the encounters would make an impact on Sam, perhaps giving him the idea that he could participate with others, at least briefly. The buddy approach might expand his range of partners if the other children eventually began contacting him more frequently and spontaneously.

PRACTICE

The clinician did not want to leave without seeing how the approach might work. She contacted Sam, pointed to him, and asked his name. He responded, "Sam." She smiled, repeated it, and pointed to herself, saying her name; he repeated it. She waved goodbye and he imitated her; less than a minute had passed.

Next, she waited for a child to approach her as she held a toy car in her lap. When one did, she took the child by the hand to Sam and the three of them took turns pushing the car back and forth, making silly car sounds. When she left this time, the two were still at it and had acquired one observer. Although there was not enough time for the staff to practice, they had observed the clinician's strategies and her success.

INTEGRATE INTO DAILY LIFE

After observing the clinician's success, the day care staff was motivated. They thought each of them could manage at least three contacts a day and would try the buddy approach as well. This meant nine or more contacts per day because there were three on the staff. The lead teacher posted a reminder for the staff which she made with a file folder and a marker: "Contact Sam three times a day." They showed that they understood the purpose of the plan by letting her know that although they already contacted Sam regularly for caregiving routines, they knew that this did not satisfy the purpose of his placement in their program. They knew he needed to benefit from the models the typical peers in his day care program provided.

The clinician made a note that the goal was for each teacher to contact Sam three times a day for brief exchanges of messages and actions in play. She made a follow-up appointment to occur in 2 weeks. At the next visit, she planned to interview this motivated staff and observe to see if the children were contacting Sam more spontaneously.

Model 3: A Group Communication Intervention Program

The teacher requested a consultation to assist her in adapting her opening group to include more communication.

ASSESS

When the clinician asked the teacher to describe her goals, she said she wanted the group to be a language experience for everyone, but currently only a few children seemed to communicate. She said her group activity consisted of calendar activity, a song, and a question-answer session on the unit of the week, such as weather, community helpers, or transportation. Two children were verbal, almost 3 years old, and communicating in single words and short phrases. The rest of the children were quiet during group, even if they had a few words or sounds they could contribute.

PLAN/EDUCATE

The clinician shared her ideas with the teacher. First, they would focus on one part of the group, the question-answer session. She suggested they make it more action oriented so the quiet children could participate through actions. She recommended that the teacher model actions and messages she thought some of the children could use in the group. The teacher could continue to ask the kinds of questions the other children appeared to respond to. In this way, she progressively matched the teacher, incorporating the teacher's present behavior in the plan and then adding something to it. It was her hope that the children would participate more if they saw models of things they could do and heard models of things they could say. The plan made sense to the teacher, but she wanted to see it in action.

PRACTICE

The unit this week was farm animals. The clinician conducted the group with a set of six plastic farm animals: a cow, horse, pig, sheep, goat, and chicken. One by one she pulled them out of a bag and named them for the children. She modeled an action with each, like walking, running, or making a sound. Then she extended an animal to a child, so that eventually every other child in the group of 12 had an animal. She went to each set of two children with one animal and had them trade it back and forth, walking or running the animal to the other child, making a silly sound, making it jump up and down. Next, she held the bag up to each set of children and had them deposit their animal in the bag, waiting for them to say or do something. If they did not, she modeled something matched to the particular child, like "bah," "sheep," "there goes the goat." She always added an attitude of fun by laughing, smiling, or varying her vocal intonation as she talked. Once all of the animals were put away, she repeated the activity so different children held the animal first and the sets of children got different animals. The routine lasted 10 minutes and was a little hectic because not everything was focused on a single teacher-child exchange. It did, however, foster the ECO outcomes of participation, balance, match, and enjoyment.

INTEGRATE INTO DAILY LIFE

The teacher liked the concept and saw its benefits. However, she decided to start small and build up her skills in this type of interaction. She thought she would devote the last 5 minutes or less of each group to the interaction; however, she wanted to wait to practice on her own before the clinician observed her in action. She asked for material to read, ideas of other activities, and a list of the strategies that seemed essential to the success of such an activity.

The strategy list included the following: Play in childlike ways, wait-signal and expect, be animated, and model actions and messages the child can imitate. The clinician also gave the teacher the ECO Guide to Communicating with Groups (Gillette, 1989, p. 190). The clinician shared some strategy descriptions for background reading material and some conversation routines to give the teacher some ideas for group routines she might conduct on her own (Gillette & MacDonald, 1989). However, the clinician assured the teacher that most of her typical activities could easily be adapted to this format. They agreed to revise their plan of action at the next consultation, scheduled in 2 weeks.

Conclusion

Early intervention legislation recognizes the two ways in which families hold the key to their child's development. First, as families interact with their child during daily routines, they shape the child's life experience, influencing the child's development and future outcomes. Second, as they make the decisions that shape the child's life outside the home, they provide additional influences. The IFSP process formalizes this decision-making process and provides advice in the form of the multidisciplinary team for the family of an eligible child.

The ECO Program provides clinicians with a systematic method to evaluate and intervene as they provide communication input to the IFSP process. Clinicians using ECO do evaluate children in the context of the family's daily life, noting the profile of their partnerships in terms of a set of ecological variables. Together, families and clinicians thus shape plans that influence the child to communicate more effectively each day, with careful attention to the pace of the child's development. ECO provides a unique vantage point from which clinicians can guide families and their children toward their communicating partnership.

References

Als, H., Tronick, E., & Brazelton, T. (1979). Affective reciprocity and the development of autonomy. *Journal of the American Academy of Child Psychiatry, 19*, 22–40.

Bandura, A. (1977). *Social learning theory*. Englewood Cliffs, NJ: Prentice Hall, 1977.

Bee, H. L., Barnard, K. E., Eyres, S. J., Gray, C. A., Hammond, M. A., Spietz, A. L., Snyder, C. & Clark,

B. (1982). Predictions of IQ and language skill from perinatal status, child performance, family characteristics, and mother-infant interaction. *Child Development, 53,* 1134–1156.

Bell, R. Q. (1968). A reinterpretation of the direction of effects in studies of socialization. *Psychological Review Developmental Psychology, 75,* 81–95.

Bell, R. Q. (1971). Stimulus control of parent or caregiver behavior by offspring. *Dev Psych, 4,* 63–72.

Bell, R. Q., & Harper, L. V. (1977). *Child effects on adults.* Hillsdale, NJ: Erlbaum.

Biklen, D. (1992). *Schooling without labels: Parents, educators and inclusive education.* Philadelphia: Temple University Press.

Bronfenbrenner, U. (1979). *The ecology of human development.* Cambridge, MA: Harvard University Press.

Bruner, J. S. (1983). *Child's talk: Learning to use language.* New York: W. W. Norton.

Buckhalt, J. A., Rutherford, R. B., & Goldberg, K. E. (1978). Verbal and nonverbal interaction of mothers with their Down syndrome and nonretarded infants. *AJMD, 82,* 337–343.

Cheseldine, S., & McConkey, R. (1979). Parental speech to young Down's syndrome children: An intervention study. *American Journal of Mental Deficiency, 83,* 612–620.

Crais, E. R. (1991). Moving from "parent involvement" to family-centered services. *American Journal of Speech-Language Pathology, 1,* 5–8.

Cunningham, C., Blackwell, J., Reuler, E., & Deck, J. (1981). Behavioral and linguistic development in the interactions of normal and retarded children with their mothers. *Child Development, 52,* 62–70.

Dunst, C. J., Wortman, L. L. & Bartholomew, P. C. (1989). Contingent social responsiveness, family ecology, and infant communicative competence. *National Student Speech Language Hearing Association Journal, 17,* 39–49.

Early Intervention Program for Infants and Toddlers with Handicaps, Final Regulations. (1989). *Federal Register, 54,* 26306–26348.

Feuerstein, R., Rand, Y., & Hoffman, M. (1979). *The dynamic assessment of retarded performers.* Baltimore: University Park Press.

Furono, S., O'Reilly, K. A., Hosaka, C. M., Inatsuka, T., Allman, T. L., & Zeisloft, B. (1985). *HELP: Hawaii Early Learning Profile: Charts.* Palo Alto, CA: Vort Corporation.

Gillette, Y. (1989). *Ecological programs for communicating partnerships: Models and cases.* Chicago: Riverside Publishing.

Gillette, Y., & MacDonald, J. D. (1989). *ECO resources: Using the ECO model for communicating partnerships.* Chicago: Riverside Publishing.

Gillette, Y. (1992). *CATCH guide to planning services with families: Coordinated transition from the hospital to the community and home.* Tucson: Communication Skill Builders.

Gillette, Y. (1993). *Communicating effectively with young children: A video-assisted training program.* Tucson, A2: Communication Skill Builders.

Goodman, J. F. (1992). *When slow is fast enough: Educating the delayed preschool child.* New York: Guilford.

Greenspan, S. (1985). *First feelings: Milestones in the emotional development of your baby and child.* New York: Viking Press.

Hunt, J. (1965). *Intelligence and experience.* New York: Ronald Press.

Jones, O. H. M. (1980). Prelinguistic communication skills in Down syndrome and normal infants. In T. M., Field, S. Golberg, D. Stern, & A. M. Sostek (Eds.), *High risk infants and children* (pp. 205–226). New York: Academic Press.

Kaye, K. (1976). Infant's effects on their mother's teaching strategies. In J. C. Glidewell (Ed.), *The social context of learning and development* (pp. 173–206). New York: Gardner Press.

Kaye, K., & Charney, R. (1980). How mothers maintain dialogue with two-year-olds. In D. Olsen (Ed.), *The social foundations of language and thought: Essays in honor of Jerome S. Bruner* (pp. 211–229). New York: W. W. Norton.

MacDonald, J. D., & Gillette, Y. (1984). Conversational engineering: A pragmatic approach to early social competence. *Seminars in Speech and Language, 5,* 171–183.

MacDonald, J. D., & Gillette, Y. (1985). Taking turns: Teaching communication to your child. *The Exceptional Parent, 15,* 49–52.

MacDonald, J. D., & Gillette, Y. (1986). Communicating with handicapped persons: Roles of parents and professionals. *The Journal of The Association for the Severely Handicapped, 11,* 255–264.

MacDonald, J. D., & Gillette, Y. (1988). Communicating partners: A conversational model for building relationships with handicapped children. In K. Marfo (Ed.), *Parent-child interaction and developmental disabilities: Theory research, and intervention* (pp. 220–241). New York: Praeger.

MacDonald, J. D. (1989). *Becoming partners: From play to conversation.* Chicago: Riverside Publishing.

MacDonald, J. D., & Gillette, Y. (1989). *The introduction to the ECO program.* Chicago: Riverside Publishing.

MacDonald, J., Gillette, Y., & Hutchinson, T. (1989). *ECO Scales.* Chicago: Riverside Publishing.

MacDonald, J. D., & Carroll, J. Y. (1992). A social partnership model for assessing early communication development: An intervention model for preconversational children. *Language Speech and Hearing Services in the Schools, 23,* 113–124.

Mahoney, G., Finger, I., & Powell, A. (1985). The relationship of maternal behavior style to the development of organically impaired mentally retarded infants. *AJMD, 90,* 292–302.

Mahoney, G. (1988). Enhancing the developmental competence of handicapped infants. In K. Marfo (Ed.), *Parent-child interaction and developmental disabilities: Theory, research, and intervention* (pp. 203–219). New York: Praeger.

Massie, H. N. (1980). Pathological interactions in infancy. In T. Field, S. Goldberg, D. Stern, & A. M. Sostek (Eds.), *High risk infants and children: Adult and peer interactions* (pp. 79–98). New York: Academic Press.

McConkey, R. (1988). Educating all parents: An approach based on video. In K. Marfo (Ed.), *Parent-child interaction and developmental disabilities: Theory, research, and intervention* (pp. 253–272). New York: Praeger.

Meisels, S. J., & Wasik, B. (1990). Who should be served? Identifying children in need of early intervention. In S. Meisels & J. Shonkoff (Eds.), *Handbook of early childhood intervention.* Cambridge: Cambridge University Press.

Merighi, J., Edison, M., & Zigler, E. (1990). The role of motivational factors in the functioning of mentally retarded individuals. In R. Hoddap, J. Burack, & E. Zigler (Eds.), *Issues in the developmental approach to mental retardation* (pp. 114–130). Cambridge, UK: Cambridge University Press.

Murray, L., & Trevarthen, C. (1986). The infant's role in mother-infant communications. *Journal of Child Language, 13,* 15–29.

Olswang, L. B., Bain, B. A., & Johnson, G. A. (1992). Using dynamic assessment with children with language disorders. In S. Warren & J. Reichle, (Eds.), *Causes and effects in communication and language intervention* (pp. 187–216). Baltimore: Paul H. Brookes.

Piaget, J. (1951). *Play, dreams, and imitation in childhood.* New York: W. W. Norton.

Stern, D. (1977). *A first relationship.* Cambridge, MA: Harvard University Press.

Stern, D. (1986). *The interpersonal world of the infant: A view from psychoanalysis and developmental psychology.* New York: Basic Books.

Stillman, R., & Battle, C. (1984). Developing prelanguage communication in the severely handicapped: An interpretation of the Van Dijk Method. *Seminars in Speech and Language, 5,* 159–169.

Tjossem, T. D. (1976). *Intervention strategies for high risk infants and young children.* Baltimore: University Park Press.

Tronick, E., Als, H., & Adamson, L. (1979). Structure of early face-to-face communicative interactions. In M. Bullowa (Ed.), *Before speech: The beginning of interpersonal communication* (pp. 349–372). Cambridge; Cambridge University Press.

Valentine, C. W. (1930). The psychology of imitation with special reference to early childhood. *British Journal of Psychology, 21,* 105–132.

Vygotsky, L. S. (1962). *Thought and language.* Cambridge, MA: MIT Press.

Weinberg, G. (1985). *The secrets of consulting: A guide to giving and getting advice successfully.* New York: Dorset.

Index